To
The ...ar of a
great future

[signature]

Long-Term Tamoxifen Treatment for Breast Cancer

LONG-TERM TAMOXIFEN TREATMENT FOR BREAST CANCER

Edited by V. Craig Jordan

The University of Wisconsin Press

The University of Wisconsin Press
114 North Murray Street
Madison, Wisconsin 53715

3 Henrietta Street
London WC2E 8LU, England

Library of Congress Cataloging-in-Publication Data
Long-term tamoxifen treatment for breast cancer /
edited by V. Craig Jordan.
310 p.   cm.
Includes bibliographical references and index.
ISBN 0-299-14070-9 (cl.)
1. Tamoxifen. 2. Breast—Cancer—Chemotherapy.
I. Jordan, V. Craig (Virgil Craig)
[DNLM: 1. Breast Neoplasms—drug therapy.
2. Tamoxifen.   WP 870 L857 1994]
RC280.B8L57   1994
616.99'449061—dc20
DNLM/DLC
for Library of Congress   93-39744

To Monica
  Who never faltered or was discouraged.
  Who made this book and the future possible.

The Editor

V. Craig Jordan, Ph.D., D.Sc., is Professor of Cancer Pharmacology, and Director of the Breast Cancer Research Program at the Robert H. Lurie Cancer Center, Northwestern University Medical School, Chicago, Illinois.

Dr. Jordan graduated with a first-class honors degree (1969) and a Ph.D. (1972) from the Department of Pharmacology, Leeds University Medical School. From 1972 to 1974, he was a visiting scientist at the Worcester Foundation for Experimental Biology in Shrewsbury, Massachusetts, where he conducted the first systematic laboratory study of the antitumor actions of tamoxifen. He then returned to the University of Leeds as a lecturer in pharmacology and headed a Leeds University–ICI Pharmaceuticals joint research scheme to investigate tamoxifen and other antiestrogens as antitumor agents. In 1979, he accepted a one-year appointment as head of the endocrinology unit at the Ludwig Institute for Cancer Research in Bern, Switzerland, before joining the faculty at the University of Wisconsin–Madison in 1980. Until 1993 Dr. Jordan was Professor of Human Oncology and Pharmacology, and Director of the Breast Cancer Research and Treatment Program at the University of Wisconsin Comprehensive Cancer Center.

Dr. Jordan is a fellow of the Royal Society of Chemistry and the American Institute of Chemists. In 1984, he was awarded a University of Wisconsin H. I. Romnes Faculty Fellowship and in a 1985 a doctor of science degree by the University of Leeds for his research contributions. Since 1985, he has been a core member of the Breast Cancer Task Force of the European School of Oncology, Milan, Italy. In 1989, Dr. Jordan was the co-recipient, with Dr. Leonard J. Lerner, of the eighth Bruce F. Cain Award for outstanding preclinical research in cancer chemotherapy from the American Association for Cancer Research.

In 1992, Dr. Jordan was the recipient of the first Brinker International Breast Cancer Award for Basic Science from the Susan G. Komen Foundation, Dallas, Texas, and in 1993, he received the Gaddum Memorial Award from the British Pharmacological Society for his research contributions to pharmacology and the American Society for Pharmacology and Experimental Therapeutics Award for Experimental Therapeutics. In December 1993 Dr. Jordan was awarded the prestigious Cameron Prize from the University of Edinburgh, Scotland for his practical contribution to therapeutics.

Dr. Jordan is a member of the editorial board of *Breast Cancer Research and Treatment, Cancer Letters, Cancer Research, European Journal of Cancer, International Journal of Oncology, Journal of the National Cancer Institute, Journal of Steroid Biochemistry and Molecular Biology, Molecular and Cellular Endocrinology, Receptor, Molecular Aspects of Medicine,* and *Reviews of the Endocrine Aspects of Cancer.*

Contents

Contributors   ix

Preface   xiii

Acknowledgments   xix

1. The Development of Tamoxifen for Breast Cancer Therapy   3
   V. Craig Jordan

2. Clinical Pharmacology and Endocrinology of Long-Term
   Tamoxifen Therapy   27
   Susan M. Langan Fahey, V. Craig Jordan, Nancy F. Fritz,
   Simon P. Robinson, David Waters, and Douglass C. Tormey

3. Multisystem Biological and Symptomatic Toxicity of
   Tamoxifen in Postmenopausal Women   57
   Richard R. Love

4. Endocrine Therapy for the Premenopausal Woman   83
   R. W. Blamey

5. The Nolvadex Adjuvant Trial Organisation (NATO) and the
   Cancer Research Campaign (CRC) Trials of Adjuvant
   Tamoxifen Therapy   93
   J. Houghton, D. Riley, and M. Baum

6. The Stockholm Adjuvant Tamoxifen Trial   115
   Lars E. Rutqvist

7. Maintenance Tamoxifen after Induction Postoperative
   Chemotherapy in Node-Positive Breast Cancer Patients   133
   D. C. Tormey, R. Gray, H. C. Falkson, K. Gilchrist, M. D.
   Abeloff, G. Falkson, and participating investigators

8. Prolonged Tamoxifen Treatment of Early Breast Cancer:
The Experience of the Italian Cooperative Group for
Chemohormonal Therapy of Early Breast Cancer   159
Francesco Boccardo, Domenico Amoroso, Alessandra
Rubagotti, Mario Capellini, Paolo Pacini, Luigi
Castagnetta, Adele Traina, Antonio Farris, Stefano
Iacobelli, Giorgio Mustacchi, Italo Nenci, Adriano
Piffanelli, Piero Sismondi, Corrado De Sanctis, Mario
Mesiti, Luigi Gallo, Eugenio Villa, Guiseppe Schieppati,
and other participants in the GROCTA studies.

9. Interactions of Tamoxifen with Cytotoxic Chemotherapy for
Breast Cancer   181
C. K. Osborne

10. Tamoxifen-Resistant Growth   199
Douglas M. Wolf, Marco M. Gottardis, and V. Craig Jordan

11. A New Approach to Breast Cancer Therapy—Total Estrogen
Ablation with Pure Antiestrogens   219
A. E. Wakeling

12. Symptomatic Side Effects of Tamoxifen Therapy   235
Michael Fritsch and Douglas M. Wolf

13. The Prevention of Breast Cancer with Tamoxifen   257
Monica Morrow and V. Craig Jordan

Appendix   281

Index   283

Contributors

Martin D. Abeloff
Johns Hopkins Oncology Center, 600 N. Wolfe Street, 1st floor, Room 124, Baltimore, Maryland 21205

Domenico Amoroso
Department of Medical Oncology II, Instituto Nazionale per la Ricerca sul Cancro, Genova, Italy

Michael Baum
Professor of Surgery, Royal Marsden Hospital, Fulham Road, London, SW3 6JJ, Great Britain

R.W. Blamey
Professor of Surgery, Professorial Unit of Surgery, City Hospital, Nottingham NG5 1PB, Great Britain

Francesco Boccardo
Chief, Department of Medical Oncology II, Instituto Nazionale per la Ricerca sul Cancro, and Instituto Scientifico per la Studio e la Cura dei Tumori, V. le Benedetto (XO), 10, 16132, Genova, Italy

Mario Cappellini
Department of Radiotherapy, USL 10/D, Ospedale di Careggi, Firenze, Italy

Luigi Castagnetta
Laboratory of Molecular Endocrinology, Instituto Nazionale per la Ricerca sul Cancro (Sede di Palermo), Chair of Oncology, University of Palermo, Italy

Corrado De Sanctis
Chair of Gynecological Oncology, Institute of Gynecology, University of Turin, Italy

Susan M. Langan Fahey
Department of Human Oncology, University of Wisconsin Medical School, University of Wisconsin Comprehensive Cancer Center, K4/649 CSC, Madison, Wisconsin 53792

Geoffrey Falkson
H.F. Verwoerd Hospital and University of Pretoria, Department of Medical Oncology, Private Bag X169, Pretoria 0001, Republic of South Africa

Hendrica Falkson
H.F. Verwoerd Hospital and University of Pretoria, Department of Medical Oncology, Private Bag X169, Pretoria 0001, Republic of South Africa

Antonio Farris
Chair of Clinical Oncology, University of Sassari, Italy

ix

Michael Fritsch
Laboratory of Biochemistry, Bldg. 37, National Cancer Institute, National Institutes of Health, Bethesda, MD

Nancy F. Fritz
158 Flint Street, Sun Prairie, Wisconsin 53590

Luigi Gallo
Oncologic Unit, Ospedale Galliera, Genova, Italty

Kennedy Gilchrist
University of Wisconsin Medical School, University of Wisconsin Comprehensive Cancer Center, K4/550 CSC, Madison, Wisconsin 53792

Marco M. Gottardis
Ligand Pharmaceuticals, 11149 North Torrey Pines Road, La Jolla, California 92034

Robert Gray
Statistical Center, Dana-Farber Cancer Institute, Division of Biostatistics, Dana II, 44 Binney Street, Boston, Massachusetts 02115

Joan Houghton
Assistant Director, Cancer Research Campaign Clinical Trials Centre, Kings College School of Medicine and Dentistry, Rayne Institute, London, SE5 9NU, Great Britain

Stephano Iacobelli
Chair of Clinical Oncology, University "G. D'Annunzio," Chieti, Italy

V. Craig Jordan
Robert H. Lurie Cancer Center, Northwestern University Medical School, 303 E. Chicago, 8250 Olson Pavilion, Chicago, Illinois 60611

Richard Love
Department of Human Oncology, University of Wisconsin Medical School, University of Wisconsin Comprehensive Cancer Center, Madison, Wisconsin 53792

Mario Mesiti
Institute of Oncology, University of Messina, Italy

Monica Morrow
Department of Surgery, Northwestern University Medical School, 250 E. Superior, WESL201, Chicago, Illinois 60611

Giorgio Mustacchi
Oncology Unit "M. Lovenati," Trieste, Italy

Italo Nenci
Institute of Pathology, University of Ferrara, Italy

C. Kent Osborne
Department of Medicine/Medical Oncology, University of Texas Health Science Center at San Antonio, San Antonio, Texas 78284

Paolo Pacini
Department of Radiotherapy, USL 10/D, Ospedale di Careggi, Firenze, Italty

Adriano Piffanelli
Chair of Nuclear Medicine, Institute of Radiology, University of Ferrara, Italy

Diana Riley
Senior Coordinator, Cancer Research Campaign Clinical Trials Centre, Kings College School of Medicine and Dentistry, Rayne Institute, London, SE5 9NU, Great Britain

Simon P. Robinson
Department of Oncology, BSAF, Bioresearch Corporation, 100 Research Drive, Worcester, Massachusetts 01605

Alessandra Rubagotti
Clinical Trial Unit, Instituto Nazionale per la Ricerca sul Cancro, Instituto di Oncologia Clinica e Sperimentale, University of Genoa, Italy

Lars E. Rutqvist
Oncologic Centre, Karolinska Hospital, S-104 01 Stockholm, Sweden

Giuseppe Schieppati
Oncologic Unit, Department of Medicine, City Hospital, Saronno (Varese), Italy

Piero Sismondi
Chair of Gynecological Oncology, Institute of Gynecology, University of Turin, Italy

Douglass C. Tormey
AMC Cancer Research Center, 1600 Pierce Street, Denver, Colorado 80214

Adele Traina
Institute of Oncology "M. Ascoli," Palermo, Italy, University of Turin, Italy

Eugenio Villa
Department of Chemotherapy and Radiotherapy, Instituto S. Raffaele, Milan, Italy

Alan E. Wakeling
Cancer Research Department, Zeneca Pharmaceuticals, Alderley Park, Macclesfield, Cheshire, SK10 4TG, Great Britain

David Waters
Department of Veterinary Medicine, School of Veterinary Medicine, Lynn Hall, Indiana University, West Lafayette, Indiana 47907

Douglas M. Wolf
Department of Medicine/Medical Oncology, University of Texas Health Sciences Center, San Antonio, Texas 78284.

Preface

THIS book is practical testimony to the memory of Dr. Harold Rusch and his dream to conquer cancer. He was a Wisconsin native who graduated from the University of Wisconsin Medical School in 1933 and spent his scientific career working in the laboratory studying how cancer cells grow and how to control their growth. He was one of the first to understand the importance of learning how cells know when and how often to divide. He also was among the first to study the role of calories in cancer growth. After a productive career as a laboratory investigator and building a world-class basic science oncology department, the McArdle Laboratory, he was instrumental in forming and establishing the Department of Human Oncology and the University of Wisconsin Comprehensive Cancer Center (UWCCC). His dream for this new center, established in 1973, was to focus on human problems.

However, he instinctively knew that in trying to conquer cancer there needs to be a close association between the laboratory investigators and clinicians. Ideas, crystalized at the bench, have to be translated into the clinic. The discovery of tamoxifen and its action against breast cancer cells, its use as a long-term therapy, and its potential role as a chemoprevention agent were based on laboratory experimental results and applied to the clinic by a team of investigators working closely together. The subject of this book is a direct result of the interactive process and milieux that Dr. Rusch wanted the UWCCC to have. Let me briefly go over some of the highlights and people involved.

In 1962 Dr. Arthur Walpole, working at the laboratories of Imperial Chemical Industries (ICI) Pharmaceuticals Division in England, tested ICI 46,474 (tamoxifen), a compound that is an antiestrogen and that was thought might be useful as a contraceptive agent. He showed that this drug would prevent implantation of the fertilized eggs in rats. Unfortunately, the early clinical trials demonstrated the opposite effect, namely the enhancement of pregnancies. Walpole understood the potential of this compound as an agent that might interfere with estrogen stimulation of human breast cancer and encouraged its testing by Cole at the Christie Hospital in the United Kingdom. Craig Jordan, a young predoctoral student was working on antiestrogents, studying their structure activity relationships in mice, for his pharmacology thesis at

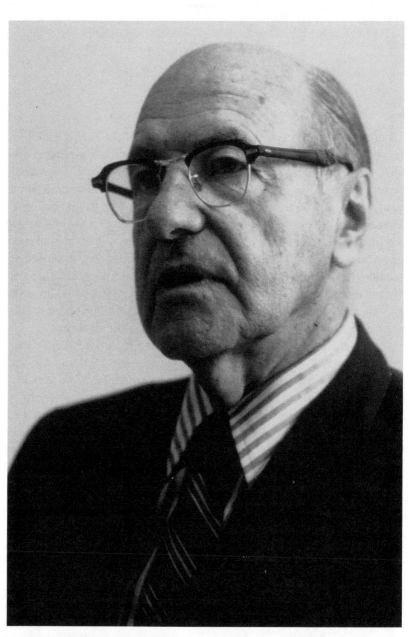

Harold P. Rusch, M.D.; Director of the McArdle Laboratory 1946–1972; Chairman of the Department of Oncology at the University of Wisconsin–Madison 1948–1972; Director of the University of Wisconsin Comprehensive Career Center 1972–1978; Chairman of the Department of Human Oncology at the University of Wisconsin–Madison 1975–1977.

Leeds University. He subsequently completed the first studies in the laboratory with tamoxifen as an antitumor agent at the Worcester Foundation for Experimental Biology. Because of his interest in this compound and the emphasis on breast cancer at the University of Wisconsin, we were able to attract him to our faculty in Madison. He continued his work and began to influence clinical studies. He and Dr. Douglass C. Tormey, actively collaborated on a series of studies improving the utility of tamoxifen to treat breast cancer as well as increasing our understanding of its full potential. Literally the ideas generated in the laboratory were put to clinical testing in a few months, and over the years the concept and safety of long-term administration of tamoxifen traveled from the bench to pilot studies in Madison and to large-scale trials in the Eastern Cooperative Oncology Group. Tamoxifen, intially restricted to use as a therapy for advanced disease, became a major tool for the treatment of node-positive as well as node-negative breast cancer.

But the interchange did not stop here. Craig Jordan had shown that, in the laboratory, rats treated with a carcinogen universally developed breast tumors. However, the tumors which had not yet become clinically visible could be prevented from developing if tamoxifen were given for extended periods of time—months rather than days. To the Wisconsin Breast Group, which had grown to include Richard Love, a medical oncologist, Dave DeMets, a statistician with experience in cardiovascular prevention trials, and Polly Newcomb, an epidemiologist, this raised the possibility that tamoxifen might be useful in preventing or suppressing the ultimate occurence of breast cancer in women at high risk. Data were becoming available from the adjuvant trials, demonstrating women who were on tamoxifen following surgery for one breast cancer were exhibiting a lower incidence of second cancers. This supported the idea that tamoxifen might be useful as a preventive.

However, caution and prudence required that, before subjecting women to therapy with antiestrogens, certain concerns be addressed. It is well known that estrogens given to women postmenopausally protect them against heart attacks and osteoporosis. Would tamoxifen both adversely affect the risks of developing heart attacks and cause excess loss of bones? These adverse actions, if they were seen, could completely ablate any positve effects of tamoxifen as a chemoprotective agent. This led to the initiation of the Wisconsin Tamoxifen Study, a study chaired by Dr. Love, involving 120 postmenopausal women with stage I breast cancer, given either tamoxifen or a placebo. The objective was to look not at survival gains but rather at the effects of tamoxifen on lipid and bone mineral density. The results were surprising. Rather than adversely affecting cardiovascular risk factors and

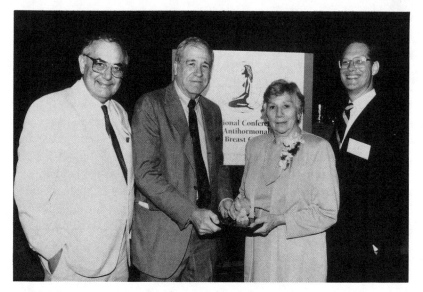

Bernard Fisher, M.D., recipient of the first Rusch Memorial Breast Cancer Award 1991, presented by Mrs. Louise Rusch. Paul P. Carbone, M.D. Director of the University of Wisconsin Comprehensive Cancer Center *(left)* and V. Craig Jordan, Ph.D., D.Sc. *(right)*.

bone density, tamoxifen appeared to lower serum cholesterol and cause calcium retention in the lumbar spine. In addition the side effects of tamoxifen, although considerable, did not prevent 85% of the women from continuing on the drug for at least two years. These data and the information from other confirmatory trials provided the impetus in 1991 for the National Cancer Institute (NCI) to initiate a trial of tamoxifen as a chemopreventive agent in women at high risk of developing breast cancer. This trial sponsored by the NCI is being run by the National Surgical Adjuvant Breast and Bowel Project and will involve 16,000 subjects. Dr. Bernard Fisher, the first recipient of the Harold Rusch Memorial Award, is leading that trial. The outcomes being assessed will be not only decreasing the incidence of breast cancer deaths but also preventing osteoporosis and cardiac mortality.

Tamoxifen use has now come full circle. At least in a research mode tamoxifen is being given to apparently healthy women and is not restricted to individuals with cancer. Women with breast cancers in all countries now have a simple, effective, adjunctive therapy that will increase their life span. The drug potentially may benefit millions of women, and major diseases may be prevented.

The Wisconsin team effort continues tackling new issues, such as why breast cancers become resistant to hormones, and looking for other useful agents to treat and prevent breast and other cancers. Other members have been added to the team, in Madison and elsewhere. These successes are in major part related to the hard work and intelligence of Jordan, Love, Tormey, and others, but they also reflect the success of the intellectual environment made possible by Dr. Harold Rusch, who wanted a center that increased the interactions between the laboratory and clinical investigators. Also important was the support of the ICI Pharma Company, which gave generously of its funds to supplement and complement the NCI and American Cancer Society to do these projects. Clinical testing of ideas is expensive in terms of both time and resources. This book is written testimony of successful progress. Today many more women are alive because of the ideas and results of these laboratory studies and clinical trials. These survivors make the hard work worthwhile, and such saving of human lives provides reason for supporting fundamental as well as applied research.

> Paul P. Carbone, M.D., D.Sc.(Hon.), FACP
> Professor of Human Oncology and Medicine
> Director, University of Wisconsin Comprehensive Cancer Center

Acknowledgments

THIS book was written at a time when the drug tamoxifen was exploding in the news media. The aim was to ask colleagues and students to provide an informed overview of progress for the physician. The text is unavoidably a personal perspective of the story of an obscure compound, ICI 46,474, becoming a first-line therapy for breast cancer *and* the first experimental preventive in normal women. The process has taken more than 20 years to complete.

First I thank Dr. E. R. Clark, formerly of the Department of Pharmacology, University of Leeds, who developed my interest in endocrine pharmacology and guided my doctoral studies. His keen interest in the studies of Elwood Jensen and Jack Gorski was catalytic in our early "quest" to crystalize the estrogen receptor with estrogens and antiestrogen 20 years ago. A few technical difficulties (somewhat of an understatement, inasmuch as no one has yet completed the task) caused us to refocus on the pharmacology of antiestrogens.

I want to thank the dozens of my students, staff, and collaborators who, over the past 20 years, helped to translate ideas into concepts of practical value for women. I also wish to thank those staff members at ICI Pharmaceuticals (now Zeneca)—Brian Newbould, Barry Furr, and Alex Pleuvry—who were more than helpful with support over the years. I am deeply grateful to Paul Carbone and Timothy Kinsella, who provided support and assistance at critical times during the development of my program in Wisconsin. The dedicated assistance of Susan Glad-Anderson, my program coordinator, Bonnie Rayho, my secretary, and Helen Jordan was essential to convert the submitted manuscripts into the final form for the publishers.

In 1970 there was no tamoxifen, but to my daughters, Helen and Alexandra, there has always been a tamoxifen. They heard about the drug every day. I hope it will make their future brighter.

V. Craig Jordan

Long-Term
Tamoxifen Treatment
for Breast Cancer

1

The Development of Tamoxifen for Breast Cancer Therapy

V. Craig Jordan

I.	Introduction	4
II.	ICI 46,474: The Early Years	5
III.	ICI 46,474 to Tamoxifen	8
IV.	Adjuvant Tamoxifen: Laboratory Studies to Clinical Trials	10
V.	Node Negative Disease and Premenopausal Women	14
VI.	Tamoxifen: The Overview	14
VII.	The Biological Basis for Prevention	16
VIII.	General Conclusion	18
	References	19

3

I. *Introduction*

Tᴀᴍᴏxɪꜰᴇɴ (ICI 46,474; Nolvadex) (Fig. 1.1), a nonsteroidal antiestrogen, is the endocrine treatment of choice for advanced breast cancer (Furr and Jordan 1984). Adjuvant therapy with tamoxifen has also proved to be effective (Early Breast Cancer Trialists' Collaborative Group 1992) because a sustained survival advantage is noted for women with node-positive and node-negative disease. The Food and Drug Administration (FDA) has approved the use of tamoxifen as an adjuvant therapy with chemotherapy (1986), as an adjuvant therapy alone (1988) in node-positive postmenopausal patients and pre- and postmenopausal node-negative patients with estrogen receptor-positive disease (1990). Tamoxifen is, however, one of those remarkable examples of a drug originally designed for one primary purpose that fails, but is then steered by dedicated scientists toward a recognized secondary application where it becomes enormously successful.

The chief credit for the discovery of tamoxifen in 1962, and its subsequent application as an anticancer agent, must be given to Dr. Arthur L. Walpole, then head of the fertility control program for Imperial Chemical Industries (ICI) Pharmaceuticals Division. Tamoxifen had been identified as an effective postcoital contraceptive in rats (Harper and Walpole 1966, 1967a,b), and there was a distinct possibility that antiestrogens could be developed as "morning-after" pills (Emmens 1970). However, the basic pharmacology and physiology of ovulation and implantation are critically different in women and rats. When tamoxifen was tested in patients in preliminary clinical studies, it was found to induce ovulation rather than reduce fertility (Klopper and Hall 1971; Williamson and Ellis 1973) and so is now marketed in some countries for the induction of ovulation in subfertile women (Furr and Jordan 1984).

The ovarian dependence of some breast cancers has long been recognized (Beatson 1896; Boyd 1900), and the first antiestrogens (Lerner et al. 1958; Holtkamp et al. 1960) were shown to be effective in their treatment, but the drugs then available were considered to be too toxic for chronic use (Kistner and Smith 1959; Herbst et al. 1964). By the end of the 1960s, the direct role of estrogen in breast cancer growth was further substantiated with the description of estrogen receptors in breast tumors (Sander 1968; Johansson et al.

4

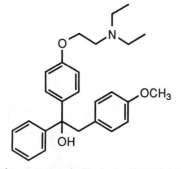

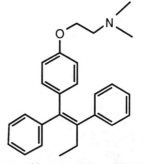

Ethamoxytriphetol (MER 25)

**Tamoxifen (ICI 46,474)
Nolvadex**

Figure 1.1. The structure of antiestrogens described in the text.

1970; Korenman and Dukes 1970) and the subsequent clinical correlation with hormone dependency (Jensen et al. 1971; McGuire et al. 1975). Consequently, Walpole encouraged the clinical testing of the antiestrogen tamoxifen at the Christie Hospital and Holt Radium Institute in Manchester.

This chapter will trace the development of tamoxifen for the treatment of advanced breast cancer in postmenopausal patients and consider the biological basis for the success of tamoxifen as a long-term adjuvant therapy in patients with node-positive and -negative disease. The contemporary fashion is to evaluate tamoxifen as a preventive in women at risk for breast cancer (Powles et al. 1989, 1990; Fisher 1992). The laboratory research that forms the rationale for this treatment strategy will be considered in this chapter, and the biological basis for the clinic studies will be reviewed in the final chapter (Morrow and Jordan, Chapter 13).

II. *ICI 46,474: The Early Years*

In 1958, Lerner and co-workers described the first nonsteroidal antiestrogen MER25 (Fig. 1.1). The drug was tested in clinical trials but proved to be toxic at the high doses required (Lerner 1981). A successor compound, clomiphene (also known as chloramiphene or MRL41), now known to be a mixture of two geometric isomers with opposing biological activities, was a postcoital contraceptive in rats but was developed only clinically as a fertility drug (Clark and Markaverich 1982). ICI 46,474 was first synthesized by Dr. Dora Richardson at ICI Ltd., Pharmaceuticals Division, and was shown to be an antifertility agent in rodents (Harper and Walpole 1967a,b). Dr. Michael Harper (Harper and

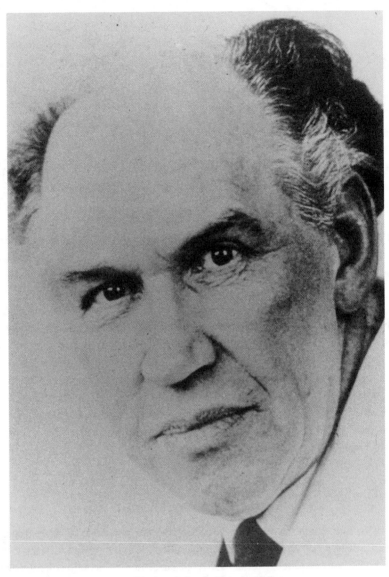

The late Arthur L. Walpole, Ph.D.

Walpole 1966) made the discovery that the geometric isomers of substituted triphenylethylenes have opposing biological properties; the *cis* isomer ICI 47,699 is an estrogen, whereas the *trans* isomer ICI 46,474 has antiestrogenic activity. Thus the structure of the drug can program the cells for estrogenic or antiestrogenic properties (Lieberman et al. 1983; Jordan et al. 1988; Murphy et al. 1990). Another observation made by Harper and Walpole was that ICI 46,474 exhibits species specificity; in short-term tests the compound is an estrogen in the mouse and an antiestrogen in the rat (Harper and Walpole 1966, 1967a). The triphenylethylene derivative blocks the binding of [^{3}H]estradiol to estrogen receptors derived from both rat and mouse target tissues (Skidmore et al. 1972; Jordan 1975a; Jordan and Dowse 1976), but no completely satisfactory subcellular mechanism for the species difference of ICI 46,474 has yet been established. In fact, the situation is probably more complex than may at first be appreciated. The long-term administration of tamoxifen to ovariectomized mice results in an initial estrogen-like effect in the vagina (Jordan 1975a) and the uterus (Jordan et al. 1990), but as treatment progresses both the uterus and vagina become refractory to the effects of exogenous estrogen, and ICI 46,474 becomes a complete antiestrogen.

Preliminary clinical studies with ICI 46,474 to treat advanced breast cancer in postmenopausal women were conducted by Mary Cole and her co-workers (Cole et al. 1971) at the Christie Hospital in Manchester. The confirmation that ICI 46,474 could be used successfully as a palliative in advanced disease but produced few side effects (Ward 1973; O'Halloran and Maddock 1974) acted as a catalyst to encourage the study of the mode of action of the drug in animal tumor models. Indeed the conversation between the laboratory and the clinic has become the hallmark for the successful development of tamoxifen.

Animal studies were first started in 1973 at the Worcester Foundation for Experimental Biology, Shrewsbury, Massachussets (Jordan 1974a,b,c; Jordan 1976; Jordan and Koerner 1975, 1976). The dimethyl-benzanthracene (DMBA)-induced rat mammary carcinoma model, originally described a decade earlier by the Nobel Laureate Professor Charles Huggins (Huggins et al. 1961), was used to study the efficacy and mode of action of ICI 46,474 under controlled laboratory conditions. The model was considered to be state of the art, because no other hormone-dependent models were then available for study. Rob Nicholson, then a graduate student at the Tenovus Institute for Cancer Research in Cardiff, Wales, also selected the DMBA-induced rat mammary carcinoma model for his study of the antitumor actions of ICI 46,474 and related compounds (Nicholson and Golder 1975). These parallel research ventures fully described the antitumor activity of the antiestrogen *in vivo* (Jordan 1975b; Jordan and Dowse 1976; Jordan and Koerner 1976; Jordan and Jaspan 1976; Nicholson et al. 1976) at a time when the efficacy of tamoxifen was being established widely in breast cancer clinical trials (Tamoxifen Workshop 1976).

III. ICI 46,474 to Tamoxifen

In 1973, Nolvadex, the ICI brand of tamoxifen (as its citrate salt), was approved for the treatment of breast cancer by the Committee on the Safety of Medicines in the United Kingdom. Similar approval was given in the United States of America for the treatment of advanced disease in postmenopausal women by the Food and Drug Administration on December 30, 1977. Nolvadex is now available in more than 110 countries as the first-line endocrine therapy for the treatment of breast cancer (Furr and Jordan 1984). To mark this achievement ICI Pharmaceuticals Division was presented with the Queen's Award for Technological Achievement by the Lord Lieutenant of Cheshire, Viscount Leverhulme, on July 6, 1978. The remarkable success of tamoxifen encouraged a closer examination of its pharmacology with a view to further development and wider applications.

The metabolism of tamoxifen in animals and patients was first described by Fromson and co-workers (Fromson et al. 1973a,b). The major metabolic route to be described was hydroxylation to form 4-hydroxytamoxifen, which was subsequently shown to have high binding affinity for the estrogen receptor and to be a potent antiestrogen in its own right (Jordan et al. 1977) with antitumor properties in the DMBA model (Jordan and Allen 1980). Indeed it is an advantage for tamoxifen to be metabolically activated to 4-hydroxytamoxifen (Allen et al. 1980), but this is not a prerequisite for antiestrogen action. The metabolite was subsequently shown to localize in target tissues after the administration of radioactive tamoxifen to rats (Borgna and Rochefort 1981). Originally, 4-hydroxytamoxifen was believed to be the major metabolite in patients (Fromson et al. 1973b), but Hugh Adam (Adam et al. 1979) at ICI Pharmaceuticals Division demonstrated that N-desmethyltamoxifen is the principal metabolite found in patients. There is usually a blood level ratio of 2:1 for N-desmethyltamoxifen:tamoxifen in patients maintained on tamoxifen therapy, because N-desmethyltamoxifen has twice the plasma half-life of tamoxifen (14 days versus 7 days) (Patterson et al. 1980). The ubiquitous use of tamoxifen in recent years has resulted in the

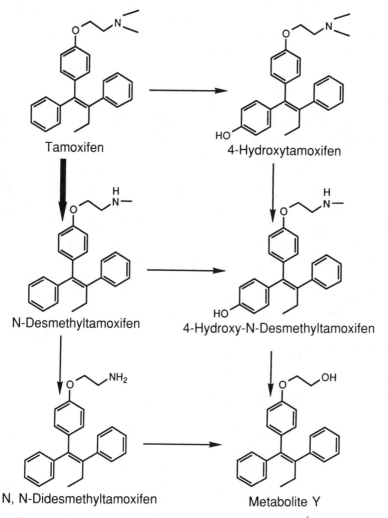

Figure 1.2. The metabolites of tamoxifen detected in patient serum. The thick arrow denotes the principal route of metabolism.

publication of numerous methods to estimate tamoxifen and its metabolites in serum (reviewed in Jordan and Murphy 1990). The metabolites that have been identified in patients are shown in Figure 1.2. The minor metabolites, metabolite Y (Jordan et al. 1983), metabolite Z (Kemp et al. 1983), and 4-hydroxy-N-desmethyltamoxifen (Lien et al. 1989), may all contribute to the antitumor actions of tamoxifen, because they are all antiestrogens which inhibit the binding of estradiol to the estrogen receptor.

The next significant advance came with the availability of hormone-dependent human breast cancer to study antitumor mechanisms in the laboratory. Marc Lippman (Lippman and Bolan 1975) was the first to describe the ability of tamoxifen to inhibit the growth of MCF-7 estrogen receptor–positive breast cancer cells (Brooks et al. 1973) in culture and to demonstrate that the addition of estrogen could reverse the action of tamoxifen. Nearly a decade later Kent Osborne (Osborne et al. 1983) and Rob Sutherland (Sutherland et al. 1983) independently described the blockade by tamoxifen of breast cancer cells at the G_1 phase of the cell cycle.

Studies with the heterotransplantation of MCF-7 cells into athymic mice demonstrate that, unlike estradiol, tamoxifen does not support the growth of tumors (Shafie and Grantham 1981). Tamoxifen (Osborne et al. 1985) and its metabolites (Gottardis et al. 1988) will block estrogen-stimulated tumor growth. However, very high circulatory levels (2300 pg/ml) of estradiol in a low tamoxifen environment (40 ng/ml) can partly reverse the inhibitory actions of tamoxifen for MCF-7 tumor growth (Iino et al. 1991). Overall, these studies of the reversibility of tamoxifen action could have implications for its extended adjuvant use in premenopausal women. A more detailed examination of the pharmacology and endocrinology of tamoxifen is to be found in Chapter 2.

IV. *Adjuvant Tamoxifen: Laboratory Studies to Clinical Trials*

The initial success of adjuvant monotherapy with L-phenylalanine mustard (Fisher et al. 1975) or combination chemotherapy (Bonadonna et al. 1976) to delay the recurrence of node-positive breast cancer helped to encourage the investigation of other, perhaps less toxic, therapies. Laboratory studies using the DMBA-induced rat mammary carcinoma model were first used to explore whether tamoxifen would be effective and whether the drug produced a tumoristatic or tumoricidal effect *in vivo*. Studies *in vitro* had previously indicated that tamoxifen could be a tumoricidal drug (Lippman and Bolan 1975), but the results from the DMBA studies *in vivo* (first reported at a breast cancer symposium at King's College, Cambridge, England, in September 1977) demonstrated that a short course of tamoxifen therapy (1 month) given 1 month after the carcinogenic insult only delayed the appearance of mammary tumors; continuous therapy (for 6 months) resulted in 90% of the animals remaining tumor-free (Figure 1.3) (Jordan 1978; Jordan et al. 1979). Indeed if tamoxifen therapy is stopped, tumors appear (Robinson et al. 1989). Thus,

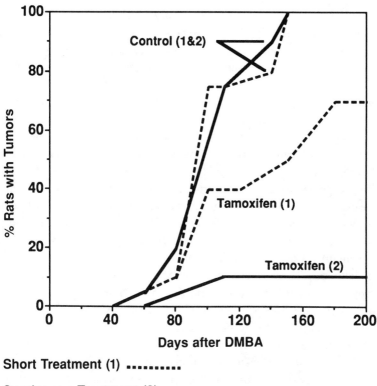

Days after DMBA

Short Treatment (1) •••••••••

Continuous Treatment (2) ━━━

Figure 1.3. The effect of short- or long-term tamoxifen treatment (50μg daily SC in 0.1 ml peanut oil) on the incidence of dimethylbenzanthracene (DMBA)-induced rat mammary tumors. Fifty-day-old, female, Sprague Dawley rats were given 20 mg DMBA in 2 ml peanut oil by gavage. Control groups were injected with 0.1 ml peanut oil alone. There were 20 animals per group.

tamoxifen was shown to have a tumoristatic component to its mode of action, and the laboratory results indicated that long-term (up to 5 years) or indefinite therapy might be the best clinical strategy for adjuvant treatment. Subsequent laboratory studies using DMBA- or N-nitrosomethylurea (NMU)-induced rat mammary tumors (Jordan et al. 1980; Gottardis and Jordan 1987) or human breast cancer cell lines inoculated into athymic mice (Osborne et al. 1985, 1987) have all supported the initial observation. However, most attention has now focused on the clinical evaluation of the laboratory concept.

Several trials of tamoxifen monotherapy as an adjuvant to mastectomy were initiated toward the end of the 1970s. The majority of clinical trial organizations selected a conservative course of 1 year of adjuvant tamoxifen (Ludwig

Breast Cancer Study Group 1984; Rose et al. 1985; Ribeiro and Palmer 1983; Ribeiro and Swindell 1985). This decision was, however, based on a number of reasonable concerns. Patients with advanced disease usually respond to tamoxifen for 1 year, and it was expected that estrogen receptor (ER) negative disease would be encouraged to grow prematurely during adjuvant therapy. If this growth was to occur, then the physician would have already used a valuable palliative drug and would have only combination chemotherapy to slow the relentless growth of recurrent disease. A related argument involved the changing strategy for the application of adjuvant combination chemotherapy. Recurrent treatment cycles (2 years) were found to be of no long-term benefit for the patient. An aggressive course of short-term treatment (6 months) with the most active cytotoxic drugs could have the best chance to kill tumor cells before the premature development of drug resistance. The same argument provided an intuitive reluctance to use long-term tamoxifen therapy because it would lead to premature drug resistance: longer might not be better.

Finally, there were sincere concerns about the side effects of adjuvant therapy and the ethical issues of treating patients who might never have recurrent disease. Although this argument primarily focused on chemotherapy and node-negative patients, it is fair to say that few women in the mid-1970s had received extended therapy with tamoxifen, so that long-term side effects were largely unknown. The majority of tamoxifen-treated patients had received only about 2 years of treatment for advanced disease before drug resistance occurred. Potential side effects of thrombosis, osteoporosis, and so on, were only of secondary importance. The use of tamoxifen in the disease-free patient would change that perspective.

In 1977, Dr. Douglass C. Tormey organized the first evaluation of long-term tamoxifen therapy in node-positive patients treated with combination chemotherapy plus tamoxifen (Tormey and Jordan 1984; Tormey et al. 1987). This pilot study was initiated to determine whether patients could tolerate 5 years of adjuvant tamoxifen therapy and whether metabolic tolerance would occur during long-term tamoxifen therapy. No unusual side effects of tamoxifen therapy were noted, and blood levels of tamoxifen and its metabolites N-desmethyltamoxifen and metabolite Y remained stable throughout the 5 years of treatment. Although this study was not a randomized trial, those patients who are receiving long-term tamoxifen therapy continue to make excellent progress, and many patients have taken the drug for more than 14 years. We have recently reported (Langan-Fahey et al. 1990) that tamoxifen does not produce metabolic tolerance during 10 years of administration. Serum levels of tamoxifen and its metabolites are maintained.

These data and the DMBA rat mammary carcinoma data (Jordan 1983) were used to support randomized Eastern Cooperative Oncology Group (ECOG) trials EST 4181 and 5181. An early analysis of EST 4181, which compares short-term tamoxifen with long-term tamoxifen (both with combination chemotherapy), has demonstrated an increase in disease-free survival with long-term tamoxifen therapy (Falkson et al. 1990). In fact, the 5-year tamoxifen arm has now gone through a second randomization either to stop the tamoxifen or to continue the antiestrogen indefinitely. These clinical studies are discussed in detail in Chapter 7. The National Surgical Adjuvant Breast and Bowel Project (NSABP) clinical trial organization has conducted a registration study of 2 years of combination chemotherapy (L-PAM, 5-FU) plus tamoxifen with an additional year of tamoxifen alone (Fisher et al. 1987) to build on the successes of these earlier trials that demonstrated the efficacy of tamoxifen in receptor-positive postmenopausal patients (Fisher et al. 1981, 1983, 1986). Overall, these investigators conclude that 3 years of tamoxifen confer a significant advantage over 2 years of tamoxifen.

A recent report from Italy has demonstrated that the addition of combination chemotherapy (CMF 6 cycles followed by 5 courses of epirubicin) to long-term (5 years) tamoxifen therapy does not seem to improve significantly the clear-cut effectiveness of tamoxifen alone to prevent recurrence in ER- and node-positive disease (Boccardo et al. 1990). Further information is presented in Chapter 8.

Although the 2-year adjuvant tamoxifen study that was conducted by the Nolvadex Adjuvant Trial Organisation (NATO) was the first to demonstrate a survival advantage for women (NATO 1985), current clinical trials are all evaluating a longer duration of tamoxifen therapy. A current update after 10 years of follow-up of this landmark study is presented in Chapter 5. A small, randomized clinical trial of 3 years of tamoxifen versus no treatment has demonstrated a survival advantage for ER-positive patients who receive tamoxifen (Delozier et al. 1986). Similarly, the Scottish trial that has evaluated 5 years of tamoxifen versus no treatment has demonstrated a survival advantage for patients who take tamoxifen (Breast Cancer Trials Committee 1987). The Scottish trial is particularly interesting because it addresses the question of whether to administer tamoxifen early as a adjuvant or to save the drug until recurrence. This comparison was possible because most patients in the control arm received tamoxifen at recurrence. Early concerns that long-term adjuvant tamoxifen would result in premature drug resistance are unjustified, because the patients have a survival advantage on the adjuvant tamoxifen arm. Indeed, a recent analysis of non-cancer-related deaths has demonstrated a significant decrease in fatal myocardial infarction for patients receiving adjuvant tamoxifen for 5 years (McDonald and Stewart 1991).

V. *Node Negative Disease and Premenopausal Women*

Tamoxifen was initially used in premenopausal women to treat menometrorrhagia (el-Sheikha et al. 1972) and to induce ovulation in infertile women (Klopper and Hall 1971; Williamson and Ellis 1973). Subsequent evaluation of the endocrine effects of tamoxifen by Groom and Griffiths (1976) revealed an increase in ovarian estrogen production. These findings have been confirmed by many groups of investigators, and their results will be discussed in Chapter 2.

Although concerns have been expressed about the potential for the reversal of tamoxifen's action in a high estrogen environment, tamoxifen can effectively control the growth of advanced breast cancer in premenopausal patients (Manni et al. 1979; Pritchard et al. 1980; Kalman et al. 1982, Planting et al. 1985; Sawka et al. 1986), and small clinical trials have demonstrated that tamoxifen and oophorectomy (Ingle et al. 1986; Buchanan et al. 1986) have similar efficacy. Nolvadex is currently available in the United States for the treatment of patients with ER-positive advanced breast cancer. Adjuvant monotherapy with tamoxifen has shown efficacy in node-positive premenopausal patients (Cancer Research Campaign Adjuvant Breast Trial Working Party 1988), but most experience has been derived from the study B_{14} of node-negative ER-positive premenopausal patients conducted by the NSABP (Fisher et al. 1989). Tamoxifen increases the disease-free survival and, perhaps most importantly, the antiestrogen is active in premenopausal women. The protocol used an initial treatment period of 5 years of adjuvant tamoxifen, but the patients will now continue tamoxifen for an additional 5-year period.

Nolvadex is currently available to treat selected patients at each stage of breast cancer, but the recent overview analysis of randomized clinical trials has precisely described the worth of antiestrogen therapy.

VI. *Tamoxifen: The Overview*

The effectiveness of adjuvant tamoxifen in both node-positive and node-negative breast cancer has recently been established in an overview analysis (Early Breast Cancer Trialists' Collaborative Group 1992). The review included 30,000 women in randomized trials of tamoxifen. Highly significant

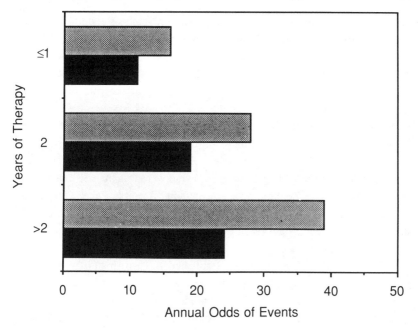

Figure 1.4. The *reduction* in the annual odds of either recurrence (shaded bars) or death (black bars) in randomized trials of adjuvant tamoxifen therapy. The duration of therapy caused a marked increase in recurrence and survival. The percentage of reduction in recurrence and survival is shown on each histogram. (Adapted from Early Breast Cancer Trialists' Collaborative Group 1992.)

reductions in the annual rates of recurrence and death are produced by tamoxifen (25% SD2 for recurrence and 17% SD2 for mortality), and tamoxifen reduced the risk of developing a contralateral breast cancer by 39% SD9 ($p <$ 0.0001). Most interestingly, the difference in survival produced by 2 years of tamoxifen therapy was greater at 10 years than at 5 years. Nevertheless, as was predicted by the laboratory data (Jordan 1983), the duration of adjuvant therapy was important for both controlling recurrence and improving mortality (Fig. 1.4). In fact, this appeared to be true for women above or below the age of 50, although postmenopausal women had a more consistent advantage. Node-negative women had a similar benefit whether they were above or below the age of 50. In contrast, the node-positive women had more benefit if they were postmenopausal and less benefit if they were premenopausal. This, in part, could be because the node-positive population also received combination chemotherapy, which is known to cause ovarian ablation. It is therefore possible that the benefit to be gained from this form of endocrine therapy (i.e., chemical oophorectomy) is optimal, and tamoxifen can add little further benefit. It is perhaps pertinent to point out that the overview analysis found that ovarian ablation below the age of 50 reduces the annual rates of recurrence (26% SD6) and decreases mortality (25% SD2, $p \leq 0.004$), i.e., to an extent similar to polychemotherapy (28% SD3 recurrence and 16% SD3 mortality, $p < 0.00001$).

Finally, there has been much controversy about the role of the ER in predicting a response to tamoxifen therapy. The FDA has approved the use of tamoxifen as an adjuvant therapy for all postmenopausal patients with node-positive disease, but the ER may improve the chances of response. The overview analysis found the percentage of reduction in annual odds of recurrence for ER-poor patients (<10 fmol/mg) who were less than 50 years old are only 3%, but 16% if the patient was more than 50 years of age. The situation improves if the ER value is >10 fmol/mg protein; under 50 years of age patients have a 19% reduction in annual odds of recurrence, but 36% if they are over 50 years of age.

These statistical studies have established the worth of tamoxifen as a valuable therapeutic agent in the armamentarium of the medical oncologist. The success of the therapy and its low incidence of side effects have increased enthusiasm to evaluate the role of tamoxifen in preventing breast cancer. The clinical strategies will be considered in the final chapter, but the laboratory rationale is well established.

VII. *The Biological Basis for Prevention*

The successful use of tamoxifen for the treatment of breast cancer, and the low reported incidence of side effects observed with the more than 4.5 million women years of clinical experience, has acted as a catalyst to support the use of tamoxifen in normal women at risk for developing breast cancer (Cuzick et al. 1986; Fentiman and Powles 1987). The past 2 decades' expanded literature on the prevention of rodent mammary cancer can be used to support the clinical use of tamoxifen to prevent breast cancer. Indeed, as early as 1936 Lacassagne predicted that a therapeutic intervention could be developed that would "prevent or antagonize the congestion of oestrone in the breast." Unfortunately, no therapeutic agent was available and all his predictions were based upon the known effect of early oophorectomy on the development of mammary cancer in high-incidence strains of mice (Lacassagne 1936). Clearly the indiscriminate oophorectomy of young women would be an inappropriate intervention.

The animal studies with tamoxifen have been undertaken for two reasons.

First, to establish the efficacy of tamoxifen in well-described models of carcinogenesis, and second, to discover whether tamoxifen would always be an inhibitor or whether the drug would ever exacerbate tumorigenesis. Two animal model systems have been used extensively: the carcinogen-induced rat mammary carcinoma model and mouse mammary tumor virus (MMTV) infected strains of mice.

The mammary carcinogens DMBA (Huggins et al. 1961) and NMU (Gullino et al. 1975) induce tumors in young female rats. The timing of the carcinogenic insult is very important, because as the animals age they become resistant to the mammary carcinogens. Tumorigenesis does not occur in oophorectomized animals, and the sooner oophorectomy is performed after the carcinogenic insult, the more effective it is in preventing the development of tumors (Dao 1962).

The administration of tamoxifen to carcinogen-treated rats prevents the initiation of carcinogenesis, and animals remain tumor-free (Jordan 1976; Turcot-Lemay and Kelley 1980). The short-term administration of tamoxifen at different times after the carcinogenic insult is effective in reducing the number of tumors that develop (Jordan et al. 1979; Jordan and Allen 1980; Wilson et al. 1982), although most animals develop at least one tumor after therapy is stopped.

Continuous tamoxifen therapy that is started at 1 month after the administration of carcinogens completely inhibits the appearance of mammary tumors (Jordan 1983; Gottardis and Jordan 1987). Under these circumstances tamoxifen is preventing promotion and suppressing the appearance of occult disease. The principle is illustrated in Figure 1.4. In fact, if treatment is stopped prematurely (i.e., a 3–4-month duration of therapy) the microfoci of transformed cells grow into palpable tumors (Robinson et al. 1989). Because the timing of initiation in human breast cancer is unknown, and unlike the laboratory model not all women will develop tumors, tamoxifen will be given to target populations to suppress and, it is hoped, reverse the promotional effects of estrogen during carcinogenesis.

Until recently there was a paucity of information about the efficacy of tamoxifen to inhibit mouse mammary tumorigenesis. This was true in part because tamoxifen is estrogenic in short-term tests in oophorectomized (Harper and Walpole 1967a) and immature mice (Terenius 1971). However, the finding that long-term tamoxifen therapy renders the oophorectomized mouse vagina (Jordan 1975a) and athymic mouse uterus (Gottardis and Jordan 1988) refractory to estrogenic stimuli prompted a reconsideration of the value of tamoxifen as a preventive in mouse mammary tumor models.

High-incidence strains of mice that develop mammary tumors are infected with MMTV, which is transferred to the offspring in the mothers' milk (Bittner 1939). Tumorigenesis appears to be ovarian dependent, because the highest incidence of tumors appears in females and tumorigenesis can be delayed or prevented depending upon the age at oophorectomy (Lathrop and Loeb 1916). Steroid hormones activate the pro-viral MMTV (Hynes et al. 1984), which in turn can initiate an increase in growth factors from the viral integration site Int. 2 (Peters et al. 1989). Promotion of the initiated cells with steroid hormones and prolactin then completes tumorigenesis.

Long-term tamoxifen therapy, after an early cycle of pregnancy and weaning to facilitate early tumorigenesis, is equivalent to an oophorectomy performed at 4 months in reducing tumorigenesis to 50% at 14 months of age. However, tamoxifen is superior to oophorectomy, even after therapy is stopped, because oophorectomized animals continue to develop tumors, whereas animals previously treated with tamoxifen do not develop any more tumors (Jordan et al. 1990).

We have followed up on initial observations with an investigation of tumorigenesis in virgin mice. In this study design, mice develop mammary tumors during their second year of life. Again, long-term tamoxifen therapy started at 3 months of age is superior to oophorectomy at 3 months. Fifty percent of the oophorectomized animals develop tumors by the third year of life, whereas 90% of tamoxifen-treated mice remain tumor-free (Jordan et al. 1991). These studies are illustrated in Figure 1.5.

Overall, the results of the studies in the mouse model are particularly interesting because they have changed our view of the interspecies pharmacology of tamoxifen. Long-term treatment with tamoxifen results in an initial classification of tamoxifen as an estrogen, but within a few weeks the pharmacology changes and tamoxifen becomes an antiestrogen. Clearly, an understanding of this process may have important implications for the long-term use of tamoxifen as an adjuvant therapy and a preventive.

VIII. *General Conclusion*

During the past 20 years tamoxifen has moved from the laboratory to become the endocrine treatment of choice for all stages of breast cancer. The drug has a remarkable profile of interesting pharmacological effects; on one hand, tamoxifen can inhibit estrogen-stimulated breast cancer growth, and on the other hand, it can mimic some of the physiological functions of estrogen to

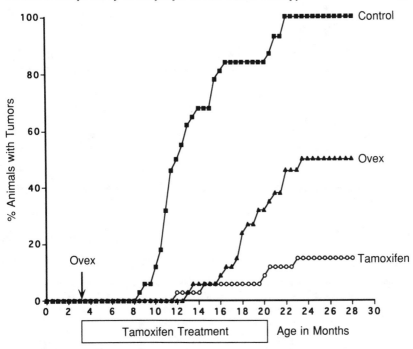

Figure 1.5. The effect of oophorectomy or the administration of long-term tamoxifen therapy on the development of mammary tumors in virgin C3H/OUJ mice. Tamoxifen was administered as a sustained-release preparation as described in Jordan et al. 1990. There were 30 animals per group. Tamoxifen, O; control, ■. (Data adapted from Jordan et al. 1991.)

support bone density and to lower circulating cholesterol (Love et al. 1991, 1992). These studies will be described in detail in Chapter 3.

Overall the following chapters in this volume are intended to provide an up-to-date appraisal of the effectiveness of long-term tamoxifen therapy and survey the pharmacology and side effects of this drug. For the future, the clinical trials to test the worth of tamoxifen as a preventive for breast cancer in normal women will provide the physician with a new therapeutic dimension that, it is hoped, will contribute to the improved health for thousands of women.

References

Adam, H. K., E. J. Douglas, and J. V. Kemp. 1979. The metabolism of tamoxifen in humans. *Biochemical Pharmacology* 28:145–147.
Allen, K. E., E. R. Clark, and V. C. Jordan. 1980. Evidence for the metabolic activation of non-

steroidal antioestrogens: a study of structure-activity relationships. *British Journal of Pharmacology* 71:83–91.

Beatson, G. T. 1896. On the treatment of inoperable cases of carcinoma of the mamma: suggestions for a new method of treatment with illustrative cases. *Lancet* 2:104–107.

Bittner, J. J. 1939. Relation of nursing to the extra chromosomal theory of breast cancer in mice. *American Journal of Cancer* 35:90–97.

Boccardo, F., A. Rubagotti, P. Bruzzi, M. Capellini, G. Isola, I. Nenci, A. Piffanelli, A. Scanni, P. Sismondi, L. Santi, F. Genta, F. Saccani, M. Sassi, P. Malacarne, D. Donati, A. Farris, L. Castagnetta, A. DiCarlo, A. Traina, L. Galletto, F. Smerieri, and F. Buzzi. 1990. Chemotherapy versus tamoxifen versus chemotherapy plus tamoxifen in node-positive, estrogen receptor–positive breast cancer patients: results of a multicentric Italian study. *Journal of Clinical Oncology* 8:1310–1320.

Bonadonna, G., E. Brusamolino, P. Valagussa, A. Rossi, L. Brugnatelli, C. Brambilla, M. De Lena, G. Tancini, E. Bajetta, R. Musumeci, and U. Veronesi. 1976. Combination chemotherapy as an adjuvant treatment in operable breast cancer. *New England Journal of Medicine* 294:405–410.

Borgna, J. L., and H. Rochefort. 1981. Hydroxylated metabolites of tamoxifen are formed *in vivo* and bound to estrogen receptor in target tissues. *Journal of Biological Chemistry* 256:859–868.

Boyd, S. 1900. On oophorectomy in cancer of the breast. *British Medical Journal* 2:1161–1167.

Breast Cancer Trials Committee, Scottish Cancer Trials Office. 1987. Adjuvant tamoxifen in the management of operable breast cancer: the Scottish trial. *Lancet* 2:171–175.

Brooks, S. C., E. R. Locke, and H. D. Soule. 1973. Estrogen receptor in a human cell line (MCF-7) from breast carcinoma. *Journal of Biological Chemistry* 248:6251–6253.

Buchanan, R. B., R. W. Blamey, K. R. Durrant, A. Howell, A. G. Paterson, P. E. Preece, D. C. Smith, C. J. Williams, and R. G. Wilson. 1986. A randomized comparison of tamoxifen with surgical oophorectomy in premenopausal patients with advanced breast cancer. *Journal of Clinical Oncology* 4:1326–1330.

Clark, J. H., and B. M. Markaverich. 1982. The agonistic-antagonistic properties of clomiphene: a review. *Pharmacology and Therapeutics* 15:467–519.

Cole, M. P., C. T. Jones, and I. D. H. Todd. 1971. A new antioestrogenic agent in late breast cancer. An early clinical appraisal of ICI 46,474. *British Journal of Cancer* 25:270–275.

CRC Adjuvant Breast Trial Working Party. 1988. Cyclophosphamide and tamoxifen as adjuvant therapies in the management of breast cancer. *British Journal of Cancer* 57:604–607.

Cuzick, J., D. Y. Wang, and R. D. Bulbrook. 1986. The prevention of breast cancer. *Lancet* 1:83–86.

Dao, T. L. 1962. The role of ovarian hormones in initiating the induction of mammary cancer in rats by polynuclear hydrocarbons. *Cancer Research* 22:973–981.

Delozier, T., J. P. Julien, P. Juret, C. Veyret, J. E. Couette, Y. Graic, J. M. Ollivier, and E. de Ranieri. 1986. Adjuvant tamoxifen in postmenopausal breast cancer: preliminary results of a randomized trial. *Breast Cancer Research and Treatment* 7:105–119.

Early Breast Cancer Trialists' Collaborative Group. 1992. Systematic treatment of early breast cancer by hormonal, cytotoxic, or immune therapy. 133 randomised trials involving 31,000 recurrences and 24,000 deaths among 75,000 women. *Lancet* 339:1–15 and 71–85.

Emmens, C. W. 1970. Postcoital contraception. *British Medical Bulletin* 26:45–51.

el-Sheikha, Z., A. Klopper, and J. S. Beck. 1972. Treatment of menometrorrhagia with an antioestrogen. *Clinical Endocrinology* 1:275–282.

Falkson, H. C., R. Gray, W. H. Wolberg, K. W. Gilchrist, J. E. Harris, D. C. Tormey, and G. Falkson. 1990. Adjuvant trial of 12 cycles of CMFPT followed by observation or continuous tamoxifen versus four cycles of CMFPT in postmenopausal women with breast cancer: an Eastern Cooperative Oncology Group phase III study. *Journal of Clinical Oncology* 8:599–607.

Fentiman, I. S., and T. J. Powles. 1987. Tamoxifen and benign breast problems. *Lancet* 2:1070–1072.

Fisher, B. 1992. The evolution of paradigms for the management of breast cancer: a personal perspective. *Cancer Research* 52:2371–2383.

Fisher, B., P. P. Carbone, S. G. Economou, R. Frelick, A. Glass, H. Lerner, C. Redmond, M. Zelen, P. Band, D. L. Katrych, N. Wolmark, and E. R. Fisher. 1975. L-Phenylalanine mustard (L-PAM) in the management of primary breast cancer. A report of early findings. *New England Journal of Medicine* 292:117–122.

Fisher, B., J. Costantino, C. Redmond, and 50 other members of the NSABP. 1989. A randomized clinical trial evaluating tamoxifen in the treatment of patients with node-negative breast cancer who have estrogen-receptor–positive tumors. *New England Journal of Medicine* 320:479–484.

Fisher, B., and National Surgical Breast and Bowel Project investigators. 1987. Prolonging tamoxifen therapy for primary breast cancer. Findings from the National Surgical Adjuvant Breast and Bowel Project clinical trial. *Annals of Internal Medicine* 106:649–654.

Fisher, B., C. Redmond, A. Brown, E. R. Fisher, N. Wolmark, D. Bowman, D. Plotkin, J. Wolter, R. Bornstein, S. Legault-Poisson, E. A. Saffer, and other NSABP investigators. 1986. Adjuvant chemotherapy with and without tamoxifen in the treatment of primary breast cancer: 5-year results from the National Surgical Adjuvant Breast and Bowel Project trial. *Journal of Clinical Oncology* 4:459–471.

Fisher, B., C. Redmond, A. Brown, D. L. Wickerham, N. Wolmark, J. Allegra, G. Escher, M. Lippman, E. Savlov, J. Wittliff, E. R. Fisher, and other NSABP investigators. 1983. Influence of tumor estrogen and progesterone receptor levels on the response to tamoxifen and chemotherapy in primary breast cancer. *Journal of Clinical Oncology* 1:227–241.

Fisher, B., C. Redmond, A. Brown, N. Wolmark, J. Wittliff, E. R. Fisher, D. Plotkin, S. Sachs, J. Wolter, R. Frelick, R. Desser, N. LiCalzi, P. Geggie, T. Campbell, E. G. Elias, D. Prager, P. Koontz, H. Volk, N. Dimitrov, B. Gardner, H. Lerner, H. Shibata, and other NSABP investigators. 1981. Treatment of primary breast cancer with chemotherapy and tamoxifen. *New England Journal of Medicine* 305:1–6.

Fromson, J. M., S. Pearson, and S. Bramah. 1973a. The metabolism of tamoxifen (ICI 46,474). 1. In laboratory animals. *Xenobiotica* 3:693–709.

Fromson, J. M., and S. Pearson, and S. Bramah. 1973b. The metabolism of tamoxifen (ICI 46,474). 2. In female patients. *Xenobiotica* 3:711–714.

Furr, B. J., and V. C. Jordan. 1984. The pharmacology and clinical uses of tamoxifen. *Pharmacology and Therapeutics* 25:127–205.

Gottardis, M. M., and V. C. Jordan. 1987. Antitumor actions of keoxifene and tamoxifen in the N-nitrosomethylurea–induced rat mammary carcinoma model. *Cancer Research* 47:4020–4024.

Gottardis, M. M., and V. C. Jordan. 1988. Development of tamoxifen stimulated growth of MCF-7 tumors in athymic mice after long-term antiestrogen administration. *Cancer Research* 48:5183–5187.

Gottardis, M. M., S. P. Robinson, and V. C. Jordan. 1988. Estradiol-stimulated growth of MCF-7 tumors implanted in athymic mice: a model to study the tumoristatic action of tamoxifen. *Journal of Steroid Biochemistry* 30:311–314.

Groom, G. V., and K. Griffiths. 1976. Effect of the antioestrogen tamoxifen on plasma levels of luteinizing hormone, follicle-stimulating hormone, prolactin, oestradiol and progesterone in normal pre-menopausal women. *Journal of Endocrinology* 70:421–428.

Gullino, P. M., H. M. Pettigrew, and F. H. Grantham. 1975. N-Nitrosomethylurea as mammary gland carcinogen in rats. *Journal of the National Cancer Institute* 54:401–414.

Harper, M. J. K., and A. L. Walpole. 1966. Contrasting endocrine activities of *cis* and *trans* isomers in a series of substituted triphenylethylenes. *Nature* (London) 212:87.

Harper, M. J. K., and A. L. Walpole. 1967a. A new derivative of triphenylethylene: effect on implantation and mode of action in rats. *Journal of Reproduction and Fertility* 13:101–119.

Harper, M. J. K., and A. L. Walpole. 1967b. Mode of action of ICI 46,474 in preventing implantation in rats. *Journal of Endocrinology* 37:83–92.

Herbst, A. L., C. T. Griffiths, and R. W. Kistner. 1964. Clomiphene citrate (NSC-35770) in disseminated mammary carcinoma. *Cancer Chemotherapy Reports* 43:39–41.

Holtkamp, D. E., S. C. Greslin, C. A. Root, and L. J. Lerner. 1960. Gonadotropin inhibiting and antifecundity effects of chloramiphene. *Proceedings of the Society for Experimental Biology and Medicine* 105:197–201.

Huggins, C., L. C. Grand, and F. P. Brillantes. 1961. Mammary cancer induced by a single feeding of polynuclear hydrocarbons and its suppression. *Nature* (London) 189:204–207.

Hynes, N. E., B. Grand, and R. Michalides. 1984. Mouse mammary tumor virus: transcriptional control and involvement in tumorigenesis. *Advances in Cancer Research* 41:155–184.

Iino, Y., D. M. Wolf, S. M. Langen-Fahey, D. A. Johnson, M. Ricchio, M. E. Thompson, and V. C. Jordan. 1991. Reversible control of oestradiol-stimulated MCF-7 tumours by tamoxifen in the athymic mouse. *British Journal of Cancer* 64:1019–1024.

Ingle, J. N., J. E. Krook, S. J. Green, T. P. Kubista, L. K. Everson, D. L. Ahman, M. N. Chang, H. F. Bisel, H. E. Windschitl, D. I. Twito, and D. M. Pfeifle. 1986. Randomized trial of bilateral oophorectomy versus tamoxifen in premenopausal women with metastatic breast cancer. *Journal of Clinical Oncology* 4:178–185.

Jensen, E. V., G. E. Block, S. Smith, K. Kyser, and E. R. DeSombre. 1971. Estrogen receptors and breast cancer response to adrenalectomy. *NCI Monographs* 34:55–67.

Johansson, H., L. Terenius, and L. Thoren. 1970. The binding of estradiol-17beta to human breast cancers and other tissues *in vitro*. *Cancer Research* 30:692–698.

Jordan, V. C. 1974a. Antitumour activity of the antioestrogen ICI 46,474 (tamoxifen) in the dimethylbenzanthracene (DMBA)-induced rat mammary carcinoma model. *Journal Steroid Biochemistry* 5:354.

Jordan, V. C. 1974b. The antiestrogen tamoxifen (ICI 46,474) as an antitumor agent. *Proceedings of the Eastern Cooperative Oncology Group*, February 11–12, Miami, Florida.

Jordan, V. C. 1974c. Tamoxifen: mechanism of antitumor activity in animals and man. *Proceedings of the Eastern Cooperative Oncology Group*, June 22–25, Jaspar, Alberta.

Jordan, V. C. 1975a. Prolonged antioestrogenic activity of ICI 46,474 in the ovariectomized mouse. *Journal of Reproduction and Fertility* 42:251–258.

Jordan, V. C. 1975b. The antitumor effect of tamoxifen in the dimethylbenzanthracene-induced mammary carcinoma model. *Proceedings of the Symposium on the Hormonal Control of Breast Cancer*, Alderly Park, pp. 11–17. Macclesfield: ICI Pharmaceuticals Division PLC.

Jordan, V. C. 1976. Effect of tamoxifen (ICI 46,474) on initiation and growth of DMBA-induced rat mammary carcinomata. *European Journal of Cancer* 12:419–424.

Jordan, V. C. 1978. Use of the DMBA-induced rat mammary carcinoma system for the evaluation of tamoxifen as a potential adjuvant therapy. *Reviews on Endocrine Related Cancer* (October Supplement):49–55.

Jordan, V. C. 1983. Laboratory studies to develop general principles for the adjuvant treatment of breast cancer with antiestrogens: problems and potential for future clinical applications. *Breast Cancer Research and Treatment* 3 (Supplement):S73–86.

Jordan, V. C., and K. E. Allen. 1980. Evaluation of the antitumor activity of the non-steroidal antioestrogen monohydroxytamoxifen in the DMBA-induced rat mammary carcinoma model. *European Journal of Cancer* 16:231–251.

Jordan, V. C., and L. J. Dowse. 1976. Tamoxifen as an antitumour agent: effect on oestrogen binding. *Journal of Endocrinology* 68:297–303.

Jordan, V. C., and T. Jaspan. 1976. Tamoxifen as an antitumour agent: oestrogen binding as a predictive test for tumour response. *Journal of Endocrinology* 68:453–460.

Jordan, V. C., and S. Koerner. 1975. Tamoxifen (ICI 46,474) and the human carcinoma 8S oestrogen receptor. *European Journal of Cancer* 11:205–206.

Jordan, V. C., and S. Koerner. 1976. Tamoxifen as an antitumour agent role of oestradiol and prolactin. *Journal of Endocrinology* 68:305–310.

Jordan, V. C., and C. S. Murphy. 1990. Endocrine pharmacology of antiestrogens as antitumor agents. *Endocrine Reviews* 11:578–610.

Jordan, V. C., K. E. Allen, and C. J. Dix. 1980. Pharmacology of tamoxifen in laboratory animals. *Cancer Treatment Reports* 64:745–759.

Jordan, V. C., C. J. Dix, and K. E. Allen. 1979. The effectiveness of long-term treatment in a laboratory model for adjuvant hormone therapy of breast cancer. In *Adjuvant therapy of cancer,* vol. 2, ed. S. E. Salmon and S. E. Jones, 19–26. New York: Grune and Stratton.

Jordan, V. C., M. K. Lababidi, and S. Langan-Fahey. 1991. Suppression of mouse mammary tumorigenesis by long-term tamoxifen therapy. *Journal of the National Cancer Institute* 83:492–496.

Jordan, V. C., M. K. Lababidi, and D. M. Mirecki. 1990. The antiestrogenic and antitumor properties of prolonged tamoxifen therapy in C3H/OUJ mice. *European Journal of Cancer* 26:718–721.

Jordan, V. C., M. M. Collins, L. Rowsby, and G. Prestwich. 1977. A monohydroxylated metabolite of tamoxifen with potent antioestrogenic activity. *Journal of Endocrinology* 75:305–316.

Jordan, V. C., R. Koch, S. Langan, and R. McCague. 1988. Ligand interaction at the estrogen receptor to program antiestrogen action: study with non-steroidal compounds *in vitro. Endocrinology* 122:2379–2386.

Jordan, V. C., R. R. Bain, R. R. Brown, B. Gosden, and M. A. Santos. 1983. Determination and pharmacology of a new hydroxylated metabolite of tamoxifen observed in patient sera during therapy for advanced breast cancer. *Cancer Research* 43:1446–1450.

Kalman, A. M., T. Thompson, and C. L. Vogel. 1982. Response to oophorectomy after tamoxifen failure in a premenopausal patient. *Cancer Treatment Reports* 66:1867–1868.

Kemp, J. V., H. K. Adam, A. E. Wakeling, and R. Slater. 1983. Identification and biological activity of tamoxifen metabolites in human serum. *Biochemical Pharmacology* 32:2045–2052.

Kistner, R. W., and O. W. Smith. 1959. Observations on the use of nonsteroidal estrogen antagonist: MER25. *Surgical Forum* 10:725–729.

Klopper, A., and M. Hall. 1971. New synthetic agent for the induction of ovulation: preliminary trials in women. *British Medical Journal* 1:152–154.

Korenman, S. G., and B. A. Dukes. 1970. Specific estrogen binding by the cytoplasm of human breast carcinoma. *Journal of Clinical Endocrinology and Metabolism* 30:639–645.

Lacassagne, A. 1936. Hormonal pathogenesis of adenocarcinoma of the breast. *American Journal of Cancer* 14:217–225.

Langan-Fahey, S. M., D. C. Tormey, and V. C. Jordan, 1990. Tamoxifen metabolites in patients on long-term adjuvant therapy for breast cancer. *European Journal of Cancer* 26:883–888.

Lathrop, A. E. C., and L. Loeb. 1916. Further investigations on the origins of tumors in mice III. On the part played by internal secretions in the spontaneous development of tumors. *Journal of Cancer Research* 1:1–16.

Lerner, L. J. 1981. The first nonsteroidal antioestrogen—MER 25. In *Non-steroidal antioestrogens: molecular pharmacology and antitumour activity,* ed. R. L. Sutherland and V. C. Jordan, 1–16. Sydney: Academic Press.

Lerner, L. J., J. F. Holthaus, and C. R. Thompson. 1958. A nonsteroidal estrogen antagonist 1-(p-2-diethylaminoethoxyphenyl)-1-phenyl-2-p-methoxyphenyl-ethanol. *Endocrinology* 63:295–318.

Lieberman, M. E., J. Gorski, and V. C. Jordan. 1983. An estrogen receptor model to describe the regulation of prolactin synthesis by antiestrogens *in vitro*. *Journal of Biological Chemistry* 258:4741–4745.

Lien, E. A., E. Solheim, O. A. Lea, S. Lundgren, S. Kvinnsland, and P. M. Ueland. 1989. Distribution of 4-hydroxy-N-desmethyltamoxifen and other tamoxifen metabolites in human biological fluids during tamoxifen treatment. *Cancer Research* 49:2175–2183.

Lippman, M. E., and G. Bolan. 1975. Oestrogen-responsive human breast cancer in long-term tissue culture. *Nature* 256:592–593.

Love, R. R., R. B. Mazess, H. S. Barden, S. Epstein, P. A. Newcomb, V. C. Jordan, P. P. Carbone, and D. L. DeMets. 1992. Effects of tamoxifen on bone mineral density in postmenopausal women with breast cancer. *New England Journal of Medicine* 326:852–856.

Love, R. R., D. A. Weibe, P. A. Newcomb, L. Cameron, H. Leventhal, V. C. Jordan, J. Feyzi, and D. L. DeMets. 1991. Effects of tamoxifen on cardiovascular risk factors in postmenopausal women. *Annals of Internal Medicine* 115:860–864.

Ludwig Breast Cancer Study Group. 1984. Randomized trial of chemoendocrine therapy, endocrine therapy and mastectomy alone in postmenopausal patients with operable breast cancer and axillary node metastases. *Lancet* 1:1256–1260.

McDonald, C. C., and H. J. Stewart. 1991. Fatal myocardial infarction in the Scottish adjuvant tamoxifen trial. The Scottish Breast Cancer Committee. *British Medical Journal* 303:435–437.

McGuire, W. L., P. P. Carbone, and E. P. Vollmer, eds. 1975. *Estrogen receptors in human breast cancer.* New York: Raven Press.

Manni, A., J. E. Trujillo, J. S. Marshall, J. Brodkey, and O. H. Pearson. 1979. Antihormone treatments of stage IV breast cancer. *Cancer* 43:444–450.

Murphy, C. S., S. M. Langan-Fahey, R. McCague, and V. C. Jordan. 1990. Structure-function relationships of hydroxylated metabolites of tamoxifen that control the proliferation of estrogen-responsive T47D breast cancer cells *in vitro*. *Molecular Pharmacology* 38:737–743.

Nicholson, R. I., and M. P. Golder. 1975. The effect of synthetic antioestrogens on the growth and biochemistry of rat mammary tumours. *European Journal of Cancer* 11:571–579.

Nicholson, R. I., M. P. Golder, P. Davis, and K. Griffiths. 1976. Effects of oestradiol-17beta and tamoxifen on total and accessible cytoplasmic oestradiol-17beta receptors in DMBA-induced rat mammary tumours. *European Journal of Cancer* 12:711–717.

Nolvadex Adjuvant Trial Organisation (NATO). 1985. Controlled trial of tamoxifen as a single adjuvant agent in the management of early breast cancer. *Lancet* 1:836–840.

O'Halloran, M. J., and P. G. Maddock. 1974. ICI 46,474 in breast cancer. *Journal of the Irish Medical Association* 67:38–39.

Osborne, C. K., E. B. Coronado, and J. P. Robinson. 1987. Human breast cancer in the athymic nude mouse: cytostatic effects of long-term antiestrogen therapy. *European Journal of Cancer and Clinical Oncology* 23:1189–1196.

Osborne, C. K., K. Hobbs, and G. M. Clark. 1985. Effect of estrogens and antiestrogens on growth of human breast cancer cells in athymic nude mice. *Cancer Research* 45:584–590.

Osborne, C. K., D. H. Boldt, G. M. Clark, and J. M. Trent. 1983. Effects of tamoxifen on human breast cancer cell cycle kinetics: accumulation of cells in early G1 phase. *Cancer Research* 43:3583–3585.

Patterson, J. S., R. S. Settatree, H. K. Adam, and J. V. Kemp. 1980. Serum concentrations of tamoxifen and major metabolite during long-term Nolvadex therapy, correlated with clinical response. *European Journal of Cancer* 1(Supplement):89–92.

Peters, G., S. Brookes, R. Smith, M. Placzek, and C. Dickson. 1989. The mouse homology of the hst/K-FGF gene is adjacent to int-2 and is activated by proviral insertion in some virally induced mammary tumors. *Proceedings of the National Academy of Sciences of the United States of America* 86:5678–5682.

Planting, A. S., J. Alexieva-Figusch, J. Blonk-v. d. Wijst, and W. L. van Putten. 1985. Tamoxifen therapy in premenopausal women with metastatic breast cancer. *Cancer Treatment Reports* 69:363–368.

Powles, T. J., C. R. Tillyer, A. L. Jones, S. E. Ashley, J. Treleaven, J. B. Davey, and J. A. McKinna. 1990. Prevention of breast cancer with tamoxifen—an update on the Royal Marsden Hospital pilot programme. *European Journal of Cancer* 26:680–684.

Powles, T. J., J. R. Hardy, S. E. Ashley, G. M. Farrington, D. Cosgrove, J. B. Davey, M. Dowsett, J. A. McKinna, A. G. Nash, H. D. Sinnett, C. R. Tillyer, and J. Treleaven. 1989. A pilot trial to evaluate the acute toxicity and feasibility of tamoxifen for prevention of breast cancer. *British Journal of Cancer* 60:126–131.

Pritchard, K. I., D. B. Thomson, R. E. Myers, D. J. Sutherland, B. G. Mobbs, and J. W. Meakin. 1980. Tamoxifen therapy in premenopausal patients with metastatic breast cancer. *Cancer Treatment Reports* 64:787–796.

Ribeiro, G., and M. K. Palmer. 1983. Adjuvant tamoxifen for operable carcinoma of the breast: report of a clinical trial by the Christie Hospital and Holt Radium Institute. *British Medical Journal* 286:827–830.

Ribeiro, G., and R. Swindell. 1985. The Christie Hospital tamoxifen (Nolvadex) adjuvant trial for operable breast carcinoma—seven-year results. *European Journal of Cancer and Clinical Oncology* 21:897–900.

Robinson, S. P., D. A. Mauel, and V. C. Jordan. 1989. Antitumor actions of toremifene in the 7, 12-dimethylbenzanthracene (DMBA)-induced rat mammary tumor model. *European Journal of Cancer and Clinical Oncology* 24:1817–1821.

Rose, C., S. M. Thorpe, K. W. Andersen, B. V. Pedersen, H. T. Mouridsen, M. Blichert-Toft, and B. B. Rasmussen. 1985. Beneficial effect of adjuvant tamoxifen therapy in primary breast cancer patients with high oestrogen receptor values. *Lancet* 1:16–19.

Sander, S. 1968. The *in vitro* uptake of oestradiol in biopsies from 25 breast cancer patients. *Acta Pathologica et Microbiologica Scandinavica* 74:301–302.

Sawka, C. A., K. I. Pritchard, A. H. Paterson, D. B. Thomson, W. E. Shelley, R. E. Myers, B. G. Mobbs, A. Malkin, and J. W. Meakin. 1986. Role and mechanism of action of tamoxifen in premenopausal women with metastatic breast carcinoma. *Cancer Research* 46:3152–3156.

Shafie, S. M., and F. H. Grantham. 1981. Role of hormones in the growth and regression of human breast cancer cells (MCF-7) transplanted into athymic nude mice. *Journal of the National Cancer Institute* 67:51–56.

Skidmore, J., A. L. Walpole, and J. Woodburn. 1972. Effect of some triphenylethylenes on oestradiol binding *in vitro* to macromolecules from uterus and anterior pituitary. *Journal of Endocrinology* 52:289–298.

Sutherland, R. L., M. D. Green, R. E. Hall, R. R. Reddel, and I. W. Taylor. 1983. Tamoxifen induces accumulation of MCF-7 human mammary carcinoma cells in the G0/G1 phase of the cell cycle. *European Journal of Cancer and Clinical Oncology* 19:615–621.

Tamoxifen Workshop. 1976. Proceedings of the Annual Spring Meeting of the Primary Breast Cancer Therapy Group, Key Biscayne, Florida, April 28. *Cancer Treatment Reports* 60:1409–1466.

Tormey, D. C., and V. C. Jordan. 1984. Long-term tamoxifen adjuvant therapy in node-positive breast cancer: a metabolic and pilot clinical study. *Breast Cancer Research and Treatment* 4:297–302.

Tormey, D. C., P. Rasmussen, and V. C. Jordan. 1987. Long-term adjuvant tamoxifen study: clinical update (Letter). *Breast Cancer Research and Treatment* 9:157–158.

Terenius, L. 1971. Structure-activity relationships of anti-oestrogens with regard to interaction with 17ß oestradiol in the mouse uterus and vagina. *Acta Endoclinologica* 66:431–447.

Turcot-Lemay, L., and P. A. Kelley. 1980. Characterization of estradiol, progesterone and prolactin receptors in nitrosomethylurea-induced mammary tumors and effects of antiestrogen treatment on the development and growth of these tumors. *Cancer Research* 40:3232–3240.

Ward, H. W. C. 1973. Antioestrogen therapy for breast cancer: a trial of tamoxifen at two dose levels. *British Medical Journal* 1:13–14.

Williamson, J. G., and J. D. Ellis. 1973. The induction of ovulation by tamoxifen. *Journal of Obstetrics and Gynaecology of the British Commonwealth* 80:844–847.

Wilson, A. J., F. Tehrani, and M. Baum. 1982. Adjuvant tamoxifen therapy for early breast cancer: an experimental study with reference to oestrogen and progesterone receptors. *British Journal of Surgery* 69:121–125.

2

Clinical Pharmacology and Endocrinology of Long-Term Tamoxifen Therapy

Susan M. Langan Fahey, V. Craig Jordan,
Nancy F. Fritz, Simon P. Robinson, David
Waters, and Douglass C. Tormey

I.	Introduction	28
II.	Metabolism	29
	a. Measurement and Identification of Tamoxifen	29
	b. Metabolic Pathways	30
	c. Species Variation	33
III.	Pharmacokinetics	36
	a. Single Dose Kinetics	36
	b. Steady State Kinetics	36
	c. Distribution into Tissues	40
IV.	Endocrinology	44
	a. Postmenopausal	44
	b. Premenopausal	45
V.	Conclusions	48
	References	50

I. *Introduction*

ADJUVANT tamoxifen therapy of greater than 2 years' duration is a relatively recent development in the treatment of breast cancer. Studies using animal models of hormone-dependent mammary cancer (Jordan et al. 1979; Jordan and Allen 1980; Gottardis and Jordan 1987; Robinson and Jordan 1987) demonstrated that short-term tamoxifen only delayed the onset of mammary tumor development after exposure to carcinogens. However, treatment for 6 months stopped the development of tumors in 90% of the animals. The observation in carcinogen-induced rat models that longer may be better was also supported by similar findings in the athymic nude mouse model of breast cancer using hormone-dependent MCF-7 cells transplanted into the mammary fat pads (Gottardis et al. 1987; Osborne et al. 1985).

The observation in animal models that tamoxifen acts as a tumoristatic rather than a tumoricidal agent led to the concept that tamoxifen might be more effective in improving survival if given for 5 years or possibly indefinitely. As a result, a pilot study of 5 years of tamoxifen therapy was initiated at the University of Wisconsin Comprehensive Cancer Center in 1977 (Tormey and Jordan 1984). The results showed that 5 years of treatment with tamoxifen were well tolerated and that no unusual side effects developed over time (Tormey and Jordan 1984). Most important, the blood levels of tamoxifen and two metabolites, N-desmethyltamoxifen and metabolite Y after reaching steady state, remained constant over the 5-year treatment course. The results of the pilot study coupled with the animal model data led to the development of two randomized Eastern Cooperative Oncology Group (ECOG) trials of long-term tamoxifen, EST 4181 and EST 5181, which reported an increase in disease-free survival in the 5-year treatment arm (Falkson et al. 1990). The concept was further developed by the National Surgical Adjuvant Breast and Bowel Project (NSABP), and 5 years of tamoxifen have become a standard of treatment (Fisher et al. 1987, 1989). Indeed, the overview analysis of adjuvant tamoxifen trials with a total accrual of nearly 30,000 women has demonstrated that both disease-free and overall survival are increased with increasing duration of tamoxifen and that the benefits are greater at 10 years than at 5 years (Early Breast Cancer Trialists' Collaborative Group 1992).

Worldwide, it has been estimated that there are 4.5 million women years of experience with tamoxifen, but now the duration of therapy has been routinely extended beyond 5 years. Consequently, information regarding the pharmacology and endocrinology of long-term tamoxifen therapy is essential toxicological information.

II. *Metabolism*

A. Measurement and Identification of Tamoxifen (ICI 46,474; *TRANS*-1-(4-BETA-DEMETHYLAMINOETHOXYPHENYL)-1,2-DIPHENYLBUT-1-ENE; MW = 371.53)

The initial work on tamoxifen metabolism and pharmacokinetics was reported by Fromson and co-workers (1973a,b) in the early 1970s. Samples of serum, urine, bile, and feces were collected from rat, mouse, rhesus monkey, and dog after oral dosing with [^{14}C]tamoxifen (Fromson et al. 1973a). In addition, samples of serum, urine, and feces from breast cancer patients treated with [^{14}C]tamoxifen were also collected for analysis (Fromson et al. 1973b). Methanol extracts of the samples were prepared, and the parent drug and metabolites were separated using thin-layer chromatography (TLC). By comparing the relative mobilities of the radioactive areas on the TLC plate with authentic standards, a tentative identification of several metabolites was accomplished.

Originally, Fromson and co-workers (1973a,b) reported 4-OH tamoxifen as the major metabolite of tamoxifen in all species examined, including the human. Subsequent work showed that 4-OH tamoxifen comigrated with N-desmethyltamoxifen in the TLC system employed by Fromson and that N-desmethyltamoxifen is the major metabolite of tamoxifen in human serum (Adam et al. 1979, Adam, Patterson, and Kemp 1980). Daniel and co-workers (1979), using gas chromatography–mass spectrometry (GC-MS), quantitated N-desmethyltamoxifen at 150% and 4-hydroxytamoxifen at 2% of the concentration of the parent drug in serum from patients receiving 20 mg BID.

Development of high-performance liquid chromatography (HPLC) to separate and quantitate tamoxifen and its metabolites was delayed because of technical difficulties with detection methods. Ultraviolet (UV) absorbance requires microgram quantities of tamoxifen and consequently could not provide the sensitivity needed to measure the nanogram levels in serum and tissues. However, this difficulty was overcome by employing a photochemical reaction of tamoxifen to form the corresponding phenanthrene when exposed

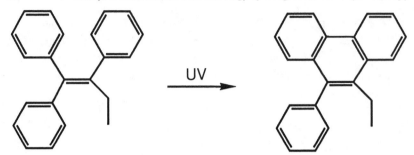

Figure 2.1. UV photocyclization of triphenylethylenes to form corresponding phenanthrenes.

to UV light (Fig. 2.1; Mendenhall et al. 1978). The resulting phenanthrene is highly fluorescent and measurable in nanogram amounts. Originally the photochemical reaction was reported as part of an HPLC assay system, but it has also been incorporated into a TLC assay system (Adam, Gay, and Moore 1980).

The metabolites of tamoxifen are also capable of forming the phenanthrene derivative, although the fluorescence level will vary with each compound, resulting in the need for a standard curve to assure correct quantitation (Mendenhall et al. 1978; Golander and Sternson 1980; Brown et al. 1983; Camaggi et al. 1983; Nieder and Jaeger 1987; Kikuta and Schmid 1989; Salamoun et al. 1990). Several methods include an internal standard to correct for extraction recoveries as well as for variations in the photochemical reaction which produces the fluorescent phenanthrenes (Wilbur et al. 1985; Lien et al. 1987; Brown et al. 1983; Langan-Fahey et al. 1990).

Techniques employing GC-MS are the most sensitive methods available and are capable of measuring picogram quantities of compound. GC-MS also has the advantage of providing positive identification of metabolites on the basis of comparing mass ion fragment patterns with those of authentic compounds (Gaskell et al. 1978; Bain and Jordan 1983; Kemp et al. 1983; Murphy et al. 1987). Consequently, further discussion of tamoxifen metabolism will be limited to those metabolites that have been identified in human patients using GC-MS.

B. Metabolic Pathways

Metabolism of tamoxifen occurs primarily in the liver and involves the microsomal P-450 system in a series of phase I–type reactions (Fig. 2.2) that result in demethylation followed by deamination and hydroxylation of key positions on the phenyl groups (Reunitz and Toledo 1980; Meltzer et al. 1984; Reunitz et al. 1984; Reunitz and Bagley 1985; Jacolot et al. 1991). The major

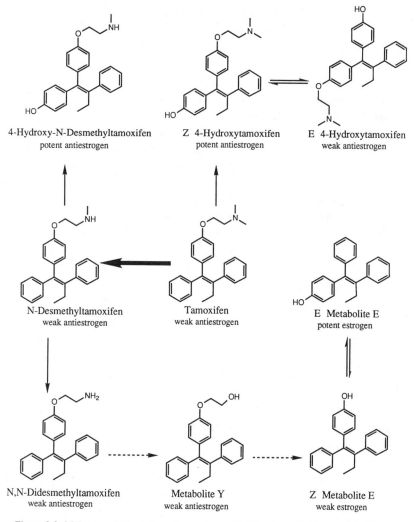

4-Hydroxy-N-Desmethyltamoxifen
potent antiestrogen

Z 4-Hydroxytamoxifen
potent antiestrogen

E 4-Hydroxytamoxifen
weak antiestrogen

N-Desmethyltamoxifen
weak antiestrogen

Tamoxifen
weak antiestrogen

E Metabolite E
potent estrogen

N,N-Didesmethyltamoxifen
weak antiestrogen

Metabolite Y
weak antiestrogen

Z Metabolite E
weak estrogen

Figure 2.2. Major metabolic routes of tamoxifen. (Modified from Robinson et al. 1984.)

metabolite of tamoxifen is N-desmethyltamoxifen (Adam et al. 1979), which results from demethylation of the tertiary amine. Further demethylation forms N,N-didesmethyltamoxifen (Kemp et al. 1983) followed by deamination to form the polar metabolite Y (Bain and Jordan 1983). Removal of the ethoxy sidechain from metabolite Y would form metabolite E (Fromson et al. 1973; Murphy et al. 1987; Wiebe et al. 1992).

Alternatively, tamoxifen may be hydroxylated at the 4-position pre- or postdemethylation of the N to generate 4-hydroxytamoxifen (Fromson et al. 1973a; Daniel et al. 1979; Robinson et al. 1989) and 4-hydroxy-N-desmethyl-tamoxifen (Lien et al. 1988, 1989; Robinson et al. 1989), respectively. Further modification by removal of the amine and resulting ethoxy sidechain would result in the production of bisphenol (Mauvais-Jarvis et al. 1986; Wiebe et al. 1992), although at this time the identification of this compound should be considered tentative.

Several drug interactions with tamoxifen have been reported. The most serious interaction involves Warfarin and has life-threatening implications (Lodwick et al. 1987; Ritchie and Grant 1989; Tenni et al. 1989). Concurrent treatment with medroxyprogesterone acetate results in significantly reduced levels of N-desmethyltamoxifen, although the half-lives of tamoxifen and N-desmethyltamoxifen are not affected (Camaggi et al. 1985). More recently, simultaneous treatment with tamoxifen and aminoglutethimide has been correlated with decreased serum tamoxifen and metabolite levels (Lien et al. 1990).

All the major metabolites of tamoxifen are believed to contribute to the antiestrogenic activity *in vivo* on the basis of their binding affinity for the estrogen receptor *in vitro* and their ability to inhibit competitively the estradiol-stimulated growth of MCF-7 breast cancer cells *in vitro*. Metabolites that are hydroxylated in the 4-position exhibit high binding affinity for the estrogen receptor (Jordan et al. 1977). 4-Hydroxytamoxifen has a relative binding affinity for the estrogen receptor that is similar to that for estradiol (Jordan et al. 1977) and is 100 times more potent than the parent compound, tamoxifen, in competing with estradiol *in vitro* to inhibit MCF-7 cell growth (Coezy et al. 1982).

Phase II, or conjugation, reactions are primarily concerned with modification of compounds by adding polar groups such as sulfate or glucuronate to increase solubility in aqueous solutions. Conjugation of metabolites of tamoxifen with glucuronic acid appears to be the most common phase II reaction (Fromson et al. 1973a). Sulfated conjugates have also been described.

In addition to the metabolic conversions described above, the metabolites of tamoxifen that are hydroxylated directly on the phenyl ring are capable of undergoing a time-temperature dependent conversion from the Z isomer to the E isomer (Katzenellebogen et al. 1985). The ethylene bond is weakened by the presence of the electron-withdrawing hydroxyl group, allowing the substituents attached to the carbons to rotate. Tamoxifen is usually described in the literature as having *cis* or *trans* configuration because of the two unsubstituted phenyl groups on adjacent carbons across the double bond. The

Z isomer and *trans* configuration of tamoxifen are identical structures. Hydroxylation of tamoxifen to form 4-hydroxytamoxifen removes the symmetry across the double bond, and consequently the *cis* and *trans* nomenclature becomes meaningless. Isomerization of 4-hydroxytamoxifen across the double bond should be correctly described by the Z and E designations (Fig. 2.2).

The configuration of the substituents on the carbons forming the double bond becomes important when discussing the antiestrogenic and estrogenic actions of the various metabolites. Both *in vivo* (Jordan et al. 1981) and *in vitro* assays (Katzenellenbogen et al. 1984) demonstrate that the Z isomer of tamoxifen is an antiestrogen, whereas the E isomer is an estrogen. However, both Z and E 4-hydroxytamoxifen are classified as antiestrogenic (Jordan et al. 1981; Lieberman, Jordan, et al. 1983; Katzenellenbogen et al. 1984). The 4-OH group is important for binding to the estrogen receptor, and consequently Z 4-hydroxytamoxifen has a binding affinity for the estrogen receptor that is similar to that of estradiol (Jordan et al. 1977). The amine sidechain is believed to be essential for antiestrogenenic activity (Jordan and Gosden 1982). Only the Z *(trans)* isomer has high binding affinity; the E *(cis)* isomer has low binding affinity (Lieberman, Jordan, et al. 1983).

Metabolite E, however, lacks the amine sidechain, retaining only a hydroxyl group in this position. Upon isomerization to the E isomer, the hydroxyl group occupies the same phenyl position as in Z 4-hydroxytamoxifen and consequently exhibits high binding affinity for the estrogen receptor. Without the amine sidechain, the E isomer of metabolite E becomes a potent estrogenic compound with high binding affinity for the estrogen receptor (Murphy et al. 1990).

C. Species Variation

The metabolic variation between species was of great interest during the late 1970s and early 1980s, because tamoxifen was found to act as an estrogen in the mouse and dog, and as a partial estrogen in the rat. Initially, it was believed that the response variation between species could be explained by preferential metabolism of tamoxifen to estrogenic compounds such as E metabolite E or bisphenol. However, such estrogenic compounds have not been reported to date in sufficient quantities to account for the pharmacological differences observed (Jordan and Robinson 1987).

Figures 2.3 and 2.4 show the metabolic variations for the mouse, dog, and rat after single and multiple dosing. Interestingly, despite the estrogenic activity of tamoxifen, the mouse and dog metabolize significant quantities of

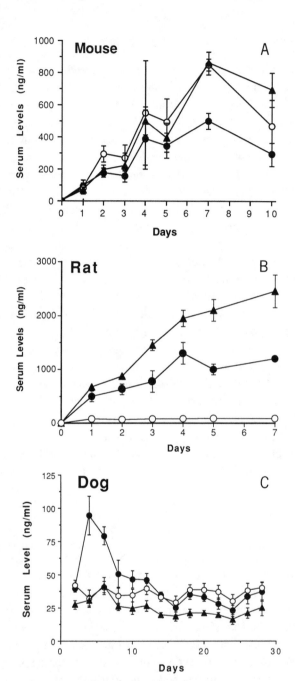

Figure 2.3. Metabolic variation between mouse, rat, and dog:
tamoxifen, ●; 4-hydroxytamoxifen, ○; N-desmethyltamoxifen,
▲. (A and B adapted from Robinson et al. 1991.)

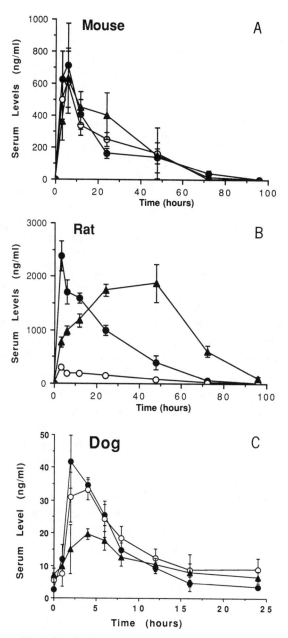

Figure 2.4. Decline in serum levels post–single dose of tamoxifen (A and B). Decay of serum levels post–14 days of treatment (C). Tamoxifen, ●; 4-hydroxytamoxifen, ○; N-desmethyltamoxifen, ▲. (A and B adapted from Robinson et al. 1991.)

35

parent compound to the more potent antiestrogen 4-hydroxytamoxifen. However, the rat, which exhibits significant antiestrogenic effects, produces smaller amounts of 4-hydroxytamoxifen and large amounts of N-desmethyltamoxifen. Currently, the estrogenicity of tamoxifen is believed to be linked to the interpretation of the estrogen receptor–ligand complex by the target tissue (Jordan and Robinson 1987).

III. *Pharmacokinetics*

A. SINGLE DOSE KINETICS

Tamoxifen is administered orally in tablet form as the citrate salt (MW = 563.6). The standard dose in the United States for all stages of breast cancer is 10 mg twice daily. Complete absorption studies have not been done because a parenteral solution of tamoxifen is not available. However, tamoxifen is believed to be well absorbed through the gut.

Fromson and co-workers (1973b) performed the initial studies of tamoxifen metabolism in women using [^{14}C]tamoxifen administered orally. Peak serum levels are reached approximately 4 hours after a single dose followed by biphasic excretion with an initial half-life of 7–14 hours. The half-life in the terminal excretion phase is approximately 7 days. Similar results have been obtained using direct chromatographic assays (Fabian et al. 1980, 1981; Guelen et al. 1987).

Work in mouse, dog, and monkey indicates that up to 90% of the radioactivity administered as tamoxifen is excreted via the feces over a 2-week period postdose. The majority of the radioactivity was present as glucuronidated conjugates (Fromson et al. 1973a). Similar observations were made in female patients (Fromson et al. 1973b). Only about 10% of the radioactivity was found in the urine. Consequently, tamoxifen is believed to undergo extensive first-pass metabolism in the liver and biliary excretion.

B. STEADY STATE KINETICS

During continuous treatment, the serum level of tamoxifen reaches steady state after approximately 4 weeks, whereas the serum level of the main metabolite, N-desmethyltamoxifen, rises more slowly and reaches steady state after approximately 8 weeks (Patterson et al. 1980). Prior to reaching steady state, differences in serum levels pre- and postdose are still evident for tamoxifen and N-desmethyltamoxifen (Fig. 2.5).

The majority of tamoxifen and metabolites are believed to be bound to

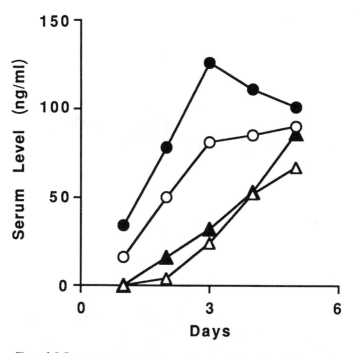

Figure 2.5. Pre–steady state levels in a patient receiving 40 mg bolus per day via gastrostomy tube. Tamoxifen, ●, ○; N-desmethyltamoxifen, ▲, △; closed symbols are levels measured predose; open symbols are levels measured 4 hours postdose.

serum proteins (Lien et al. 1989; Shah and Parsons 1991) with approximately 2% in the unbound state. Unpublished observations of two kidney dialysis patients show that there is neither a substantial loss of tamoxifen when pre- or postdialysis serum levels are analyzed (54 vs 51 ng/ml and 55 vs 66 ng/ml) nor a substantial loss of N-desmethyltamoxifen (61 vs 63 ng/ml and 92 vs 129 ng/ml). Further evidence of the extent of protein binding comes from consideration of almost nonexistent levels of tamoxifen in cerebral spinal fluid (CSF) (Jordan et al. 1983; Noguchi et al. 1988). In one breast cancer patient, even with dose escalation from 20 mg/day (serum tamoxifen = 85 ng/ml, N-desmethyltamoxifen = 64 ng/ml) to 40 mg/day (serum tamoxifen = 234 ng/ml, N-desmethyltamoxifen = 515 ng/ml), tamoxifen and metabolites measured <1 ng/ml in CSF. Only tamoxifen in an unbound state would be able to cross the blood brain barrier and equilibrate with CSF. Finally, one breast cancer patient with diabetes incipidus had a serum tamoxifen level of 105 ng/

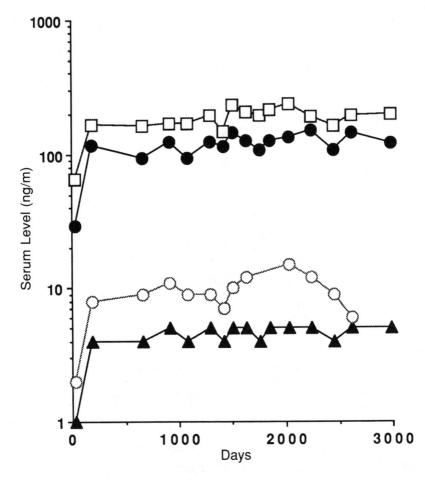

Figure 2.6. Serum levels measured in a patient receiving 10 mg BID for 8 years. Tamoxifen, ●; 4-hydroxytamoxifen, ▲; N-desmethyltamoxifen, □; metabolite Y, ○. (Adapted from Langan-Fahey et al. 1990.)

ml and serum N-desmethyltamoxifen of 148 ng/ml after 6 months of tamoxifen therapy (10 mg BID) despite the increased output of urine due to the disease state.

When treatment is stopped, serum tamoxifen levels decline more quickly (t ½ = 7 days; Fabian et al. 1981; Camaggi et al. 1985) than those of N-desmethyltamoxifen (t ½ = 14 days; Patterson 1980; Camaggi et al. 1985. However, it may take several weeks to clear the parent compound and metabolites completely from serum (Lien et al. 1991) and several months from tissues (Lien et

Table 2.1. Serum levels in breast cancer patients receiving tamoxifen for at least 60 days

Source	Dose (mg/day)	N	Serum level (ng/ml)					
			TAM	4-OH	N-dMT	4-OH N-dMT	Z	Y
Langan-Fahey et al. 1990	20	35	148	NR	290	NR	NR	NR
Bratherton et al. 1984	20	77	159	NR	NR	NR	NR	NR
Milano et al. 1987	30	5	145	6.5	343	NR	55	35
Stevenson et al. 1988	30	12	113	<5	242	NR	33	26
Lien et al. 1989	30	5	141	3.5	220	9.3	51	34
Daniel et al. 1981	40	5	361	7.9	552	NR	NR	NR
Kemp et al. 1983	40	15	310	NR	481	NR	NR	49
Bratherton et al. 1984	40	75	273	NR	NR	NR	NR	NR
McVie et al. 1986	40	8	214	NR	246	NR	NR	NR

NR = not reported.

al. 1991). Once steady state is achieved, the serum levels of tamoxifen and its metabolites remain constant during 10 years of treatment (Fig. 2.6; Langan-Fahey et al. 1990).

There are numerous reports in the literature showing steady state serum levels of breast cancer patients receiving various doses of tamoxifen (Table 2.1). Breast cancer patients at steady state receiving 10 mg BID have a mean serum tamoxifen level of 100–150 ng/ml. Patients receiving high doses, 150–170 mg BID, maintain serum levels of 1200–1500 ng/ml (Jordan et al. 1983). Extremely high doses of tamoxifen have been used in an attempt to reverse multidrug resistance, and serum levels as high as 3500 ng/ml have been achieved after 12 days of dosing with 260 mg/sqm BID (Trump et al. 1992).

Individuals, however, vary greatly in their metabolic handling of the drug, as is evidenced by the wide ranges reported (Fig. 2.7). Individuals who are believed to be compliant appear to maintain constant blood levels and tamoxifen:N-desmethyltamoxifen ratios when serial serum samples are analyzed even after 8–11 years (Fig. 2.8). It has been proposed that monitoring the serum tamoxifen:N-desmethyltamoxifen ratio provides an accounting of compliance for a given patient (Bratherton et al. 1984); i.e., upon cessation of treatment, tamoxifen levels would fall, resulting in a change in the ratio of parent:metabolite. However, because of the wide individual variation, serial sampling would be necessary to establish the patient's steady state levels.

Several parameters have been examined in an attempt to explain the serum level variation between individuals. We examined 35 postmenopausal patients who had received tamoxifen for at least 6 months and found that

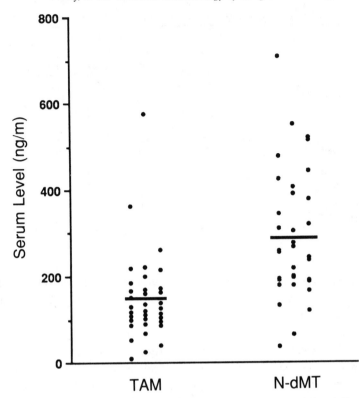

Figure 2.7. The variation in serum tamoxifen and N-desmethyltamoxifen levels in 35 postmenopausal women who received 10 mg BID for at least 6 months. Solid bars indicate mean values: tamoxifen, 148 ng/ml ± 16.9; and N-desmethyltamoxifen, 290 ± 24.5. (Adapted from Langan-Fahey et al. 1990.)

serum levels are not correlated with weight, height, or body surface area (Langan-Fahey et al. 1990). Furthermore, despite the wide variation, steady state serum levels do not predict treatment response (Bratherton et al. 1984; Watkins 1988). Interestingly, however, there is anecdotal evidence that an increase in the dose of tamoxifen may result in a response where none was observed previously (Manni and Arafah 1981; Watkins 1988).

C. DISTRIBUTION INTO TISSUES

Animal data suggest that tissue levels of tamoxifen and metabolites are substantially higher than serum levels. Rat and mouse data show that liver and uterus accumulate high levels of tamoxifen when compared with muscle following daily oral gavage of tamoxifen citrate in peanut oil. Metabolites

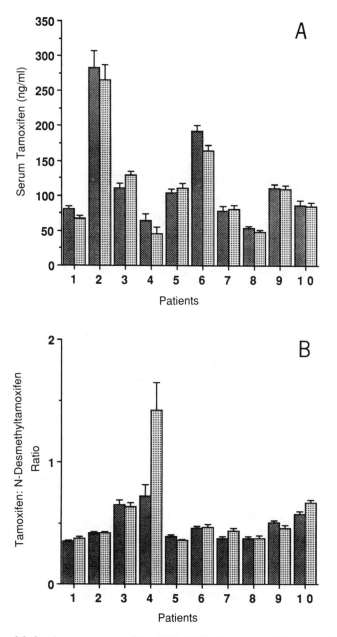

Figure 2.8. Steady state serum profiles of 10 individual patients receiving tamoxifen for at least 8 years. At least two samples were measured in each year. (A) Comparison of mean serum level for the first 4 years of therapy (▨) with the level after at least 4 additional years (▨). (B) Comparison of the mean ratio of serum tamoxifen to N-desmethyltamoxifen. Values are calculated from the serum levels reported in A. *Note*: Patient #4 was withdrawn for 3 months during year 6. (Adapted from Langan-Fahey et al. 1990.)

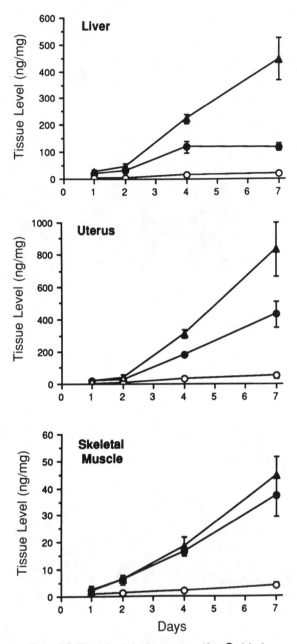

Figure 2.9. Tissue levels in the rat: tamoxifen, ●; 4-hydroxy-tamoxifen, ○; N-desmethyltamoxifen, ▲. (Adapted from Robinson et al. 1991.)

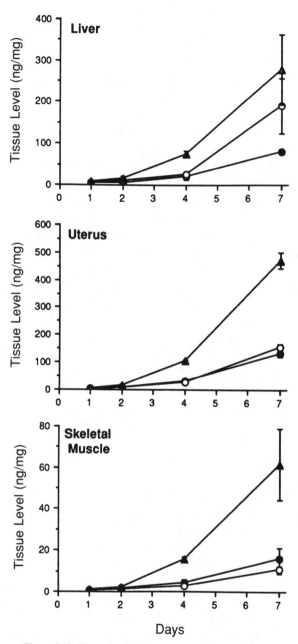

Figure 2.10. Tissue levels in the mouse: tamoxifen, ●; 4-hydroxytamoxifen, ○; N-desmethyltamoxifen, ▲. (Adapted from Robinson et al. 1991.)

follow a similar accumulation pattern (Robinson et al. 1991; Figs. 2.9, 2.10). Studies of MCF-7 human tumor explants grown in the athymic nude mouse show that tumor tamoxifen levels increase 25–70-fold above serum levels when concentrations similar to those measured in patients are achieved (De-Gregorio et al. 1989; Iino et al. 1991).

Limited information is available to describe the tissue distribution of tamoxifen in patients, because it is difficult to obtain adequate biopsy samples for analysis. Work by Lien and co-workers (1991) demonstrates that tamoxifen and metabolites accumulate in tissues 8–70-fold above serum levels in patients receiving 40 mg/day for at least 30 days, i.e., steady state. Daniel and co-workers (1981) measured tamoxifen and N-desmethyltamoxifen levels in breast tumor homogenates and found that N-desmethyltamoxifen was present at about twice the level of tamoxifen and 4-hydroxytamoxifen was present at about 2% of the level of the parent drug. Although they reported the tumor levels on the basis of a per milligram of protein, the amount accumulated when compared with the serum levels is similar to that reported by Lien when tissue water content is considered. Trump and co-workers (1992) reported that the levels in melanoma were increased 4-fold (9100 ng/gm vs 2294 ng/ml) above the serum level in one high dose patient and 6-fold (9500 ng/gm vs 1646 ng/ml) in a squamous cell head/neck tumor from a second high dose patient.

IV. Endocrinology

A. POSTMENOPAUSAL

The majority of breast cancer patients receiving tamoxifen therapy are postmenopausal, and consequently most endocrine studies have examined the impact of tamoxifen in the presence of a low estrogen environment. The effects of tamoxifen on serum hormones and sex hormone–binding globulin (SHBG) are summarized in Figure 2.11. In the presence of low-serum estrogens, circulating tamoxifen decreased levels of follicle-stimulating hormone (FSH) and luteinizing hormone (LH) (Manni et al. 1979; Jordan et al. 1987a,b). This would indicate that tamoxifen is acting as an estrogen on the hypothalamus-pituitary axis. Estrogenic actions of tamoxifen are observed in other tissues as well. Serum levels of SHBG, a protein synthesized in the liver, rise in response to tamoxifen therapy (Sakai et al. 1978; Szamel et al. 1986; Jordan et al. 1987a,b). Prolactin levels are unchanged (Manni et al. 1979) or decreased (Jordan et al. 1987a,b). Decreased levels of prolactin are

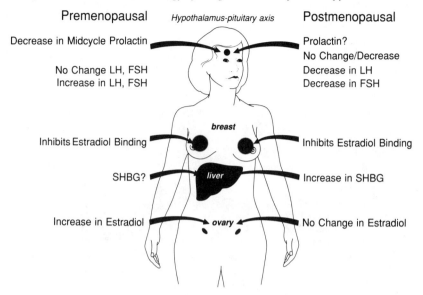

Figure 2.11. Endocrine changes in premenopausal and postmenopausal women receiving tamoxifen. (Adapted from Jordan et al. 1986.)

an antiestrogen effect of tamoxifen on pituitary lactotrophs *in vitro* (Lieberman, Gorski, and Jordan 1983) and, as a result, provide evidence for a direct effect of tamoxifen on the pituitary. Serum levels of estrogens and progesterone remain the same, an indication that tamoxifen is unable to reactivate the postmenopausal ovary (Manni et al. 1979; Jordan et al. 1987a,b).

B. PREMENOPAUSAL

Endocrine changes in response to tamoxifen by premenopausal patients are more complex than those of postmenopausal patients because of the presence of functioning ovaries. The situation is further complicated by the use of chemotherapy, which can ablate ovarian function, particularly in women over age 40. Serum estrogens increase in response to tamoxifen and reach levels that exceed the upper limit of the range for normal women (Sherman et al. 1979; Jordan et al. 1987b; Ravdin et al. 1988; Jordan et al. 1991). The response of the gonadotrophins, FSH and LH, is more difficult to characterize because of the pulsatile secretion in the premenopausal patient. Some studies report no change in LH and FSH (Groom and Griffiths 1976; Sherman et al. 1979; Manni and Pearson 1980; Jordan et al. 1991), whereas other studies report increases in FSH (Manni and Pearson 1980; Jordan et al. 1987b; Ravdin et al. 1988).

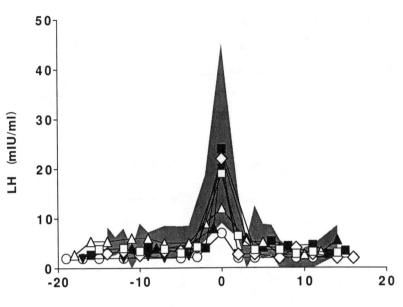

Figure 2.12. Serum LH levels in premenopausal breast cancer patients receiving 10 mg BID tamoxifen. Shaded area represents the normal range; each symbol represents serial samples from one patient. (Adapted from Jordan et al. 1991.)

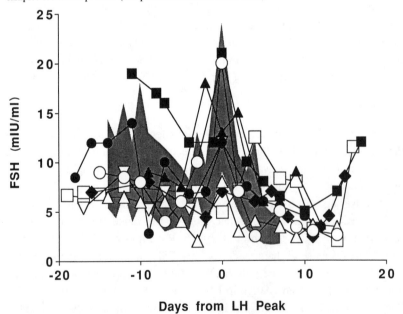

Figure 2.13. Serum FSH levels in premenopausal breast cancer patients receiving 10 mg BID tamoxifen. Shaded area represents the normal range; each symbol represents serial samples from one patient.

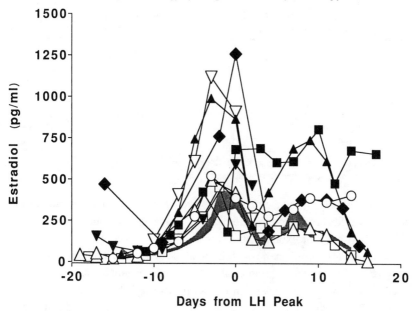

Figure 2.14. Serum estradiol levels in premenopausal breast cancer patients receiving 10 mg BID tamoxifen. Shaded area represents the normal range; each symbol represents serial samples from one patient.

Some of the contradictory results may be partly explained by the effect of chemotherapy on the ovary of the premenopausal patient. Patients treated with chemotherapy only (no tamoxifen) exhibited increased LH and FSH to postmenopausal levels with decreased serum estradiol. Patients who received tamoxifen with chemotherapy had increased levels of the gonadotrophins but not to postmenopausal levels. Cessation of tamoxifen therapy in these patients resulted in a further increase of LH and FSH to postmenopausal levels (Jordan et al. 1987b). Patients treated with chemotherapy who maintained ovarian function as evidenced by high circulating levels of estradiol also had paradoxically high FSH levels, but patients treated with only tamoxifen maintained normal levels of FSH and LH in the presence of high levels of estradiol (Figs. 2.12, 2.13, 2.14; Jordan et al. 1987b, 1991). The same study reported no change in SHBG despite increased serum levels of estradiol. An increase in estradiol without a concomitant increase in SHBG could lead to increased free estradiol in the serum with potentially adverse effects on tumor control.

Because the tumoristatic action of tamoxifen is believed to result from competition with estradiol for the estrogen receptor, an increase in serum estradiol could overcome the action of tamoxifen. Are the supraphysiological

Table 2.2. Response rate to castration in premenopausal patients who initially respond to tamoxifen therapy and then experience treatment failure

Source	Dose (mg BID)	Prior response[a] to tamoxifen	Response[a] to subsequent castration
Ingle et al. 1986	10	15	5 (33%)
Planting et al. 1985	20	12	6 (50%)
Hoogstraten et al. 1982	10	16	2[b] (13%)
Sawka et al. 1986	20	20	9 (45%)

[a]Designation of response requires at least stable disease.
[b]Patients continued tamoxifen therapy postcastration.

levels of estradiol that have been observed high enough to overcome the antiestrogenic activity of tamoxifen? Work in the athymic nude mouse model using MCF-7 tumor explants shows that in the presence of high circulating estradiol (>900 pg/ml) the growth inhibitory action of tamoxifen (40 ng/ml) may be partly overcome (Iino et al. 1991). Some patients described in studies had serum estradiol levels in excess of 900 pg/ml (Fig. 2.14; Sherman et al. 1979; Ravdin et al. 1988; Jordan et al. 1991) and may have been at risk for renewed tumor growth if serum tamoxifen levels were low (<100 ng/ml). Several studies show that some premenopausal patients who initially respond to tamoxifen and fail will respond to oophorectomy (Table 2.2). Perhaps patients that subsequently respond to oophorectomy had serum estradiol levels that were high and tamoxifen levels that were too low, resulting in estrogen-stimulated growth.

Currently there is interest in the use of synthetic luteinizing hormone–releasing hormone (LHRH) superagonists (e.g., goserelin; trademark Zoladex, ICI 118,630) in clinical trials to prevent LH and FSH release from the pituitary, thus inhibiting ovarian function and resulting in castrate serum estrogen levels. Concurrent treatment with tamoxifen does not result in increased serum estrogen concentrations. Figure 2.15 shows the serum estradiol profile of a premenopausal breast cancer patient who received Zoladex while taking tamoxifen. Initially, serum estradiol levels increased, but declined while therapy continued. Tamoxifen levels remained constant once steady state was achieved.

Conclusions

Tamoxifen undergoes extensive metabolism in the liver after absorption, although the pattern of metabolites and pharmacokinetics varies greatly among species. All the major metabolites identified to date have anti-

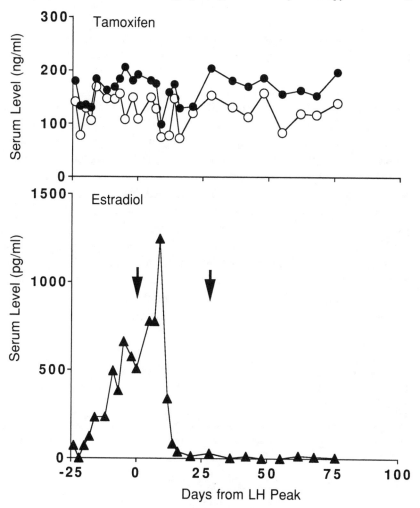

Figure 2.15. Serum levels of estradiol (lower panel) and tamoxifen (upper panel) in a pre-menopausal patient treated with goserelin, indicated by arrows at 0 and 28 days post–LH peak. Estradiol, ▲; tamoxifen, ○; N-desmethyltamoxifen, ●.

estrogenic activity and may contribute to the total antitumor action of tamoxifen. Minor metabolites with estrogenic potential have been identified, but their role in the pharmacological profile of tamoxifen remains controversial.

Postmenopausal breast cancer patients receiving tamoxifen therapy of greater than 2 years' duration do not exhibit alterations in the metabolism or pharmacokinetics of the parent drug and its main metabolites. Serum estrogen levels remain low, and there is no evidence that tamoxifen reactivates the ovary.

Premenopausal women present a challenge to the clinician for breast cancer treatment because of ongoing steroidogenesis by the ovary. Although chemotherapy may ablate the ovary and destroy its capacity for steroidogenesis, there are many reports of returning ovarian function and the resulting production of estrogen that may cause renewed tumor growth in the noncompliant patient. Close monitoring of the hormone status as well as serum tamoxifen levels is indicated for the premenopausal patient. The use of LHRH superagonists, such as Zoladex, or oophorectomy may provide a useful method of lowering serum estrogen levels in those patients deemed at risk for treatment failure because of an unfavorable serum estrogen and tamoxifen profile. These approaches are however experimental and should be considered in the context of a clinical trial.

Tamoxifen is effective in the control of premenopausal breast cancer. However, more information is needed on the serum hormone and tamoxifen profiles in patients who experience a treatment failure. Although tamoxifen has been shown to remain metabolically stable in postmenopausal patients who receive treatment for as long as 10 years, such information is not available for the premenopausal patient. Significant changes in steroidogenesis, which take place during menopause, could affect tamoxifen metabolism.

Acknowledgments

We thank Drs. Peter Ravdin, Scott Sedlacek, and Timothy Griffiths for supplying patient samples for some of the clinical results that were presented; Jane Wegenke and JoAnne Barrix for maintaining the University of Wisconsin Comprehensive Cancer Center Sample Bank that supplied patient samples from current and past clinical studies; and Bonnie Rayho for expert manuscript preparation. We also thank the family of Eileen Henrich for their gift to the UWCCC to provide equipment for the measurement of tamoxifen.

References

Adam, H. K., E. J. Douglas, and J. V. Kemp. 1979. The metabolism of tamoxifen in humans. *Biochemical Pharmacology* 27:145–147.

Adam, H. K., M. A. Gay, and R. H. Moore. 1980. Measurement of tamoxifen in serum by thin-layer densitometry. *Journal of Endocrinology* 84:35–42.

Adam, H. K., J. S. Patterson, and J. V. Kemp. 1980. Studies on the metabolism and pharmacokinetics of tamoxifen in normal volunteers. *Cancer Treatment Reports* 64:761–764.

Bain, R. R., and V. C. Jordan. 1983. Identification of a new metabolite of tamoxifen in patient serum during breast cancer therapy. *Biochemical Pharmacology* 32:373–375.

Bratherton, D. G., C. H. Brown, R. B. Buchanan, V. Hall, E. M. K. Pillers, T. K. Wheeler, and C. J. Williams. 1984. A comparison of two doses of tamoxifen (Nolvadex) in postmenopausal women with advanced breast cancer: 10 mg bd versus 20 mg bd. *British Journal of Cancer* 50:199–205.

Brown, R. R., R. Bain, and V. C. Jordan. 1983. Determination of tamoxifen and metabolites in human serum by high-performance liquid chromatography with post-column fluorescence activation. *Journal of Chromatography* 272:351–358.

Camaggi, C. M., E. Strocchi, N. Canova, and F. Pannuti. 1983. High performance liquid chromatographic analysis of tamoxifen and major metabolites in human plasma. *Journal of Chromatography* 275:436–442.

Camaggi, C. M., E. Strocchi, N. Canova, B. Costanti, and F. Pannuti. 1985. Medroxyprogesterone acetate (MAP) and tamoxifen (TMX) plasma levels after simultaneous treatment with "low" TMX and "high" MAP doses. *Cancer Chemotherapy and Pharmacology* 14:229–231.

Coezy, E., J. L. Borgna, and H. Rochefort. 1982. Tamoxifen and metabolites in MCF7 cells: correlation between binding to estrogen receptor and inhibition of cell growth. *Cancer Research* 42:317–323.

Daniel, P., S. J. Gaskell, H. Bishop, C. Campbell, and R. I. Nicholson. 1979. Determination of tamoxifen and an hydroxylated metabolite in plasma from patients with advanced breast cancer using gas chromatography–mass spectrometry. *Journal of Enocrinology* 83:401–408.

Daniel, P., S. J. Gaskell, H. Bishop, C. Campbell, and R. I. Nicholson. 1981. Determination of tamoxifen and biologically active metabolites in human breast tumours and plasma. *European Journal of Clinical Oncology* 17:1183–1189.

DeGregorio, M. W., E. Coronado, and C. K. Osborne. 1989. Tumor and serum tamoxifen concentrations in the athymic nude mouse. *Cancer Chemotherapy and Pharmacology* 23:68–70.

Early Breast Cancer Trialists' Collaborative Group. 1992. Systemic treatment of early breast cancer by hormonal, cytotoxic, or immune therapy. *Lancet* 339:1–15, 71–85.

Fabian, C., L. Sternson, and M. Barnett. 1980. Clinical pharmacology of tamoxifen in patients with breast cancer: comparison of traditional and loading dose schedules. *Cancer Treatment Reports* 64:765–773.

Fabian, C., L. Sternson, M. el-Serafi, L. Cain, and E. Hearne. 1981. Clinical pharmacology of tamoxifen in patients with breast cancer: correlation with clinical data. *Cancer* 48:876–882.

Falkson, H. C., R. Gray, W. H. Wolberg, K. W. Gilchrist, J. E. Harris, D. C. Tormey, G. Falkson. 1990. Adjuvant trial of 12 cycles of CMFPT followed by observation or continuous tamoxifen versus four cycles of CMFPT in postmenopausal women with breast cancer: an ECOG Phase III study. *Journal of Clinical Oncology* 8:599–607.

Fisher, B., A. Brown, N. Wolmark, and other members of the NSABP. 1987. Prolonging tamoxifen therapy for primary breast cancer. *Annals of Internal Medicine* 106:649–654.

Fisher, B., J. Costantino, C. Redmond, and other members of the NSABP. 1989. A randomized clinical trial evaluating tamoxifen in the treatment of patients with node-negative breast cancer who have estrogen receptor positive tumors. *New England Journal of Medicine* 32:479–484.

Fromson, J. M., S. Pearson, and S. Bramah (nee Meek). 1973a. The metabolism of tamoxifen (ICI 46,474). Part 1. In laboratory animals. *Xenobiotica* 3:693–709.

Fromson, J. M., S. Pearson, and S. Bramah (nee Meek). 1973b. The metabolism of tamoxifen (ICI 46,474). Part 2. In female patients. *Xenobiotica* 3:711–714.

Gaskell, S. J., C. P. Daniel, and R. I. Nicholson. 1978. Determination of tamoxifen in rat plasma by gas chromatography–mass spectrometry. *Journal of Endocrinology* 78:293–294.

Golander, Y., and L. A. Sternson. 1980. Paired-ion chromatographic analysis of tamoxifen and two major metabolites in plasma. *Journal of Chromatography* 181:41–49.

Gottardis, M. M., and V. C. Jordan. 1987. Antitumor actions of keoxifene and tamoxifen in the *N*-nitrosomethylurea induced rat mammary carcinoma model. *Cancer Research* 47:4020–4024.

Gottardis, M. M., M. K. Martin, and V. C. Jordan. 1987. Long-term tamoxifen therapy to control transplanted human breast tumor growth in athymic mice. In *Adjuvant Therapy of Cancer,* vol. 5, ed. S. E. Salmon, 447–454. New York: Grune and Stratton.

Groom, G. V., and K. Griffiths. 1976. Effect of the anti-oestrogen tamoxifen on plasma levels of luteinizing hormone, follicle-stimulating hormone, prolactin, oestradiol and progesterone in normal pre-menopausal women. *Journal of Endocrinology* 70:421–428.

Guelen, P. J. M., D. Stevenson, R. J. Briggs, and D. de Vos. 1987. The bioavailability of tamoplex (tamoxifen). Part 2. A single dose cross-over study in healthy male volunteers. *Methods and Findings in Experimental Clinical Pharmacology* 9:685–690.

Hoogstraten, B., W. S. Fletcher, N. Gad-el-Mawla, T. Maloney, S. J. Altman, C. B. Vaughn, and M. A. Foulkes. 1982. Tamoxifen and oophorectomy in the treatment of recurrent breast cancer. *Cancer Research* 42:4788–4791.

Iino, Y., D. M. Wolf, S. M. Langan-Fahey, D. A. Johnson, M. Ricchio, M. E. Thompson, and V. C. Jordan. 1991. Reversible control of oestradiol-stimulated growth of MCF-7 tumours by tamoxifen in the athymic mouse. *British Journal of Cancer* 64:1019–1024.

Ingle, J. N., J. E. Krook, S. J. Green, T. P. Kubista, L. K. Everson, D. L. Ahmann, M. N. Chang, H. F. Bisel, H. E. Windschitl, D. I. Twito, and D. M. Pfeifle. 1986. Randomized trial of bilateral oophorectomy versus tamoxifen in premenopausal women with metastatic breast cancer. *Journal of Clinical Oncology* 4:178–185.

Jacolot, F., I. Simon, Y. Dreano, P. Beaune, C. Riche, and F. Berthou. 1991. Identification of the cytochrome p450 IIIa family as the enzymes involved in the N-demethylation of tamoxifen in human liver microsomes. *Biochemical Pharmacology* 41:1911–1919.

Jordan, V. C., and K. E. Allen. 1980. Evaluation of the antitumour activity of the non-steroidal antioestrogen monohydroxytamoxifen in the DMBA-induced rat carcinoma model. *European Journal of Cancer and Clinical Oncology* 16:239–251.

Jordan, V. C., and B. Gosden. 1982. Importance of the alkylaminoethoxy side chain for the estrogenic and antiestrogenic actions of tamoxifen and trioxifene in the immature rat uterus. *Molecular and Cellular Endocrinology* 27:291–306.

Jordan, V. C., and S. Robinson. 1987. Species-specific pharmacology of antiestrogens: role of metabolism. *Federation Proceedings* 46:1870–1874.

Jordan, V. C., C. J. Dix, and K. E. Allen. 1979. The effectiveness of long-term treatment in a laboratory model for adjuvant hormone therapy of breast cancer. In *Adjuvant Therapy of Cancer,* vol. 2, ed. S. E. Salmon and S. E. Jones, 19–26. New York: Grune and Stratton.

Jordan, V. C., N. F. Fritz, and D. C. Tormey. 1987a. Long-term adjuvant therapy with tamoxifen: effects on sex hormone binding globulin and antithrombin III. *Cancer Research* 47:4517–4519.

Jordan, V. C., N. F. Fritz, and D. C. Tormey. 1987b. Endocrine effects of adjuvant chemotherapy and long-term tamoxifen administration on node-positive patients with breast cancer. *Cancer Research* 47:624–630.

Jordan, V. C., B. Haldemann, and K. E. Allen. 1981. Geometric isomers of substituted triphenylethylenes and antiestrogen action. *Endocrinology* 108:1353–1361.

Jordan, V. C., M. M. Collins, L. Rowsby, and G. Prestwich. 1977. A monohydroxylated metabolite of tamoxifen with potent antioestrogenic activity. *Journal of Endocrinology* 75:305–316.

Jordan, V. C., R. R. Bain, R. R. Brown, B. Gosden, and M. A. Santos. 1983. Determination and pharmacology of a new hydroxylated metabolite of tamoxifen observed in patient during therapy for advanced breast cancer. *Cancer Research* 43:1446–1450.

Jordan, V. C., N. F. Fritz, S. M. Langan-Fahey, M. Thompson, and D. C. Tormey. 1991. Alterations of endocrine parameters in premenopausal women with breast cancer during long-term adjuvant therapy with tamoxifen as the single agent. *Journal of the National Cancer Institute* 83:1488–1491.

Jordan, V. C., N. F. Fritz, M. M. Gottardis, D. M. Mirecki, P. M. Ravdin, and W. V. Welshons. 1986. Laboratory and clinical research on the hormone dependence of breast cancer: current studies and future prospects. In *Estrogen/Antiestrogen Action and Breast Cancer Therapy,* ed. V. C. Jordan, 501–522. Madison: University of Wisconsin Press.

Katzenellenbogen, J. A., K. E. Carlson, and B. S. Katzenellenbogen. 1985. Facile geometric isomerization of phenolic non-steroidal estrogens and antiestrogens: limitations to the interpretation of experiments characterizing the activity of individual isomers. *Journal of Steroid Biochemistry* 22:31–36.

Katzenellenbogen, B. S., M. J. Norman, R. L. Eckert, S. W. Peltz, and W. F. Mangel. 1984. Bioactivities, estrogen receptor interactions, and plasminogen activator–inducing activities of tamoxifen and hydroxytamoxifen isomers in MCF-7 human breast cancer cells. *Cancer Research* 44:112–119.

Kemp, J. V., H. K. Adam, A. E. Wakeling, and R. Slater. 1983. Identification and biological activity of tamoxifen metabolites in human serum. *Biochemical Pharmacology* 32:2045–2052.

Kikuta, C., and R. Schmid. 1989. Specific high performance liquid chromatographic analysis of tamoxifen and its major metabolites by "on-line" extraction and post-column photochemical reaction. *Journal of Pharmaceutical and Biomedical Analysis* 7:329–337.

Langan-Fahey, S. M., D. C. Tormey, and V. C. Jordan. 1990. Tamoxifen metabolites in patients on long-term adjuvant therapy for breast cancer. *European Journal of Cancer* 25:883–888.

Lieberman, M. E., J. Gorski, and V. C. Jordan. 1983. An estrogen receptor model to describe the regulation of prolactin synthesis by antiestrogens *in vitro. Journal Biological Chemistry* 258:4741–4745.

Lieberman, M. E., V. C. Jordan, M. Fritsch, M. A. Santos, and J. Gorski. 1983. Direct and reversible inhibition of estradiol-stimulated prolactin synthesis by antiestrogens *in vitro. Journal of Biological Chemistry* 258:4734–4740.

Lien, E. A., E. Solheim, and P. M. Ueland. 1991. Distribution of tamoxifen and its metabolites in rat and human tissues during steady-state treatment. *Cancer Research* 51:4837–4844.

Lien, E. A., Solheim, S. K. Kvinnsland, and P. M. Ueland. 1988. Identification of 4-hydroxy-N-desmethyltamoxifen as a metabolite of tamoxifen in human bile. *Cancer Research* 48:2304–2308.

Lien, E. A., P. M. Ueland, E. Solheim, and S. Kvinnsland. 1987. Determination of tamoxifen and four metabolites in serum by low-dispersion liquid chromatography. *Clinical Chemistry* 33:1608–1614.

Lien, E. A., G. Anker, P. E. Loonning, E. Solheim, and P. M. Ueland. 1990. Decreased serum concentrations of tamoxifen and its metabolites induced by aminogluthethimide. *Cancer Research* 50:5851–5857.

Lien, E. A., E. Solheim, O. A. Lea, S. Lundgren, S. Kvinnsland, and P. M. Ueland. 1989. Distribution of 4-hydroxy-N-desmethyltamoxifen and other tamoxifen metabolites in human biological fluids during tamoxifen treatment. *Cancer Research* 49:2175–2183.

Lodwick, R., B. McConkey, and A. M. Brown. 1987. Life threatening interaction between tamoxifen and warfarin. *British Medical Journal* 295:1141.

McVie, J. G., G. P. C. Simonetti, D. Stevenson, R. J. Briggs, P. J. M. Guelen, and D. de Vos. 1986. The bioavailability of tamoplex (tamoxifen). Part 1. A pilot study. *Methods and Findings in Experimental Clinical Pharmacology* 8:505–512.

Manni, A., and B. M. Arafah. 1981. Tamoxifen-induced remission in breast cancer by escalating the dose to 40 mg daily after progression on 20 mg daily: a case report and review of the literature. *Cancer* 48:873–875.

Manni, A., and O. H. Pearson. 1980. Antiestrogen-induced remissions in premenopausal women with stage iv breast cancer: effects on ovarian function. *Cancer Treatment Reports* 64:779–785.

Manni, A., J. E. Trujillo, J. S. Marshall, J. Grodkey, and O. H. Pearson. 1979. Antihormone treatment of stage iv breast cancer. *Cancer* 43:444–450.

Mauvais-Jarvis, P., N. Baudot, D. Castaigne, P. Banzet, and F. Kuttenn. 1986. Trans-4-hydroxy-tamoxifen concentration and metabolism after local percutaneous administration to human breast. *Cancer Research* 46:1521–1525.

Meltzer, N. M., P. Stang, L. A. Sternson, and A. Wade. 1984. Influence of tamoxifen and its N-desmethyl and 4-hydroxy metabolites on rat liver microsomal enzymes. *Biochemical Pharmacology* 33:115–123.

Mendenhall, D. W., H. Kobayashi, F. M. L. Shih, L. A. Sternson, T. Higuchi, and C. Fabian. 1978. Clinical analysis of tamoxifen, an anti neoplastic agent, in plasma. *Clinical Chemistry* 24:1518–1524.

Milano, G., M. C. Etienne, M. Frenay, R. Khater, J. L. Formento, N. Renee, J. L. Moll, M. Rancoual, M. Berto, and M. Namer. 1987. Optimized analysis of tamoxifen and its main metabolites in the plasma and cytosol of mammary tumours. *British Journal of Cancer* 55:509–512.

Murphy, C., T. Fotsis, P. Pantzar, H. Adlercreutz, and F. Martin. 1987. Analysis of tamoxifen and its metabolites in human plasma by gas chromatography–mass spectrometry (gc-ms) using selected ion monitoring (sim). *Journal of Steroid Biochemistry* 26:547–555.

Murphy, C. M., S. Langan-Fahey, R. McCague, and V. C. Jordan. 1990. Structure function relationships of hydroxylated metabolites of tamoxifen that control the proliferation of estrogen-responsive T47D breast cancer cells *in vitro*. *Molecular Pharmacology* 38:737–743.

Nieder, M., and H. Jaeger. 1987. Quantification of tamoxifen and N-desmethyltamoxifen in human plasma by high-performance liquid chromatography, photochemical reaction and fluorescence detection, and its application to biopharmaceutic investigations. *Journal of Chromatography* 413:207–217.

Noguchi, S., K. Miyauchi, S. Imaoka, and H. Koyama (Osaka). 1988. Inability of tamoxifen to penetrate into cerebrospinal fluid. *Breast Cancer Research and Treatment* 12:317–318.

Osborne, C. K., F. K. Hobbs, and G. M. Clark. 1985. Effect of estrogens and antiestrogens on growth of human breast cancer cells in athymic nude mice. *Cancer Research* 45:584–590.

Osborne, C. K., E. Coronado, D. C. Allred, V. Wiebe, and M. DeGregorio. 1991. Acquired tamoxifen resistance: correlation with reduced breast tumor levels of tamoxifen and isomerization of trans-4-hydroxytamoxifen. *Journal of the National Cancer Institute* 83:1477–1482.

Osborne, C. K., V. J. Wiebe, W. L. McGuire, D. R. Ciocca, and M. W. DeGregorio. 1992. Tamoxifen and the isomers of 4-hydroxytamoxifen in tamoxifen-resistant tumors from breast cancer patients. *Journal of Clinical Oncology* 10:304–310.

Parr, I. B., R. McCague, G. Leclercq, and S. Stoessel. 1987. Metabolism of tamoxifen by isolated rat hepatocytes. *Biochemical Pharmacology* 36:1513–1519.

Patterson, J. S., R. S. Settatree, H. K. Adam, and J. V. Kemp. 1980. Serum concentration of tamoxifen and major metabolite during long-term Nolvadex therapy, correlated with clinical response. In *Breast Cancer—Experimental and Clinical Aspects,* ed. H. T. Mouridsen and T. Palshof, 89–92. Oxford: Pergamon Press.

Pearson, O. H., A. Manni, and B. M. Arafah. 1982. Antiestrogen treatment of breast cancer: an overview. *Cancer Research* 42(Supplement):3424s–3429s.

Planting, A. S. T., J. Alexieva-Figusch, J. Blonk-v.d. Wijst, and W. L. J. van Putten. 1985. Tamoxifen therapy in premenopausal women with metastatic breast cancer. *Cancer Treatment Reports* 69:363–368.

Ravdin, P. M., N. F. Fritz, D. C. Tormey, and V. C. Jordan. 1988. Endocrine status of premenopausal node-positive breast cancer patients following adjuvant chemotherapy and long-term tamoxifen. *Cancer Research* 48:1026–1029.

Riippa, P., A. Kauppila, H. Sundstrom, and R. Vihko. 1984. Hepatic impairment during simultaneous administration of medroxyprogesterone acetate and tamoxifen in the treatment of endometrial and ovarian carcinoma. *Anticancer Research* 4:109–112.

Ritchie, L. D., and S. M. T. Grant. 1989. Tamoxifen-warfarin interaction: the Aberdeen hospitals drug file. *British Medical Journal* 298:1253.

Robinson, S. P., and V. C. Jordan. 1987. Reversal of the antitumor effects of tamoxifen by progesterone in the 7,12 dimethylbenzanthracene-induced rat mammary carcinoma model. *Cancer Research* 47:5386–5390.

Robinson, S. P., S. M. Langan-Fahey, and V. C. Jordan. 1989. Implications of tamoxifen metabolism in the athymic mouse for the study of antitumor effects upon human breast cancer xenografts. *European Journal of Clinical Oncology* 25:1769–1776.

Robinson, S. P., S. M. Langan-Fahey, D. A. Johnson, and V. C. Jordan. 1991. Metabolites, pharmacodynamics, and pharmacokinetics of tamoxifen in rats and mice compared to the breast cancer patient. *Drug Disposition and Metabolism* 19:36–43.

Ruenitz, P. C., and J. R. Bagley. 1985. Comparative fates of clomiphene and tamoxifen in the immature female rat. *Drug Metabolism and Disposition* 13:582–586.

Ruenitz, P. C., and M. M. Toledo. 1980. Inhibition of rabbit liver microsomal oxidative metabolism and substrate binding by tamoxifen and the geometric isomers of clomiphene. *Biochemical Pharmacology* 29:1583–1587.

Ruenitz, P. C., J. R. Bagley, and C. W. Pape. 1984. Some chemical and biochemical aspects of liver microsomal metabolism of tamoxifen. *Drug Metabolism and Disposition* 12:478–483.

Sakai, F., F. Cheix, M. Clavel, J. Colon, M. Mayer, E. Pannata, and S. Saez. 1978. Increases in steroid binding globulins induced by tamoxifen in patients with carcinoma of the breast. *Journal of Endocrinology* 76:219–226.

Salamoun, J., M. Macka, M. Nechvatal, M. Matousek, and L. Knesel. 1990. Identification of products formed during uv irradiation of tamoxifen and their use for fluorescence detection in high performance liquid chromatography. *Journal of Chromatography* 514:179–187.

Sawka, C. A., K. I. Pritchard, A. H. G. Paterson, D. J. A. Sutherland, D. B. Thomson, W. E. Shelley, R. E. Myers, B. G. Mobbs, A. Malkin, and J. W. Meakin. 1986. Role and mechanism of action of tamoxifen in premenopausal women with metastatic breast carcinoma. *Cancer Research* 46:3152–3156.

Shah, I. G., and D. L. Parsons. 1991. Human albumin binding of tamoxifen in the presence of a perfluorochemical erythrocyte substitute. *Journal of Pharmacy and Pharmacology* 43:790–793.

Sherman, B. M., F. K. Chapler, K. Crickard, and D. Wycoff. 1979. Endocrine consequences of continuous antiestrogen therapy with tamoxifen in premenopausal women. *Journal of Clinical Investigations* 64:398–404.

Soininen, K., T. Kleimola, I. Elomaa, M. Salmo, and P. Rissanen. 1986. The steady-state pharmacokinetics of tamoxifen and its metabolites in breast cancer patients. *Journal of Internal Medicine Research* 14:162–165.

Stevenson, D., R. J. Briggs, D. J. Chapman, and D. de Vos. 1988. Determination of tamoxifen and five metabolites in plasma. *Journal of Pharmaceutical and Biomedical Analysis* 6:1065–1068.

Szamel, I., B. Vincze, I. Hindy, I. Hermann, J. Borvendeg, and S. Eckhardt. 1986. Hormonal changes during a prolonged tamoxifen treatment in patients with advanced breast cancer. *Oncology* 43:7–11.

Tenni, P., D. L. Lalich, and M. J. Byrne. 1989. Life threatening interaction between tamoxifen and warfarin. *British Medical Journal* 298:93.

Tormey, D. C., and V. C. Jordan. 1984. Long-term tamoxifen adjuvant therapy in node-positive breast cancer: a metabolic and pilot clinical study. *Breast Cancer Research and Treatment* 4:297–302.

Trump, D. L., D. C. Smith, P. G. Ellis, M. P. Rogers, S. C. Schold, E. P. Winer, T. J. Ponella, V. C. Jordan, and R. L. Fine. 1992. Vinblastine and high dose tamoxifen, a potential multidrug resistance reversal agent: a phase I trial in combination with vinblastine. *Journal of the National Cancer Institute* 84:1811–1816.

Turner III, M. J., C. E. Fields, and D. B. Everman. 1991. Evidence for superoxide formation during hepatic metabolism of tamoxifen. *Biochemical Pharmacology* 41:1701–1705.

Watkins, S. M. 1988. The value of high dose tamoxifen in postmenopausal breast cancer patients progressing on standard doses: a pilot study. *British Journal of Cancer* 57:320–321.

Wiebe, V. J., K. C. Osborne, W. L. McGuire, and M. W. DeGregorio. 1992. Identification of estrogenic tamoxifen metabolite(s) in tamoxifen-resistant human breast tumors. *Journal of Clinical Oncology* 10:990–994.

Wilbur, B. J., C. C. Benz, and M. W. DeGregorio. 1985. Quantitation of tamoxifen, 4-hydroxytam-oxifen, and N-desmethyltamoxifen in human plasma by high performance liquid chromatography. *Analytical Letters* 18:1915–1924.

Wolf, D. M., and V. C. Jordan. 1992. Gynecologic complications associated with long-term adjuvant tamoxifen therapy for breast cancer. *Gynecologic Oncology* 45:118–128.

3

Multisystem Biological and Symptomatic Toxicity of Tamoxifen in Postmenopausal Women

RICHARD R. LOVE

I. INTRODUCTION 58
II. METHODS 59
III. RESULTS 60
   A. CARDIOVASCULAR RISK FACTOR EFFECTS 62
   B. OSSEOUS SYSTEM EFFECTS 67
   C. SYMPTOM TOXICITY 69
IV. DISCUSSION 73
   A. RESULTS COMPARED WITH THOSE IN OTHER STUDIES 73
   B. DIRECT IMPLICATIONS OF RESULTS 75
   C. BROADER IMPLICATIONS FOR LONG-TERM ADJUVANT THERAPY
     AND PREVENTION 78
V. SUMMARY 78
   REFERENCES 79

I. *Introduction*

THE successful application of therapy with tamoxifen for periods of years, particularly as adjuvant treatment, has increased interest in understanding in great detail the full breadth of its biological and symptomatic effects (Lerner and Jordan 1990; Early Breast Cancer Trialists' Collaborative Group 1988) Further, these clinically useful results in the adjuvant setting, combined with data from laboratory carcinogenesis experiments showing that long-term tamoxifen can usually suppress the majority of expected mammary cancers (Welsch et al. 1982; Jordan and Allen 1980; Gottardis and Jordan 1987), have suggested the possibility that tamoxifen might be given to healthy women at risk for breast cancer to suppress preclinical mammary malignancies and "prevent" clinical breast cancer. Tamoxifen prevention trials are now recruiting volunteers in the United Kingdom, Italy, and the United States.

In 1986 my colleagues and I began the study whose results are the focus of this chapter. At that time only limited data had been reported on the breadth of biological effects which we felt warranted rigorous investigation; there were only incomplete data describing the details of symptoms and patients' reactions consequent to tamoxifen therapy, and there were no clinical data on major disease endpoints associated with tamoxifen therapy, other than those with respect to the original breast cancer. Data regarding effects of tamoxifen on disease-free and overall survival in women with axillary node-negative breast cancer were very preliminary. Finally, the preponderance of adjuvant tamoxifen data at the time, as now, was from studies in postmenopausal women. In this context then, rigorous evaluation of tamoxifen's biological and symptomatic effects in a 2-year toxicity study appeared appropriate and ethical. The specific aims of this study were to evaluate the effects of tamoxifen on (1) cardiovascular risk factors, including, in particular, lipids, lipoproteins, and fibrinogen, as well as coagulation proteins and platelets; (2) bone metabolism and bone mineral density; and (3) symptoms and quality of life. The data to be summarized here do appear to be clinically useful, and like many such data they suggest more questions than they answer.

II. Methods

We evaluated 140 women participating in the Wisconsin Tamoxifen Study, a double-blind randomized, placebo-controlled, biological and clinical toxicity study of tamoxifen, 10 mg orally, twice daily. Volunteers were recruited to this single institution study over 20 months. Patients were postmenopausal (no menstrual periods in the preceding 12 months with both ovaries and uterus intact, or older than 50 years with a history of hysterectomy), under 65 years of age (46–64), and had a diagnosis of axillary node-negative breast cancer. Seventy patients were assigned to receive tamoxifen and 70 to receive placebo. Women were considered eligible for the study if they had been diagnosed with breast cancer up to 10 years previously and if they were disease-free, as confirmed by physical, radiological, and laboratory findings. Patients were receiving no lipid-lowering or hormonal drugs. Complete blood and platelet counts were normal, and patients had no clinical or biochemical evidence of liver disease. Fasting plasma levels of cholesterol had to be 8.06 mmol/l (310 mg/dl) or less, and fasting plasma levels of triglycerides had to be 2.147 mmol/l (190 mg/dl) or less.

Bone mineral densitometry in the radius (measured by single photon absorptiometry [SPA]) and in the lumbar spine (measured by dual photon absorptiometry [DPA]) had to be greater than 80% of age-corrected normal values. After baseline evaluations that included physical examination, bone densitometry, and blood sampling, patients were reevaluated at 3, 6, 12, 18, and 24 months. Participants received no specific nutritional counseling. All subjects provided written informed consent according to an institutionally approved protocol.

Each patient completed a detailed questionnaire about health behaviors at each visit with the assistance of a study staff member. The questionnaire included specific questions about smoking, exercise, and physical work (in hours per week).

Additional detailed questions concerned hot flashes, flushed face, gynecological symptoms (one or more of the following: vaginal discharge, irritation, or bleeding), fatigue, joint pains, upset stomach or nausea, depression, and headache. Questions concerning the occurrence of each of these symptoms over the previous 3 months requested a response on an 11-point scale of 0–10, with 0 for "did not have it" or 1–10 for a severity rating of the symptom at its worst. For each symptom, responses were classified into severity groupings of "no symptom" (a 0 rating), "mild" (ratings of 1 to 3), "moderate" (ratings of 4 to 6), and "severe" (ratings of 7 to 10).

A subject with "significant overall toxicity" was defined as follows: any subject with a moderate or severe rating for hot flashes, flushed face, or gynecological symptoms, or with a baseline rating of 2 or lower with an increase of at least 2 scale units on subsequent interviews, or a subject who dropped out of the study because of adverse reactions. These criteria were selected a priori to enhance our abilities to detect symptom changes meriting concern by our medical staff: (1) moderate or severe symptom levels; (2) the appearance of symptoms that had not been present before therapy; and (3) the subject's perception of reactions of sufficient adversity to warrant termination of study participation.

Patients were weighed at each visit using a beam scale. Systolic and diastolic blood pressures were obtained at each visit using a standard or large cuff with the patient in the sitting position. A single determination was made on one or both arms.

Total cholesterol, HDL cholesterol, and triglycerides were measured within 2 days of each visit using 12-hour fasting plasma specimens. Anticoagulated blood samples were used for platelet determinations, which were made within a few hours of sampling.

Plasma or citrated blood glucose, apolipoprotein A, apolipoprotein B, osteocalcin, parathyroid hormone, 1,25 dihydroxy vitamin D, antithrombin III, fibrinogen, protein C, and protein S determinations were made in batches on coded samples stored for up to 2.5 years. These plasma specimens were maintained at −80°C and were thoroughly mixed after thawing.

Bone mineral density measurements were made at the one-third radial shaft site and at the lumbar spine (L_2–L_4) and analyzed as described in detail elsewhere. Further details of the study methods, including all laboratory methods, are available in journal publications (Love et al. 1990; Love, Cameron, et al. 1991; Love, Surawicz, and Williams 1992; Love, Wiebe, et al. 1991; Love, Mazess, et al. 1992).

Statistical analyses included standard procedures: paired t-tests, two-sample t-tests, rank sum tests, Wilcoxon sign rank test, chi-square tests, and a more elaborate approach for the bone mineral density data (Wei and Lachin 1984; Laird and Ware 1982).

III. *Results*

Treatment groups were well balanced with respect to various important characteristics, mean age and body mass for examples (Table 3.1), with the exception that women randomly assigned treatment with tamoxifen had lower

Table 3.1. Patient characteristics and history

Characteristic	Placebo (n = 70)	Tamoxifen (n = 70)
Mean age (yrs)	57.8 ± 4.0	57.6 ± 4.5
Mean time since menopause (yrs)	9.0 ± 6.3	9.6 ± 7.3
Subjects <4 years since menopause (%)	13	14
Subjects <5 years since menopause (%)	18	19
Mean body mass (kg/m)^2	27.6 ± 6.0	26.2 ± 4.3
Mean tumor size (cm)[a]	1.96 ± 1.1	1.88 ± 1.1
History (%)		
Premenopausal at diagnosis	17	19
Hysterectomy	37	40
Surgical oophorectomy	25	17
Radiotherapy	17	12
Hot flashes	43	45
Lumpectomy	10	7
Current smokers (%)	11	10
Mean aerobic exercise (hrs/wk)	3.2 ± 5.1	3.0 ± 2.8
Mean physical activity (hrs/wk)	5.5 ± 8.6	6.2 ± 9.0

Note: Mean values are ± SD.
[a]Determined by pathological examination.

Table 3.2. Number of subjects who stopped study treatment
(N = 140 entered on study)

	Tamoxifen	Placebo
Adverse reaction		
Year 1	6	2
Year 2	0	2
Other reasons	5	8
Total attrition	11	12
	23 (16.4%)	

baseline levels of cholesterol: 5.619 mmol/l (95% CI 5.430–5.809), or 216 mg/dl (209–223), versus 5.950 mmol/l (5.731–5.169), or 229 mg/dl (220–237). Twenty-three women stopped taking the assigned tablets during the 2-year study (Table 3.2). Three of these 11 placebo participants, and 6 of the 12 tamoxifen participants had most of the determinations made through 24 months; data from these women are included in the results presented. A balance of women in the two treatment groups less than 4 years since menopause was achieved by the stratification and randomization procedure (Table 3.1). Compliance with tablet consumption, assessed by pill counts and serological evidence of tamoxifen and its metabolites, was excellent (Love et al. 1990); all women randomized to placebo showed no evidence of tamoxifen

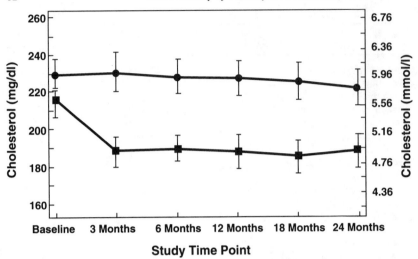

Figure 3.1. Mean fasting levels of total cholesterol over time in patients receiving tamoxifen or placebo. Control patients, ●; n = 70 at baseline and n = 70, 68, 67, 64, and 62 patients at 3, 6, 12, 18, and 24 months, respectively. Patients receiving tamoxifen, ■; n = 70 at baseline and n = 66, 66, 65, 64, and 64 patients at 3, 6, 12, 18, and 24 months, respectively. Bars indicate 95% CIs. Cholesterol levels decreased significantly at all time points in patients receiving tamoxifen ($p <$ 0.001). (Reproduced, with permission, from Love, Wiebe, et al., "Effects of tamoxifen on cardiovascular risk factors in postmenopausal women," *Annals of Internal Medicine* 115 [1991]:860–864.)

in blood samples taken at all time points in the study, and all tamoxifen-treated subjects showed evidence of these compounds.

A. CARDIOVASCULAR RISK FACTOR EFFECTS

Although lipid-lowering drug treatment was proscribed, one participant did take two drugs for a several-month period. The reported use of diuretic and antihypertensive medication was similar in the two groups. At the 3-month evaluation and persisting through evaluations at 6, 12, 18, and 24 months, tamoxifen-treated women demonstrated a decrease from baseline in total cholesterol that was significantly different ($p <$ 0.001) from the change seen in placebo-treated women (Fig. 3.1). The changes in total cholesterol values in tamoxifen-treated women from baseline to 3, 6, 12, 18, and 24 months were also statistically significant ($p <$ 0.001). The mean decrease from baseline in total cholesterol was approximately 12%. When tamoxifen-treated subjects were grouped in quintiles according to baseline levels of total cholesterol, there was a greater percentage of decrease in total cholesterol for each successive quintile (Table 3.3). The table shows these data for 6 months.

Table 3.3. Change from baseline in mean total cholesterol levels at
6 months in five groups of women treated with tamoxifen

Quintile	Number of patients	Mean baseline cholesterol level mmol/l (mg/dl)	Percent change at 6 months
1	13	4.55 (176)	−4.2
2	14	5.12 (198)	−7.4
3	13	5.48 (212)	−11.0
4	12	6.02 (233)	−13.9
5	14	6.70 (259)	−17.2

The pattern was the same at 3, 12, 18, and 24 months. Of 70 tamoxifen-treated subjects, 12 subjects developed cholesterol increases of >0.26 mmol/l (10 mg/dl), and 6 subjects developed increases of >0.52 mmol/l (20 mg/dl) at any point during the study.

During the first year there was a suggestion of greater decreases in HDL cholesterol in tamoxifen-treated subjects at 3 and 6 months, and a statistically significant decrease at 12 months ($p < 0.01$) (Fig. 3.2). At 18 and 24 months, however, the differences in mean HDL cholesterol in the two groups were not statistically significant. Triglyceride levels were modestly increased in tamoxifen-treated subjects (e.g., mean increase 0.319 mmol/l [28.2 mg/dl] at

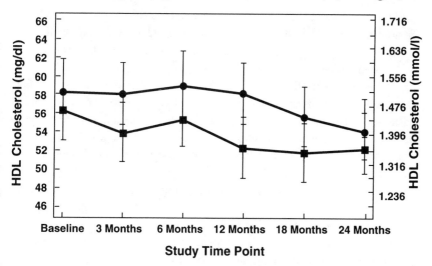

Figure 3.2. Mean fasting levels of HDL cholesterol over time in patients receiving tamoxifen or placebo. Control patients, ●; n = 70 at baseline and n = 70, 68, 67, 64, and 62 patients at 3, 6, 12, 18, and 24 months, respectively. Patients receiving tamoxifen, ■; n = 70 at baseline and n = 66, 66, 65, 64, and 64 patients at 3, 6, 12, 18, and 24 months, respectively. Bars indicate 95% CIs. The difference between the two groups is significant only at 12 months ($p = 0.01$).

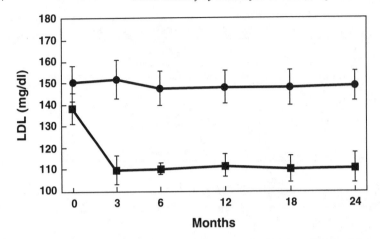

Figure 3.3. Mean fasting levels of LDL cholesterol over time in patients receiving tamoxifen or placebo. Control patients, ●; n = 70 at baseline and n = 70, 68, 67, 64, and 62 patients at 3, 6, 12, 18, and 24 months, respectively. Patients receiving tamoxifen, ■; n = 70 at baseline and n = 66, 66, 65, 64, and 64 patients at 3, 6, 12, 18, and 24 months, respectively. Bars indicate 95% CIs. The mean change (decrease) from baseline at all points in time is highly significant in patients receiving tamoxifen ($p < 0.001$).

24 months); however, no single subject had an increase to greater than 3.729 mmol/l (330 mg/dl). LDL cholesterol levels derived by indirect methods were decreased approximately 20% in tamoxifen-treated patients for the duration of the study (Friedewald et al. 1972) (Fig. 3.3).

Ratios of LDL:HDL cholesterol (Fig. 3.4) and total:HDL cholesterol (Fig. 3.5) fell by 3 months in the tamoxifen-treated group, and the decreases were sustained at the same levels for the duration of the study. Fibrinogen levels were assessed at baseline and 6 months, and showed a significant 15% decrease in the tamoxifen-treated group at the latter time point ($p = 0.0003$) (Fig. 3.6).

Apolipoprotein A-I levels, assessed at baseline and at 3 and 12 months, increased significantly at the last two time points in patients receiving tamoxifen compared with those receiving placebo ($p = 0.02$). Apolipoprotein B levels, also assessed at baseline and at 3 and 12 months, decreased significantly at the last two time points in the tamoxifen as compared with placebo subjects ($p = 0.005$). Although mean weight was slightly greater at baseline in patients receiving placebo, no significant changes in weight occurred during the 24 months of study. Patients in the placebo group had a mean increase of 1.4 kg over 2 years, and those in the tamoxifen group showed an increase of 1.0 kg ($p > 0.05$) (Fig. 3.7).

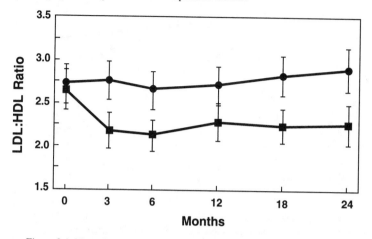

Figure 3.4. Mean fasting levels of LDL to HDL cholesterol ratios over time in patients receiving tamoxifen or placebo. Control group, ●; patients receiving tamoxifen, ■. Bars indicate 95% CIs. The differences between the groups are significant at all study time points after baseline ($p = 0.002$).

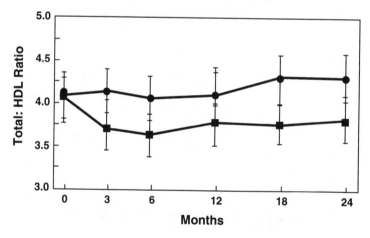

Figure 3.5. Mean fasting levels of total to HDL cholesterol ratios over time in patients receiving tamoxifen or placebo. Control group, ●; patients receiving tamoxifen, ■. Bars indicate 95% CIs. The differences between the groups are significant at all study time points after baseline ($p = 0.06$).

Fasting plasma glucose levels were similar in the two groups at baseline and showed no significant change in either group at 12 months (placebo group, +0.1 mmol/l [1.8 mg/dl]; tamoxifen group, 0.06 mmol/l [1.0 mg/dl]; $p = 0.42$). Our sample size gave 93% power to detect an average change of 10 mm Hg in systolic blood pressure and 87% power to detect a change of 5 mm

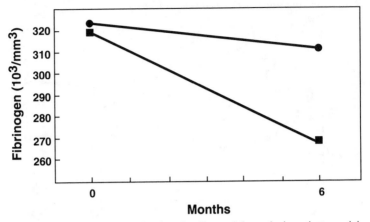

Figure 3.6. Mean fibrinogen levels at baseline and 6 months in patients receiving tamoxifen or placebo. Control patients, ●; n = 70 at baseline and n = 67 at 6 months. Tamoxifen-treated patients, ■; n = 69 at baseline and n = 65 at 6 months. The difference in the change in the two groups is highly significant (p = 0.0003).

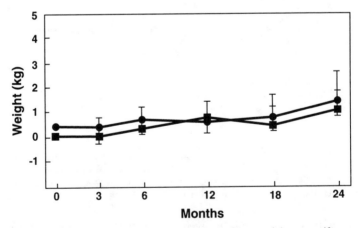

Figure 3.7. Mean weight change over time in patients receiving tamoxifen or placebo. Symbols and bars indicate mean values ± 2 SE. Control patients, ●; n = 70 at baseline and n = 69, 68, 67, 63, and 62 at 3, 6, 12, 18, and 24 months, respectively. Tamoxifen patients, ■; n = 70 at baseline and n = 66, 63, 65, 64, and 64 at 3, 6, 12, 18, and 24 months, respectively. At none of the study time points is the cumulative change in weight different between groups.

Hg in diastolic blood pressure. No significant changes in systolic or diastolic blood pressure were seen in our patients through 24 months. Reported hours per week of exercise and work activity and the number of patients who smoked did not differ or change significantly in either group during the 2-year study period (for example, at 12 months, patients in the placebo group reported a mean aerobic exercise and work time of 10 hours per week, compared with a mean of 11 hours per week for patients receiving tamoxifen). Sixteen percent of patients in the placebo group were smokers, compared with 14% in the tamoxifen group (Table 3.1).

Although detailed 3-day dietary records were obtained from each participant at each evaluation visit, these data were not analyzed. The similar modest weight gain seen in each treatment group, in light of similar exercise and work levels, suggests similar caloric consumption in both groups.

Antithrombin III (ATIII) levels were elevated at baseline in all subjects. The values at 6 months showed statistically significant falls for both placebo- and tamoxifen-treated subjects ($p = 0.001$ for each), although the decline for the tamoxifen group was greater and significantly different ($p = 0.0001$). No single subject had a decline of ATIII to clinically significant levels (less than 70%).

Platelet numbers declined significantly in tamoxifen-treated subjects by 7% at 3 months, and this fall persisted through evaluations at 6, 12, 18, and 24 months ($p = 0.04$ to 0.002 at different time points) (Fig. 3.8). The range of changes in platelet numbers was +134,000 to –196,000. No subject had a platelet count fall to lower than 149,000/mm^3.

One tamoxifen-treated subject developed superficial thrombophlebitis. This woman had no previous history and no elicited precipitating causes for this problem. Her ATIII, fibrinogen, and platelet values and changes were all in the midranges of those for the tamoxifen-treated subjects.

B. OSSEOUS SYSTEM EFFECTS

In interpreting these data, the balance at baseline in the two treatment groups for mean body mass, history of surgical oophorectomy, reported hours per week of aerobic exercise or physical activity, subjects less than 4 and 5 years since menopause, and the numbers of current smokers are important.

The mean baseline lumbar spine and radial bone mineral density (BMD) were not significantly different for the two treatment groups. Over the 2-year study, as estimated by simple linear regression, tamoxifen-treated women showed a significant BMD loss at the radius from baseline value (–0.878%/year, $p = 0.0002$), but appeared to have a BMD increase at the lumbar spine

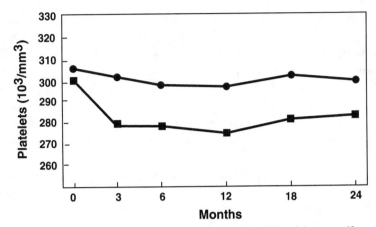

Figure 3.8. Mean levels of platelets over time in patients receiving tamoxifen or placebo. Control patients, ●; n = 70 at baseline and n = 69, 68, 67, 63, and 62 at 3, 6, 12, 18, and 24 months, respectively. Tamoxifen patients, ■; n = 70 at baseline and n = 66, 63, 65, 64, and 64 at 3, 6, 12, 18, and 24 months, respectively. After baseline, the differences between the groups are least significant at 18 months ($p = 0.04$) and most significant at 24 months ($p = 0.002$).

(0.611%/year, $p = 0.04$) (Fig. 3.9). In contrast, placebo-treated women had significant losses from baseline of BMD at both sites (radius, –1.292.%/year, $p = 0.0001$; spine, -0.996%/year, $p = 0.0008$). Tamoxifen-treated women increased their BMD at the lumbar spine by approximately 0.6% per year, whereas placebo subjects decreased their lumbar spine BMD by 1% per year; this difference in rates of change between groups was highly significant ($p = 0.0001$) using an intention-to-treat analysis (Fig. 3.9). Although there was a possible trend for preservation of BMD, there were no significant differences between the two groups' change in BMD over 2 years at the radial site. Results were similar using the Laird and Ware (1982) model. Additional analyses which included or excluded specific small subgroups, an analysis of covariance including as covariates major factors believed to influence BMD and changes in this parameter, and an efficacy analysis, all gave results which were qualitatively no different from those of the main analysis presented.

In the first 70 subjects entered on study, osteocalcin levels were measured at baseline and at 12 and 24 months. In this subset, the osteocalcin levels in tamoxifen-treated women fell to half the baseline levels, whereas there were no significant changes over time in the similarly studied half of the placebo group. Differences in changes between these two subset treatment groups at 12 and 24 months were highly significant ($p = 0.0001$).

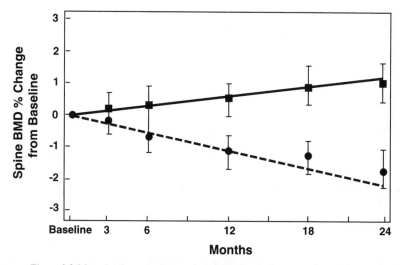

Figure 3.9. Mean lumbar spine bone mineral density changes over time with tamoxifen and placebo treatments. Symbols and bars indicate mean values ± 1 SE. Control group, ●; n = 67 at baseline and 67, 67, 66, 63, and 61 at 3, 6, 12, 18, and 24 months, respectively. Tamoxifen group, ■; n = 66 at baseline, 66, 66, 65, 64 and 64 at 3, 6, 12, 18, and 24 months, respectively. The solid and dashed lines represent the mean regression lines, respectively, as determined from the individual patient regression lines. (Love, Mazess, et al. 1992; reprinted by permission of the *New England Journal of Medicine* 326 [1992]:854.)

Parathyroid hormone and 1,25 dihydroxy vitamin D levels were similar and did not change significantly in the two subsets over the 2 years of the study. Levels of these markers for studied patients were within normal limits, consistent with no effect of sample storage.

Alkaline phosphatase levels, studied in all subjects, fell by 21% in tamoxifen-treated women at 12 months; this also was a significant change from baseline and as compared with that in the placebo group ($p = 0.0001$), which fell by 2%.

Five subjects, although clinically postmenopausal, were endocrinologically premenopausal with baseline follicle-stimulating hormone levels of 30 IU/l or less. Removal of these five subjects from any of the previously presented analyses did not significantly change our results.

C. Symptom Toxicity

Adverse reactions, attributed to the treatment and leading to its cessation, occurred in 6 of 70 tamoxifen-treated subjects (9%) and 4 of 70 placebo subjects (6%) (Table 3.2). Among these six tamoxifen subjects, five stopped

Table 3.4. Proportions of subjects reporting severe hot flashes at baseline and 3-, 6-, and
          12-month visits

	Baseline[a]	Month of visit[a]		
		3	6	12
Placebo				
subjects	0/70 (0.0)	2/69 (3.0)	5/66 (7.6)	2/64 (3.1)
Tamoxifen				
subjects	0/70 (0.0)	13/66 (20.0)	13/64 (20.3)	8/60 (13.3)
p		<0.01	<0.04	<0.04

Modified from the *Archives of Internal Medicine* 151(1991): 1843, copyright 1991, American
Medical Association.
[a]Data are arranged as: number of subjects reporting symptom/number of subjects in group (% of
subjects reporting symptom).

treatment in the first 6 months (hot flashes, 2; edema, 1; rash, 1; other, 1). The
sixth patient developed serious depression, which in retrospect might have
been recognized during the first 6 months but was diagnosed only during the
second 6 months of treatment. This patient had no personal or family history
of depressive illness. Among the four placebo subjects who stopped treatment, the reason was edema in three.

Forty-three percent of placebo subjects and 45% of tamoxifen-treated
women reported hot flashes at baseline. The proportion increased modestly
in tamoxifen-treated women, but was significantly increased only at 6 months
(67% vs 45% for placebo, $p < 0.01$). Severe hot flashes, however, did increase
significantly with tamoxifen treatment (Table 3.4); the drop in the proportion
of subjects at 12 months may reflect the absence of subjects who stopped
treatment for adverse reactions. Mild face flushes and moderate to severe face
flushes increased by 10–15% in tamoxifen-treated subjects ($p < 0.12$ to $p <
0.01$ for each at different time points).

Gynecological symptoms (vaginal discharge, vaginal dryness, bleeding,
or genital pruritus) increased modestly but significantly in tamoxifen-treated
subjects (Table 3.5). These symptoms were, however, predominantly mild.

Of particular note is the fact that we found *no* significant differences in
proportions of tamoxifen recipients who developed other common side
effects, in particular nausea, difficulty sleeping, depression, fatigue, or joint
pains. We did find an apparent and persistent decrease in the frequency of
headache reported in tamoxifen recipients (Table 3.6).

We found a delay in reported symptom increases and a high level of
situational fluctuation in symptom reports. For these reasons, we attempted to
identify those subjects who developed *persistent* side effects by dividing the

Table 3.5 Proportions of subjects reporting gynecological symptoms at baseline and 3-, 6-, and 12-month visits

	Baseline[a]	Month of visit[a]		
		3	6	12
Placebo subjects	5/70 (7.1)	7/69 (10.1)	10/66 (15.1)	9/64 (14.1)
Tamoxifen subjects	7/70 (10.0)	14/66 (21.2)	19/64 (29.7)	16/60 (26.7)
p	<0.55	<0.08	<0.05	<0.08

Modified from the *Archives of Internal Medicine* 151(1991):1844, copyright 1991, American Medical Association.
[a]Data are arranged as: number of subjects reporting symptom/number of subjects in group (% of subjects reporting symptom).

Table 3.6. Proportion of subjects reporting headache at baseline and 3-, 6-, and 12-month visits

	Baseline[a]	Month of visit[a]		
		3	6	12
Placebo subjects	32/70 (45.7)	35/69 (50.7)	33/66 (50.0)	26/64 (40.6)
Tamoxifen subjects	26/70 (37.1)	27/66 (40.9)	21/65 (32.3)	15/60 (25.5)
p	<0.30	<0.25	<0.04	<0.06

Modified from the *Archives of Internal Medicine* 151(1991):1845, copyright 1991, American Medical Association.
[a]Data are arranged as: number of subjects reporting symptom/number of subjects in group (% of subjects reporting symptom).

treatment groups into those who exhibited significant overall toxicity at both the 6- and 12-month follow-up interviews (see "Methods" section for definition of significant overall toxicity). In general, 48.5% (32/66) of tamoxifen recipients and 21.2% (14/66) of placebo subjects experienced persistent toxicity, i.e., significant overall toxicity at both the 6-month and 12-month intervals ($p < 0.001$). Sixty-one percent (40/66) of tamoxifen-treated women reported significant overall toxicity levels at 12 months.

Scores pertaining to general quality of life and anxiety about trial participation did not differ between tamoxifen and placebo groups at any of the study measurement time points.

An analysis of covariance assessed differences between tamoxifen subjects with and without persistent toxicity in trial participation anxiety scores. Baseline trial participation anxiety scores were entered as a covariate to control for potentially disproportionate levels of baseline anxiety in the high-

Table 3.7. Mean scores of anxiety about trial participation among tamoxifen recipients with and without persistent toxic effects

	Baseline[a]	Month of visit[a]		
		3	6	12
Subjects *without* persistent toxicity levels	2.02 (34)	2.05 (34)	1.89 (34)	2.11 (34)
Subjects *with* persistent toxicity levels	1.91 (32)	2.96 (31)	2.92 (26)	2.72 (26)
p	<0.82	<0.01	<0.01	<0.19

Modified from the *Archives of Internal Medicine* 151(1991):1847, copyright 1991, American Medical Association.

[a]Data are arranged as: score (number of subjects in group).

persistent toxicity group causing significantly high scores at follow-up interviews. This covariate was significantly related to trial participation anxiety scores at 3 months ($p < 0.0001$), 6 months ($p < 0.0001$), and 12 months ($p < 0.001$). The baseline mean trial participation anxiety scores and the mean scores for the follow-up interviews, adjusted for baseline trial anxiety, are presented in Table 3.7. Tamoxifen recipients with persistent toxicity levels reported higher anxiety about study participation at 3 and 6 months, even after controlling for baseline trial anxiety levels. However, the difference between tamoxifen recipients with and without persistent toxicity levels was not significant at 12 months, possibly owing to the absence of tamoxifen subjects who dropped because of toxic effects. The absence of differences between the persistent toxicity groups in baseline trial participation anxiety suggests that a priori trial anxiety is *not* associated with the development of persistent toxicity levels in response to tamoxifen.

Analyses of covariance were also conducted on scores of beliefs about experiencing unpleasant side effects, using as a covariate the baseline scores of beliefs about tamoxifen side effects in order to control for the potential differences between the persistent toxicity groups in expectations for side effects. As shown in Table 3.8, baseline scores of beliefs about tamoxifen's potential for causing side effects were *not* significantly associated with subsequent beliefs of having experienced side effects. The results indicate that subjects experiencing persistent toxicity levels *were* more likely to believe their pills were causing unpleasant side effects by the 6-month and 12-month intervals. These subjects appear to have developed stronger beliefs that tamoxifen was responsible for their adverse symptoms. This effect was independent of baseline expectations about tamoxifen side effects; these a priori

Table 3.8. Mean scores of beliefs that therapy is causing side effects among tamoxifen subjects with and without persistent toxic effects

		Month of visit[a]		
	Baseline[a]	3	6	12
Subjects *without* persistent toxicity levels	3.79 (34)	2.13 (34)	1.43 (34)	1.30 (34)
Subjects *with* persistent toxicity levels	4.41 (32)	3.37 (31)	5.14 (26)	3.84 (26)
p	<0.40	<0.14	<0.001	<0.001

Modified from the *Archives of Internal Medicine* 151(1991):1847, copyright 1991, American Medical Association.

[a]Data are arranged as: score (number of subjects in group).

expectations did not determine subsequent beliefs about adverse symptom experiences.

IV. *Discussion*

In this prospective, double-blind, controlled trial in postmenopausal women, we have found strong evidence for non–breast cancer–related biological and symptomatic effects which are themselves important and are also likely to affect major clinical endpoints. The balance of patient characteristics in the randomized groups, high compliance in consumption of assigned tablets as assessed serologically, low study drop-out rates, and absence of significant confounding factors support the study's major conclusions.

A. RESULTS COMPARED WITH THOSE IN OTHER STUDIES

In articles (Love 1989, 1991) and in detailed reports on this study we have reviewed the available cardiovascular (Love et al. 1990; Love, Wiebe, et al. 1991), coagulation (Love, Surawicz, and Williams 1992), osseos (Love, Mazess, et al. 1992), and symptomatic effects data from other investigators. In the lipid and lipoprotein area, our results are generally consistent with reported studies with respect to total and LDL cholesterol decreases. The absence of impact of tamoxifen on HDL cholesterol found in this study is at variance with some findings; differences in study sizes and major population characteristics may account for these discrepant results. Specific previous data about lipid:lipoprotein ratios, apolipoproteins AI and B, fasting glucose exercise, blood pressure, weight, fibrinogen, and platelet number changes have been very limited or absent. To date, as in this study, investigators have not found specific changes to explain fully the apparent pro-coagulant effect of tamoxifen, which results in increases in cases of thrombophlebitis at rates of 1/800 woman treatment years (Fisher et al. 1989). Antithrombin III decreases similar to those observed in this study have been seen (Jordan, Fritz, and Tormey 1987).

With respect to osseos effects, animal studies suggest that tamoxifen is an antiresorptive agent, like estrogen, and preserves trabecular and, perhaps to a lesser extent, compact bone (Jordan, Phelps, and Lindgren 1987; Turner et al. 1987a,b; Wakley et al. 1988). The results reported here are consistent with these animal studies and small, previously reported, human studies (Love et al. 1988; Fentiman et al. 1989; Fornander et al. 1990; Godfredsen et al. 1984; Turken et al. 1989; Ryan et al. 1991). Our study showed that there was significant loss of BMD for tamoxifen-treated subjects at the radial shaft site, a site composed mainly of compact bone. The decline in bone mass associated with cessation of ovarian estrogen production involves mainly the more metabolically active trabecular bone found in the spine and to a lesser degree in the hip. A longer-term study may be necessary to show a significant difference in BMD with tamoxifen treatment at the radius shaft site. In human studies, with therapeutic agents for osteoporosis, greater effects are seen in preservation of spinal BMD than peripheral BMD (Lindsay and Tohme 1990; Civitelli et al. 1988; Watts et al. 1990). Unfortunately in this study, because of the multiplicity of assessments made on each subject and the associated time commitments of subjects, as well as cost, bone density in the femur was not assessed. Some antiresorptive agents, such as calcitonin or bisphosphonates, have little or no effect on peripheral bone (Civitelli et al. 1988; Watts et al. 1990). The 3% difference in spine BMD between tamoxifen-treated and control patients at the end of 2 years in this study was identical with the difference induced by etidronate treatment in osteoporosis (Watts et al. 1990), but was lower than the 5–10% difference induced over the same period by calcitonin or estrogen (Lindsay and Tohme 1990; Civitelli et al. 1988). Estrogen also has a stabilizing effect on radial bone, an effect our short-term data do not show.

There are only limited published human data on bone metabolism. In this study, the reduction in osteocalcin and alkaline phosphatase associated with tamoxifen presumably reflects decreased bone turnover or bone remodeling.

The symptom toxicity data reported in this study differ significantly from those in other reports in many respects. In large adjuvant studies, 4–5% of subjects are reported to stop treatment because of side effects (NATO 1985;

Breast Cancer Trials Committee 1987). This study's modestly higher fraction of subjects stopping treatment for toxicity (9% in the tamoxifen group) may reflect the specific nature of the study (a toxicity, not a therapeutic, study) or a more accurate assessment of reasons for treatment cessation. (For example, subjects were aware that serological compliance monitoring was occurring; in adjuvant studies it is possible that true noncompliance is in fact significantly greater than the quoted drop-out figures indicate.) The magnitudes of vaso-motor, gynecological, and overall significant toxicity effects reported in this study are much greater than have been suggested in adjuvant trial data.

It is critical to take into account our patient population and the specific methodologies when interpreting these results and their generalizability to other studies of symptoms associated with medical treatments. Possible critical features of this study are the volunteer nature of the highly motivated subjects, the long time since menopause for most subjects, the frequent periodicity of the symptom reports, the comprehensive and standardized manner in which the information was elicited and recorded, the specific wording of the questions (notably the request for grading of symptoms at their *worst*), and the inclusion of both general and specific measures of psychological well-being. Some broad rather than specific conclusions thus seem more appropriate.

B. Direct Implications of Results

Although the precise effects of tamoxifen on all cardiovascular disease (CVD) risk factors have not been completely defined by this and other studies, and although the significance of different cardiovascular risk factors in women is poorly understood, we can make some extrapolations of available data to clinical endpoints (Manolio et al. 1991). In hypercholesterolemic men the relationship of the percentage of reduction in total cholesterol to the percentage of reduction in coronary heart disease (CHD) (sudden death and fatal and nonfatal myocardial infarction) is described by the line in Figure 3.10. A 10–15% reduction in cholesterol in intervention studies has been associated with a 20% drop in CHD (Yusuf et al. 1988). By extrapolation, then, from results of the current study, a 20–25% drop in CHD endpoints might be expected with long-term tamoxifen treatment (Fig. 3.10). In men from one trial, the relationship between lowering LDL cholesterol and reduc-tion in CHD suggests that the 20% reduction seen with tamoxifen might be accompanied by a reduction of 31% in CHD (Fig. 3.11). The uncertainty regarding an effect of tamoxifen on HDL cholesterol raised by our study requires resolution by examination of a larger population of subjects.

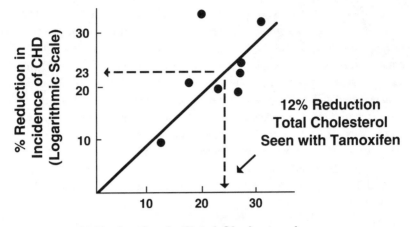

% Reduction in Total Cholesterol

Figure 3.10. Each symbol (●) represents the results from one of eight cholesterol-lowering trials in men. (Adapted from the *Journal of the American Medical Association* 251[1984]:365–374.)

In the Framingham study, lower levels of fibrinogen were associated with decreased risk of stroke in women (Kannel et al. 1987), suggesting a possible favorable effect on incidence of cardiovascular thrombosis with tamoxifen. Absence of a major effect of tamoxifen on glucose metabolism is particularly reassuring, because diabetes-associated silent myocardial infarction is significantly more common in women. Similarly, absence of major effects on systolic or diastolic blood pressure is important. For both glucose and blood pressure parameters, however, careful studies of larger numbers of subjects are needed.

Retrospectively obtained data from the Scottish tamoxifen adjuvant study and through the Early Breast Cancer Trialists' Collaborative Group have supported these suggested levels of favorable impact in CHD and CVD rates (McDonald and Stewart 1991; Early Breast Cancer Trialists' Collaborative Group 1992). In the Collaborative Trialists' data a decrease of 27% in vascular deaths has been found (Early Breast Cancer Trialists' Collaborative Group 1992). It must be emphasized, however, that these data are reassuring. Specific benefits of long-term tamoxifen on CVD endpoints need demonstration in prospectively designed trials.

The benefits of tamoxifen in stabilizing and perhaps increasing bone mineral density in the lumbar spine should be replicated in the femoral head and neck, also a trabecular bone site. If so, and the results here are supported by further data from other studies, reduction in fracture risk should be

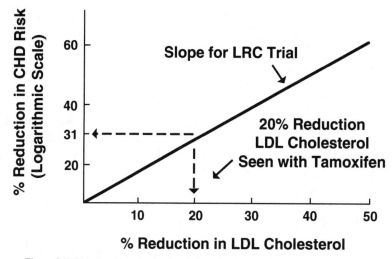

Figure 3.11. Relationship of reduction in low-density lipoprotein cholesterol (LDL-C) to reduction in coronary heart disease (CHD) risk (logarithmic scale). Adapted from the *Journal of the American Medical Association* 251(1984):365–374.

expected. By extrapolation from BMD preservation and fracture risk reduction studies with estrogen, a 25%–30% reduction in fracture risk might be expected with long-term tamoxifen (Weiss et al. 1980).

This study is reassuring in that some previously reported side effects of tamoxifen therapy were not seen: joint pain, evidence of depression in other than one treated subject, nausea, and fatigue. In addition, the suggested reduction in frequency of headache supports results in a previous study (Powles 1986). However, the significant proportions of tamoxifen recipients who developed chronic, moderate to severe vasomotor symptoms and/or mild gynecological symptoms demand clinicians' attention. Management of vasomotor symptoms has received only limited investigation, and an algorithm for evaluation and management of gynecological complaints, which lead to limited iatrogenic symptoms, may be less than optimally employed.

The heightened anxiety about trial participation, and beliefs that tamoxifen is producing adverse side effects among subjects with persistent toxicity levels, raises concern about the effects of tamoxifen on psychological well-being. Presumably, long-term tamoxifen therapy should be more acceptable to postmenopausal women, who may experience less extreme reactions to tamoxifen and who have high motivations for therapy due to a history of breast cancer. While the absence of an effect of adverse symptoms on general quality of life ratings supports this contention, the effects of tamoxifen-induced toxicity on trial anxiety, cancer worry, and beliefs of therapy-induced side effects suggest that tamoxifen carries some "costs" to specific aspects of well-being.

Most significantly for clinicians, this study suggests that, in a population of postmenopausal women with a history of axillary node-negative breast cancer, almost half the tamoxifen-treated women will report moderate or greater levels of symptoms. Both the magnitude of this toxicity and its impact on psychological well-being demand clinicians' understanding and discussion with patients so that the overall costs and benefits of tamoxifen therapy are honestly recognized.

C. Broader Implications for Long-Term Adjuvant Therapy and Prevention

The detailed data obtained in this study show that tamoxifen has organ site–specific effects which are variably estrogenic or antiestrogenic in postmenopausal women. The mixed response with blood lipids and lipoproteins warrants further careful evaluation not only in postmenopausal but also in premenopausal populations. In general, these data should raise caution, for they do show powerful effects of tamoxifen on the cardiovascular and skeletal systems.

The modest thrombocytopenia found in this study is intriguing, suggesting a growth factor–mediating effect of tamoxifen. The decreased numbers of hematopoietic cancers seen with adjuvant therapy may be a manifestation of a similar change, as also may be the apparent beneficial effect of tamoxifen in estrogen receptor–negative tumor-bearing women (Early Breast Cancer Trialists' Collaborative Group 1992). Again, these suggested effects may also herald adverse consequences.

Probably the most important data from this study, however, are those describing the frequency and magnitude of adverse side effects, greater than commonly appreciated. Although difficult to predict, there are several reasons for believing that these side effects will lead to dropping out of treatment with long-term adjuvant courses and with prevention. In the prevention trial setting, this will make completion of a study difficult.

V. *Summary*

Data from the Wisconsin Tamoxifen Study show major, likely favorable effects overall on lipids and lipoproteins and on the skeleton. Major symptomatic toxicity found in this study is greater than is commonly acknowledged. These findings should prompt more detailed study of this therapy while we struggle to improve the control of breast cancer.

Acknowledgments

Co-investigators for this study were Howard Barden, Paul Carbone, Linda Cameron, Brad Connell, David DeMets, Jan Feyzi, V. Craig Jordan, Howard Leventhal, Richard Mazess, Polly Newcomb, Tanya Surawicz, and Donald Wiebe.

Outstanding technical assistance was provided by Joy Kurt, Ruth Diaz de Leon, LouAnn Stittleburg, Betty Buckmaster, Charlene Luchterhand, Kristine Knudson, Cathy Knudsen, and Heidi Sahel.

These investigations were supported by grants PDT302A and PDT302B from the American Cancer Society; by grants from the ICI Pharmaceuticals Division of ICI Americas, Inc., Wilmington, Delaware; and by a grant from the National Institutes of Health, National Cancer Institute RO1 CA 50243.

References

Breast Cancer Trials Committee, Scottish Cancer Trials Office. 1987. Adjuvant tamoxifen in the management of operable breast cancer: the Scottish trial. *Lancet* 2:171–175.

Civitelli, R., S. Gonnelli, F. Zacchei, S. Bigazzi, A. Vattimo, L. V. Avioli, and C. Gennari. 1988. Bone turnover in postmenopausal osteoporosis. Effect of calcitonin treatment. *Journal of Clinical Investigation* 82:1268–1274.

Early Breast Cancer Trialists' Collaborative Group. 1988. The effects of adjuvant tamoxifen and of cytotoxic therapy on mortality in early breast cancer: an overview of 61 randomized trials among 28,896 women. *New England Journal of Medicine* 319:1681–1692.

Early Breast Cancer Trialists' Collaborative Group. 1992. Systematic treatment of early breast cancer by hormonal, cytotoxic, or immune therapy. 133 randomised trials involving 31,000 recurrences and 24,000 deaths among 75,000 women. *Lancet* 339:1–15.

Fentiman, I. S., M. Caleffi, A. Rodin, B. Murby, and I. Fogelman. 1989. Bone mineral content of women receiving tamoxifen for mastalgia. *British Journal of Cancer* 60:262–264.

Fisher, B., J. Costantino, C. Redmond, and 50 other members of the NSABP. 1989. A randomized clinical trial evaluating tamoxifen in the treatment of patients with node-negative breast cancer who have estrogen-receptor–positive tumors. *New England Journal of Medicine* 320:479–484.

Fornander, T., L. E. Rutqvist, H. E. Sjoberg, L. Blomqvist, A. Mattsson, and U. Glas. 1990. Long-term adjuvant tamoxifen in early breast cancer: effect on bone mineral density in postmenopausal women. *Journal of Clinical Oncology* 8:1019–1024.

Friedewald, W. T., R. I. Levy, and D. S. Fredrickson. 1972. Estimation of the concentration of low-density lipoprotein cholesterol in plasma, without use of the preparative ultracentrifuge. *Clinical Chemistry* 18:499–502.

Gotfredsen, A., C. Christiansen, and T. Palshof. 1984. The effect of tamoxifen on bone mineral content in premenopausal women with breast cancer. *Cancer* 53:853–857.

Gottardis, M. M., and V. C. Jordan. 1987. Antitumor actions of keoxifene and tamoxifen in the

N-nitrosomethylurea–induced rat mammary carcinoma model. *Cancer Research* 47:4020–4024.

Jordan, V. C., and K. E. Allen. 1980. Evaluation of the antitumour activity of the nonsteroidal antioestrogen monohydroxytamoxifen in the DMBA-induced rat mammary carcinoma model. *European Journal of Cancer* 16:239–251.

Jordan, V. C., N. F. Fritz, and D. C. Tormey. 1987. Long-term adjuvant therapy with tamoxifen: effects on sex hormone binding globulin and antithrombin III. *Cancer Research* 47:4517–4519.

Jordan, V. C., E. Phelps, and J. U. Lindgren. 1987. Effects of antiestrogens on bone in castrated and intact female rats. *Breast Cancer Research and Treatment* 10:31–35.

Kannel, W. B., P. A. Wolf, W. P. Castelli, and R. B. D'Agostino. 1987. Fibrinogen and risk of cardiovascular disease. The Framingham study. *Journal of the American Medical Association* 258:1183–1186.

Laird, N. M., and J. H. Ware. 1982. Random effects models for longitudinal data. *Biometrics* 38:963–974.

Lerner, L. J., and V. C. Jordan. 1990. Development of antiestrogens and their use in breast cancer: eighth Cain Memorial Award Lecture. *Cancer Research* 50:4177–4189.

Lindsay, R., and J. F. Tohme. 1990. Estrogen treatment of patients with established postmenopausal osteoporosis. *Obstetrics and Gynecology* 72(2):290–295.

Love, R. R. 1989. Antiestrogens as chemopreventive agents in breast cancer: promise and issues in evaluation. *Preventive Medicine* 18:661–671.

Love, R. R. 1991. Antiestrogen chemoprevention of breast cancer: critical issues and research. *Preventive Medicine* 20:64–78.

Love, R. R., T. S. Surawicz, and E. C. Williams. 1992. Antithrombin III level, fibrinogen level, and platelet count changes with adjuvant tamoxifen therapy. *Archives of Internal Medicine* 152:317–320.

Love, R. R., L. Cameron, B. L. Connell, and H. Leventhal. 1991. Symptoms associated with tamoxifen treatment in postmenopausal women. *Archives of Internal Medicine* 151:1842–1847.

Love, R. R., R. B. Mazess, D. C. Tormey, H. S. Barden, P. A. Newcomb, and V. C. Jordan. 1988. Bone mineral density in women with breast cancer treated with adjuvant tamoxifen for at least two years. *Breast Cancer Research and Treatment* 12:297–302.

Love, R. R., P. A. Newcomb, D. A. Wiebe, T. S. Surawicz, V. C. Jordan, P. P. Carbone, and D. L. DeMets. 1990. Effects of tamoxifen therapy on lipid and lipoprotein levels in postmenopausal women with node-negative breast cancer. *Journal of the National Cancer Institute* 82:1327–1332.

Love, R. R., R. B. Mazess, H. S. Barden, S. Epstein, P. A. Newcomb, V. C. Jordan, P. P. Carbone, and D. L. DeMets. 1992. Effects of tamoxifen on bone mineral density in postmenopausal women with breast cancer. *New England Journal of Medicine* 326:852–856.

Love, R. R., D. A. Wiebe, P. A. Newcomb, L. Cameron, H. Leventhal, V. C. Jordan, J. Feyzi, and D. L. DeMets. 1991. Effects of tamoxifen on cardiovascular risk factors in postmenopausal women. *Annals of Internal Medicine* 115:860–864.

McDonald, C. C., and H. J. Stewart. 1991. Fatal myocardial infarction in the Scottish adjuvant tamoxifen trial. The Scottish Breast Cancer Committee. *British Medical Journal* 303:435–437.

Manolio, T. A., T. A. Pearson, N. K. Wenger, E. Barrett-Connor, G. H. Payne, and W. R. Harlan. 1992. Cholesterol and heart disease in older persons and women: overview of a NHLBI workshop. *Annals of Epidemiology* 2:161–176.

Nolvadex Adjuvant Trial Organisation (NATO). 1985. Controlled trial of tamoxifen as a single adjuvant agent in the management of early breast cancer. Analysis at six years. *Lancet* 1:836–840.

Powles, T. J. 1986. Prevention of migrainous headaches by tamoxifen. *Lancet* 2:1344.

Ryan, W. G., J. Wolter, and J. D. Bagdade. 1991. Apparent beneficial effects of tamoxifen on bone mineral content in patients with breast cancer: preliminary study. *Journal of Bone and Mineral Research* 3(1):S130.

Turken, S., E. Siris, D. Seldin, E. Flaster, G. Hyman, and R. Lindsay. 1989. Effects of tamoxifen on spinal bone density in women with breast cancer. *Journal of the National Cancer Institute* 81:1086–1088.

Turner, R. T., G. K. Wakley, K. S. Hannon, and N. H. Bell. 1987a. Tamoxifen inhibits osteoclast-mediated resorption of trabecular bone in ovarian hormone–deficient rats. *Endocrinology* 122:1146–1150.

Turner, R. T., G. K. Wakley, K. S. Hannon, and N. H. Bell. 1987b. Tamoxifen prevents the skeletal effects of ovarian hormone deficiency in rats. *Journal of Bone and Mineral Research* 2(5):449–456.

Wakley, G. K., B. L. Baum, K. S. Hannon, and R. T. Turner. 1988. The effects of tamoxifen on the osteopenia induced by sciatic neurotomy in the rat: a histomorphometric study. *Calcified Tissue International* 43:383–388.

Watts, N. B., S. T. Harris, H. K. Genant, R. D. Wasnich, P. D. Miller, and R. D. Jackson. 1990. Intermittent cyclical etidronate treatment of postmenopausal osteoporosis. *New England Journal of Medicine* 323:73–79.

Wei, L. J., and J. M. Lachin. 1984. Two-sample asymptotically distribution-free test for incomplete multivariate observation. *Journal of the American Statistics Association* 79:653–661.

Weiss, N. S., C. L. Ure, J. H. Ballard, A. R. Williams, and J. R. Daling. 1980. Decreased risk of fractures of the hip and lower forearm with postmenopausal use of estrogen. *New England Journal of Medicine* 303:1195–1198.

Welsch, C. W., M. Goodrich-Smith, C. K. Brown, D. Mackie, and D. Johnson. 1982. 2-Bromo-alpha-ergocryptine (CB-154) and tamoxifen (ICI 46,474) induced suppression of the genesis of mammary carcinomas in female rats treated with 7,12-dimethylbenzanthracene (DMBA): a comparison. *Oncology* 39(2):88–92.

Yusuf, S., J. Wittes, and L. Friedman. 1988. Overview of results of randomized clinical trials in heart disease. 2. Unstable angina, heart failure, primary prevention with aspirin and risk factor modification. *Journal of the American Medical Association* 260:2259–2263.

4

Endocrine Therapy for the Premenopausal Woman

R. W. BLAMEY

I.   INTRODUCTION   84
II. THE HORMONAL TREATMENT OF BREAST CANCER   87
III. ADVANCES IN ENDOCRINE TREATMENT FOR ADVANCED BREAST CANCER IN THE
     PREMENOPAUSAL WOMAN   87
     A. PREDICTION OF RESPONSE   90
     B. MEASUREMENT OF RESPONSE   90
IV. ADJUVANT HORMONE THERAPY IN PREMENOPAUSAL WOMEN   91
V.   FURTHER DEVELOPMENT IN ENDOCRINE THERAPY   91
     REFERENCES   91

I. *Introduction*

T̲HE question initially posed is, does breast cancer differ in pre- and post-menopausal women? That might be considered an easy question to answer, but the results from trials of adjuvant therapy, as at present published (Early Breast Cancer Trialists' Collaborative Group 1992), indicate the effectiveness of CMF in postmenopausal women differs from that in premenopausal women.

The important parameters in breast cancer in pre- and postmenopausal women are essentially the same; these are disease-free interval (DFI) (Fig. 4.1) and survival; also, survival from the time of recognition of advanced disease (Fig. 4.2) does not differ.

Histological grade is a major prognostic factor underlying the survival curves and there is no significant difference in the overall distribution of grade, dependent on whether women are pre- or postmenopausal (Table 4.1). There are some differences (and these reflect on clinical care); women under the age of 40 tend to have more aggressive tumors—Table 4.2 shows a higher proportion of grade III tumors, some of which are very poorly differentiated indeed with very high mitotic rates. There is a difference in the histology of the parenchyma surrounding the cancer; this reflects on breast cancer screening from which premenopausal women have not been demonstrated to receive benefit. The reason for this is that a cancer showing as a small density is not easily picked out against a dense background of epithelial tissue. There are differences in estrogen receptor status (Table 4.3), in the amount of ductal carcinoma *in situ* both within and around invasive tumors and in the rate in which lymphovascular invasion is seen within the tumor. The last is a factor which codes for local recurrence both after mastectomy and after treatment with breast conservation.

In the first 250 women treated in Nottingham City Hospital by breast conservation surgery, without very wide excision, followed by intact breast irradiation, we did have a considerable recurrence rate within the treated breast (local recurrence, LR). The factors which correlated most strongly with LR were vascular invasion, size, and young age (Locker et al. 1989); unfortunately the younger the patient, the more likely that she might suffer recurrence in the treated breast (Table 4.4). Age itself cannot be a factor, but it

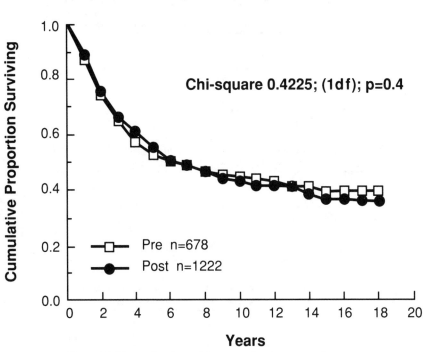

Figure 4.1. Disease-free interval in pre- and postmenopausal women.

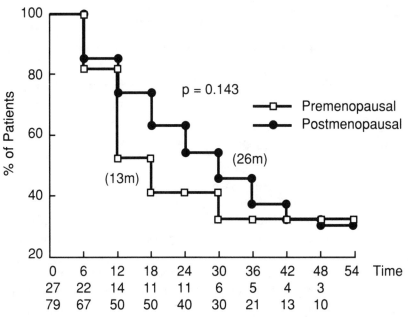

Figure 4.2. Survival time analyzed by age from starting systematic endocrine therapy.

Table 4.1. Histological grade, in pre- and postmenopausal women

	Grade (Elston)		
	I	II	III
Premenopausal	58	108	180
Postmenopausal	101	236	244

$\chi^2 = 3.2$; (2 degrees of freedom); NS

Table 4.2. Distribution of invasive carcinoma, by histological grade, in women aged 40 or less compared with those aged 41 and over

		Grade (Elston)	
Age	n	I and II	III
≤40	259	95	144
41+	2024	1066	833

$\chi^2 = 22.97$ (1 degree of freedom); $p = 0.000$

Table 4.3. Number of tumors, estrogen receptor positive and negative, in women with breast cancer in the pre- and postmenopausal series

	Estrogen receptor status	
	Positive	Negative
Premenopausal (≤50)	292	500
Postmenopausal (51–70)	654	793

$\chi^2 = 14.21$; (1 d.f.); $p < 0.002$

Table 4.4. Number of patients following treatment with breast conservation, by status of local recurrence and age (N = 263)

Age	LR	No LR
≤50	54	171
>50	2	36

Fisher's exact $p < 0.005$

predictably reflects a combination of poor differentiation, ductal carcinoma *in situ* within and around the tumor and lymphovascular invasion. The findings of other series (Fourquet et al. 1989) with regard to LR after breast conservation have been similar, with young age emerging as a strong risk factor for LR.

In summary, there is no important difference in survival or distant DFI, but there are differences that reflect on diagnosis and on surgical treatment of the primary tumor.

II. *The Hormonal Treatment of Breast Cancer*

In a publication in the *Lancet* in 1896 entitled "The treatment of inoperable cases of the mamma," a suggestion for a new method of treatment was advanced by George Beatson (1896). I quote from this article a referral letter received on May 6, 1895, which said "Dear Dr. Beatson, The bearer of this letter is and has been suffering I fear from a malignant breast. My own opinion is that nothing can be done for her." Beatson described the woman, who had a local recurrence following mastectomy which was beyond further surgery. He went on to talk about his research. He had decided to work on lactation in the sheep, and he came to some very important conclusions indeed. First, he showed that lactation was not controlled through the central nervous system. Second, he found that the ovaries could control lactation and said that this demonstrated that one organ could hold control over the secretion of another, without working through the central nervous system. This was in 1896, before the first description of a hormone—a remarkable discovery. Third, he noticed that both in lactation and in cancer there was a proliferation of epithelium, and he went on to reason that, perhaps, if you could control proliferation of the one then you could control proliferation of the other by removing the ovaries. On June 15, 1895, he carried out the first oophorectomy for breast cancer; the patient had a very good response. This was the first description of any successful systemic therapy for breast cancer, another remarkable discovery. Beatson should be saluted for two outstanding medical findings, either of which was of a magnitude worthy of a Nobel Prize.

Thus oophorectomy became the standard treatment for the premenopausal woman developing advanced breast cancer, and it is easily demonstrated that the chances of a reasonable survival duration and a reasonable quality of life at that stage of the disease depend entirely on the response to first-line endocrine treatment (Williams, Todd, et al. 1986) (Fig. 4.3). Nonresponders to first-line endocrine treatment have a median survival of less than 1 year, and the use of cytotoxic chemotherapy has not overridden this.

III. *Advances in Endocrine Treatment for Advanced Breast Cancer in the Premenopausal Woman*

Before describing this work our definition of menopausal status is given. A perimenopausal group is not recognized; the endocrine event of cessation of ovarian function is defined by an endocrine means; if a woman is menstruat-

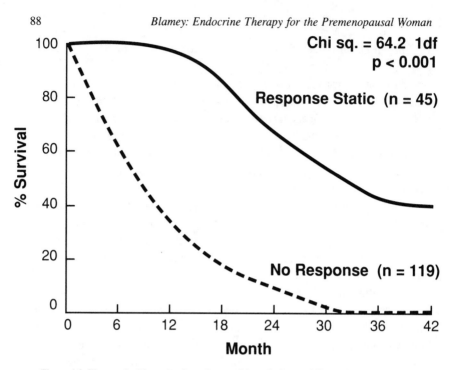

Figure 4.3. The survival from the time of recognition of advanced disease in patients showing a response to primary endocrine treatment compared with those not responding to primary endocrine treatment.

ing she is premenopausal, otherwise the follicle-stimulating hormone (FSH) is measured, and if it is less than 20 the woman is regarded as premenopausal. The work presented here is all in premenopausal women with advanced disease and previously untreated in any way.

The first study was a multicenter trial (Buchanan et al. 1986) (to which Nottingham entered around 30 patients), comparing tamoxifen as the initial treatment with surgical oophorectomy in a crossover trial. The initial response in 117 evaluable patients showed the response rate as very much the same, whether starting with tamoxifen or oophorectomy. Neither did the survival curves from the time of initial therapy show a difference, but it has to be remembered that patients received both treatments.

This trial demonstrated that initial treatment with tamoxifen was as suitable as with oophorectomy; however, the numbers in the trial were relatively small and confidence intervals quite wide. It was at that point that the new agent, the luteinizing hormone–releasing hormone (LHRH) agonist 118,630, was brought in by Imperial Chemical Industries (Macclesfield, U.K.) and subsequently named Zoladex. This agent blocks gonadotropin release and there-

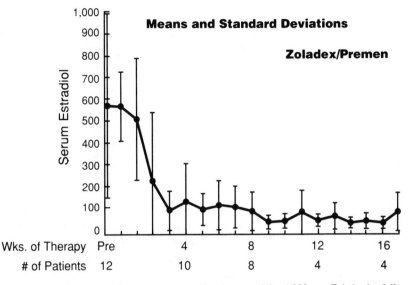

Figure 4.4. Serum estradiol in premenopausal patients receiving 1,000 mcg Zoladex by daily injection, measured over 16 weeks of therapy.

fore reduces plasma estradiol, and in fact carries out a medical oophorectomy whilst it is being administered. We tested this concept in a phase I study; initially, we began with subcutaneous daily therapy and later used the depot monthly formulation. Blood samples were taken at regular intervals and assayed by Dr. R. Nicholson from the Tenovus Institute in Cardiff for FSH, estradiol, and progesterone. We were able to demonstrate that there was a very clear blockade of the ovary; Figure 4.4 shows the serum estradiol measured over 16 weeks of therapy, which was reduced to levels comparable to the postmenopausal women or to the oophorectomized women.

Careful clinical follow-up was carried out with assessment of response according to the UICC criteria, with the added definition that we have always applied in Nottingham: that a response should have a minimum of 6 months' duration. Under these circumstances the overall response in 45 patients was 31% (Williams, Walker, et al. 1986), much the same as one would expect with oophorectomy. The side effects were minimal, being essentially those of the menopause. Initially, because this was a phase I study, we had to carry out oophorectomy after tumor progression. However, after 24 patients this was no longer done, because complete ovarian suppression had been demonstrated with Zoladex. Our early conclusions were that clinical and endocrinological responses were similar to those found after oophorectomy, that there was no serious toxicity and the drug was tolerated well.

Subsequently we have carried out studies of 75 patients on Zoladex alone, and more recently we have introduced Zoladex together with tamoxifen; we have even more recently established a multicenter clinical trial comparing Zoladex alone (Z) with Zoladex plus tamoxifen (Z + T). This was a good opportunity to reexamine the idea of giving two hormonal agents at once. Much of the previous literature in which two hormonal therapies have been given together has relied upon studies in which the side effects of treatment have been considerable, for example, comparison of oophorectomy with oophorectomy plus adrenalectomy. Here we had the chance to compare a combined hormone therapy, where the side effects were the same, whether the patient received one drug or two.

In making the historical comparison between Z and Z + T the series were comparable in patient age, site of metastatic disease, and estrogen receptor status. Tamoxifen alone raises the serum estradiol; however, it did not do so when combined with Zoladex, and there was no difference in estradiol levels between Z and Z + T, even in long-term studies.

Looking at survival of patients assessed as disease progressors, no difference was seen; but in those who had complete response, partial response, or static disease, durations of response and survival were better with the combination (Dixon and Blamey 1991). Numbers were small, but this was an interesting finding and provided a basis for the randomized trial. Recruitment for this trial is now complete; it is multicountry as well as multicenter (including 90 from Germany, 69 from Scandinavia, 32 from Nottingham, and cases from Australia). The early results of this trial were presented at the Nottingham International Breast Cancer Meeting in September 1992.[1]

A. Prediction of Response

We have found, using the estrogen receptor radio immune assay (ERICA) in the primary tumors, that metastases from tumors judged estrogen receptor–negative have a very low chance of response. At the present time we are using ERICA to determine which patients with advanced disease should receive endocrine therapy and which not.

B. Measurement of Response

We are now measuring response by biochemical means. Using CEA, CA 15.3, and erythrocyte sedimentation rate (ESR) calibrated to a carefully designed index, which we have been developing for some years, we gain, by serum assay, a very good biochemical measure of response (Robertson et al.

1991), which should replace UICC assessment and is very much easier to apply.

IV. *Adjuvant Hormone Therapy in Premenopausal Women*

It was considered for many years that the trials of ovarian ablative therapy used as adjuvant treatment after mastectomy, did not show a long-term advantage in survival. When the nine trials which were admissible were put together in metanalysis (Early Breast Cancer Trialists' Collaborative Group 1992), in women under 50 there was a clear odds reduction of death for those who received ovarian ablation. The magnitude was very much the same as with the use of CMF in the premenopausal woman or tamoxifen in the postmenopausal woman. Further analysis of the data shows that the use of tamoxifen alone in the premenopausal woman has much the same advantage over using no adjuvant therapy. It does appear that the use of either of these endocrine therapies as an adjuvant is of advantage in the premenopausal woman.

Zoladex would seem to be the ideal agent for this; not only does it produce a block of the ovaries whilst it is being administered, but there is also rapid recovery of the ovaries after the course of treatment; the woman can regain her premenopausal status without the side effects of the menopause if she so wishes. There is a multicenter randomized trial in Europe which has been set up by Jonat and Kaufman for node-positive, premenopausal women in order to look at Zoladex given for 2 years as an adjuvant compared with CMF given in 6 cycles. There will be subgroup analysis for ER status.

V. *Further Development in Endocrine Therapy*

Finally, there is the emergence of Imperial Chemical Industries' 182,780, a pure antiestrogen described elsewhere in this book. At present this agent is undergoing clinical testing in Manchester Christie Hospital and Nottingham City Hospital. It is possible that the very high affinity of this agent for ER will render ovarian suppression unnecessary.

References

Beatson, G. T. 1896. Treatment of inoperable cases of carcinoma of the mamma: suggestions for a new method of treatment, with illustrative cases. *Lancet* 2:104–107 and 162–165.

Buchanan, R. B., R. W. Blamey, K. R. Durrant, A. Howell, A. G. Paterson, P. E. Preece, D. C. Smith, C. J. Williams, and R. G. Wilson. 1986. A randomized comparison of tamoxifen with surgical oophorectomy in premenopausal patients with advanced breast cancer. *Journal of Clinical Oncology* 4:1326–1330.

Dixon, A. R., and R. W. Blamey. 1991. Zoladex and Nolvadex in premenopausal advanced breast cancer. *European Journal of Gynaecology and Oncology* 7:247.

Early Breast Cancer Trialists' Collaborative Group. 1992. Systemic treatment of early breast cancer by hormonal, cytotoxic or immune therapy. 133 randomised trials involving 31,000 recurrences and 24,000 deaths among women. *Lancet* 339:1–15 and 71–85.

Fourquet, A., F. Campana, B. Zafrani, V. Mosseri, P. Vielh, J. Durand, and J. R. Vilcoq. 1989. Prognostic factors of breast cancer recurrence in the conservative management of early breast cancer: a 25 year follow-up. *International Journal of Radiation Oncology and Biological Physics* 17:719–725.

Locker, A. P., I. O. Ellis, D. A. Morgan, A. Mitchell, C. W. Elston, and R. W. Blamey. 1989. Factors influencing local recurrence after excision and radiotherapy for primary breast cancer. *British Journal of Surgery* 76:890–894.

Robertson, J. F., D. Pearson, M. R. Price, C. Selby, J. Pearson, R. W. Blamey, and A. Howell. 1991. Prospective assessment of the role of five tumour markers in breast cancer. *Cancer Immunology and Immunotherapy* 33:403–410.

Williams, M. R., K. J. Walker, A. Turkes, R. W. Blamey, and R. I. Nicholson. 1986. The use of an LH-RH agonist (ICI 118630, Zoladex) in advanced premenopausal breast cancer. *British Journal of Cancer* 53:629–636.

Williams, M. R., J. H. Todd, R. I. Nicholson, C. W. Elston, R. W. Blamey, and K. Griffiths. 1986. Survival patterns in hormone treated advanced breast cancer. *British Journal of Surgery* 73:752–755.

5

The Nolvadex Adjuvant Trial Organisation (NATO) and the Cancer Research Campaign (CRC) Trials of Adjuvant Tamoxifen Therapy on Behalf of the CRC Breast Cancer Trials Group

J. HOUGHTON, D. RILEY, AND M. BAUM

I.	INTRODUCTION	94
II.	DESIGN OF THE NATO TRIAL	94
III.	DESIGN OF THE CRC ADJUVANT TRIAL	95
IV.	CURRENT STATUS OF THE NATO TRIAL	96
V.	CURRENT STATUS OF THE CANCER RESEARCH CAMPAIGN TRIAL	98
VI.	DISCUSSION	104
VII.	SUMMARY	111
	REFERENCES	112

I. *Introduction*

IN the 1970s and 1980s the outstanding issue in the treatment of early breast cancer was the role of adjuvant therapy. In the United States and parts of Europe the use of cytotoxic therapy was paramount, whereas in the United Kingdom and northern Europe preference was for less aggressive therapy. Availability of the antiestrogen tamoxifen (Nolvadex) renewed interest in hormonal maneuvers in the treatment of breast cancer. The activity of tamoxifen in metastatic and locally advanced disease, where worthwhile tumor responses were obtained, led to use as an adjuvant following surgery.

Two major trials of adjuvant tamoxifen therapy were carried out between 1977 and 1985 in the United Kingdom by a large group of collaborating clinicians. Both of these have subsequently made a significant contribution to the world overview, but more than this, they have generated new questions, both clinical and biological, that need to be addressed in further studies. This chapter gives a brief review of the current status of these two trials but concentrates on those results which diverge from the received wisdom about the role of adjuvant tamoxifen.

II. *Design of the NATO Trial*

The Nolvadex Adjuvant Trial Organisation (NATO) launched a study in 1977 to investigate whether tamoxifen would have any benefit for women undergoing mastectomy for early breast cancer (NATO 1983).

Over a period of 3½ years, 1131 patients were recruited. Included were premenopausal node-positive cases and postmenopausal node-positive and node-negative cases. Following local therapy, women were randomized either to a group receiving tamoxifen, 10 mg twice daily for 2 years, or to an untreated control group. A second-order hypothesis, that the women most likely to benefit were those whose primary tumor was rich in estradiol receptor (ER) content, was included. Therefore, in a parallel study, attempts were made to collect samples of tumors from all patients entered into the trial. For logistic reasons, however, this was achieved in only about 50% of the cases.

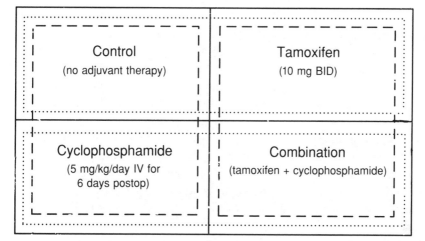

Figure 5.1. Two-by-two factorial design used in CRC Adjuvant Trial for Early Breast Cancer. The main effect for tamoxifen is determined by adding the result of the comparison of control versus tamoxifen to that of cyclophosphamide versus combination (i.e., adding the two results from the two dotted boxes). Similarly, differences due to cyclophosphamide therapy are determined by adding the two comparisons, cyclophosphamide versus control and tamoxifen versus combination (dashed boxes).

III. *Design of the CRC Adjuvant Trial*

The Cancer Research Campaign Adjuvant Trial for Early Breast Cancer (CRC trial) began recruitment in 1980. This trial was designed to repeat both the NATO trial of adjuvant tamoxifen and the Scandanavian Adjuvant Chemotherapy Study Group's trial of perioperative cyclophosphamide (Nissen-Meyer et al. 1971). Thus patients were randomized to four groups: control, tamoxifen (20 mg daily for 2 years), perioperative cyclophosphamide (5 mg/kg for 6 days following surgery), and both of the treatments. Thus, half the patients in the study received tamoxifen, and half received perioperative cyclophosphamide, commencing within 24 hours of surgery. Figure 5.1 illustrates the two-by-two factorial design of this study, which allowed an analysis for the "main effect" of perioperative cyclophosphamide and the "main effect" of adjuvant tamoxifen. A four-way comparison was also possible, although the smaller numbers and the potential for multiple subset analyses weaken the statistical power of this kind of analysis. A more detailed description of the trial design has been published (CRC Adjuvant Breast Trial Working Party 1988).

Estrogen receptor measurements were not a prerequisite for entry into this trial, but the inclusion of all operable cases of early breast cancer irrespective of menopausal or nodal status makes this trial unique.

From May 1, 1984, following data published by the NATO tamoxifen trial (Baum et al. 1983), clinicians were given the option to prescribe tamoxifen for all patients, with randomization only into the cyclophosphamide part of the trial. This left 1912 patients out of 2230 eligible for the tamoxifen main effect analysis.

The CRC trial is now in its tenth year of follow-up, and this chapter concentrates on three important areas: the role of tamoxifen in premenopausal women; the relative risk reduction amongst node-negative and node-positive patients; and the possible interaction between menopausal status and incidence of contralateral breast cancer in patients on long-term tamoxifen therapy.

IV. Current Status of the NATO Trial

An updated analysis of the NATO trial at a maximum follow-up of 11 years has demonstrated no material difference from the already published data (NATO 1988). Table 5.1 describes the overall analysis of events, with a highly significant relative risk of 0.74 (0.62–0.87) in favor of the tamoxifen-treated group. Table 5.2 presents an analysis of survival, again showing a highly significant relative risk of 0.79 (0.66–0.94) in favor of the tamoxifen-treated group. An analysis of survival divided into subgroups according to menopausal and nodal status is given in Table 5.3. It can be seen that the hazard ratios are very close to each other in all three groups, as with previous analyses.

Analysis of event-free survival or actual survival according to estradiol receptor content of the primary tumor, using cutoff points between 5 and 30 fmol/mg cytosolic protein, has failed to demonstrate a subgroup that is qualitatively different in its response to adjuvant tamoxifen. For example, Table 5.4 illustrates the analysis for survival using a cutoff of 30 fmol/mg (which is close to the median value for this study), with the observed:expected ratios in both the receptor-rich and the receptor-poor group being remarkably similar.

An analysis performed for the first time within this trial describes the log hazard ratios for both events and death in 2-year blocks within the first 8 years of this study. These analyses are illustrated in Figure 5.2 and Figure 5.3. It is clear that the significant reduction in the number of events appears only in the first 2 years (during which time the patients are on tamoxifen), whereas

Table 5.1. NATO trial: overall analysis of events

Group	Number in group	Observed events	Expected events	Ratio of observed to expected	Hazard ratio
Tamoxifen	564	259	301.5	0.86	
					0.74
No treatment	567	310	267.5	1.16	

$\chi^2 = 12.750$
Significance level = 0.0004

Table 5.2. NATO trial: overall analysis of survival

Group	Number in group	Observed events	Expected events	Ratio of observed to expected	Hazard ratio
Tamoxifen	564	223	252.0	0.88	
					0.79
No treatment	567	265	236.0	1.12	

$\chi^2 = 6.930$
Significance level = 0.0085

Table 5.3. NATO trial: analysis of survival, by menopausal and nodal status

Group	Number in group	Observed events	Expected events	Ratio of observed to expected	Hazard ratio
		Premenopausal node-positive			
Tamoxifen	72	37	40.9	0.91	
					0.69
No treatment	57	33	29.1	1.31	
		Postmenopausal node-negative			
Tamoxifen	300	83	92.2	0.90	
					0.82
No treatment	305	99	89.8	1.10	
		Postmenopausal node-positive			
Tamoxifen	181	97	115.6	0.84	
					0.72
No treatment	190	125	106.4	1.17	

Table 5.4. NATO trial: Analysis of survival, by estrogen receptor status (cutoff point, 30 fmols/mg protein. Analysis was stratified by premenopausal and nodal status.)

Group	Number in group	Observed events	Expected events	Ratio of observed to expected	Hazard ratio
		ER unknown			
Tamoxifen	296	120	130.4	0.92	
					0.85
No treatment	296	134	123.6	1.08	
		ER <30 fmols			
Tamoxifen	138	52	64.9	0.80	
					0.64
No treatment	122	65	52.1	1.25	
		ER ≥30 fmols			
Tamoxifen	119	45	53.7	0.84	
					0.71
No treatment	134	58	49.3	1.18	

the significant reduction in the number of deaths occurs only in the third and fourth years in the period immediately after cessation of treatment. There is no suggestion of a rebound phenomenon after withdrawal of therapy.

V. Current Status of the Cancer Research Campaign Trial

Between 1980 and 1985, 1912 patients were recruited to the trial, including 932 node-negative patients and 676 premenopausal patients. The groups were well matched according to major known prognostic factors (CRC Adjuvant Breast Trial Working Party 1988).

Earlier publications failed to demonstrate any significant impact on perioperative cyclophosphamide in overall survival, although there was a transient improvement in the disease-free interval (Houghton et al. 1989). The most recent analysis confirms this lack of effect, and further analyses of these results will not be included in this publication.

There are two possible ways of analyzing the data for patients receiving tamoxifen, either a main effect analysis which includes patients taking tamoxifen alone or tamoxifen plus perioperative cyclophosphamide, or a single strata analysis comparing patients taking tamoxifen only with untreated controls.

Figure 5.4A shows the main effect analysis for disease-free survival, which included all 1912 patients, whereas Figure 5.4B shows the disease-free

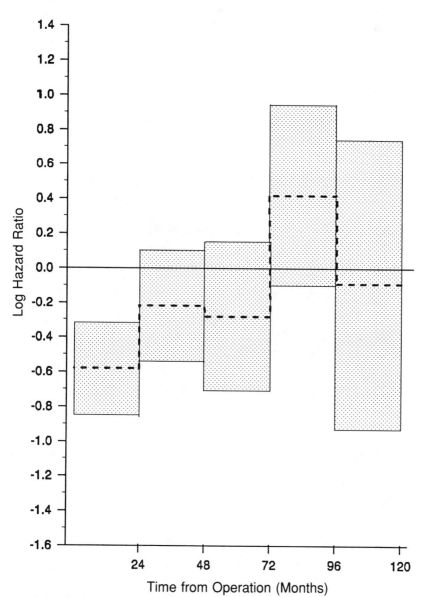

Figure 5.2. Two yearly log hazard ratios and 95% confidence intervals for events within the NATO trial.

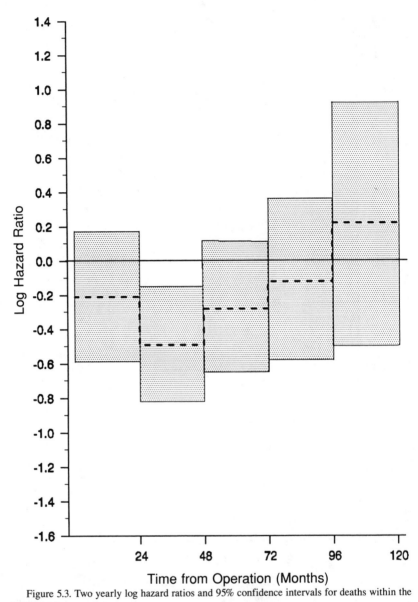

Figure 5.3. Two yearly log hazard ratios and 95% confidence intervals for deaths within the NATO trial.

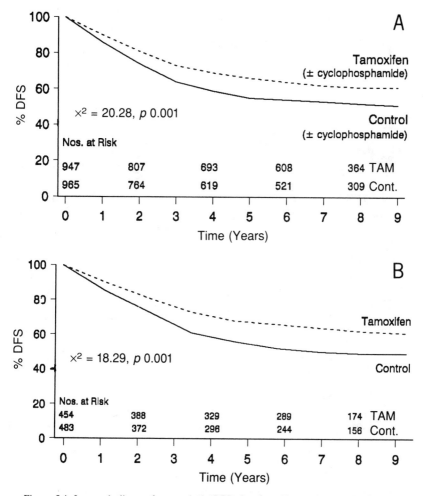

Figure 5.4. Log rank disease-free survival (DFS) for tamoxifen versus control within the CRC trial. (A) All patients (i.e., half within each group received perioperative cyclosphamide). (B) Only patients not randomized to receive cyclophosphamide.

survival for the tamoxifen versus control analysis, which contains data from only 937 patients but is more directly comparable to the NATO data. The results for these comparisons are nearly identical, as were the results for overall survival, illustrated in Figures 5.5A and 5.5B. For this reason all further analyses consider the main effect of tamoxifen (which includes the tamoxifen plus perioperative cyclophosphamide group against the two control groups, half of whom were exposed to perioperative cyclophosphamide).

Unlike the NATO trial, the CRC trial has not demonstrated a survival

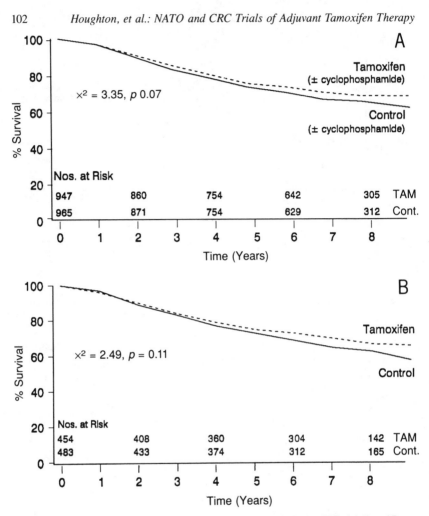

Figure 5.5. Log rank survival for tamoxifen versus control within the CRC trial (A and B are the same as for Fig. 5.4).

advantage; although in the current analysis the relative risk is decreased (0.87 [0.74–1.01], $\chi^2 = 3.35$, $p = 0.07$), this does not reach conventional levels of statistical significance. The disease-free survival of the tamoxifen-treated group was significantly increased (RR = 0.73 [0.63 - 0.85] $\chi^2 = 20.28$, $p < 0.001$).

Subgroup main effect analyses were carried out for patients divided according to nodal status, age, menopausal status, and tumor size categories. These results are illustrated in Table 5.5 and Figures 5.6 and 5.7, which show life tables according to menopausal and nodal status. Table 5.5 also gives the

Table 5.5. Stratified analysis of disease-free survivals

	RR	χ^2	p	χ^2(int)	p
All patients	0.73 (0.63–0.85)	20.28	<0.001		
Nodal status					
Negative	0.60 (0.47–0.77)	16.96	<0.001		
Positive	0.76 (0.63–0.92)	7.88	<0.01	2.41	0.12
Age					
<50	0.84 (0.64–1.08)	1.86	0.17		
≥50	0.68 (0.58–0.81)	20.19	<0.001	1.60	0.20
Menstrual status					
Premenopausal	0.72 (0.57–0.91)	7.52	<0.01		
Postmenopausal	0.72 (0.59–0.87)	11.88	<0.001	0.00	1.00
Tumor size					
<2 cm	0.71 (0.42–1.18)	1.77	0.18		
≥2 cm	0.75 (0.64–0.87)	13.49	<0.001	0.04	0.84

RR = relative risk.
χ^2(int) = χ^2 test for interaction.

statistical tests for interaction within these subgroups. Figure 5.6 clearly illustrates the significant effect of tamoxifen on prolonging the disease-free interval in both premenopausal women and postmenopausal women with no material difference in this outcome based on menopausal status.

Figure 5.7 shows the two subgroups on the basis of nodal status. Again a significant increase in the time to relapse is seen in both node-negative and node-positive patients. The impact of adjuvant tamoxifen for node-negative cases appears to be greater than for node-positive patients, as demonstrated by the relative risks; however, formal statistical tests for interaction are not significant.

Table 5.6 describes the incidence of contralateral breast cancers in the main effect analysis for all patients, and Figure 5.8 shows the life table analysis for the patients stratified according to menopausal status. Amongst patients taking tamoxifen the significant reduction in contralateral breast cancers that emerged at the 3-year follow-up (Cuzick and Baum 1985) has disappeared with time; however, a trend persists amongst postmenopausal patients. In contrast, the incidence of contralateral breast cancers amongst premenopausal women receiving tamoxifen has increased, although not significantly so. Figure 5.9 illustrates the comparison of the relative risks for developing contralateral breast cancer according to age or menstrual status. The possibility of a treatment interaction favoring the postmenopausal women cannot be ignored, because the statistical test just fails to reach conventional levels of significance.

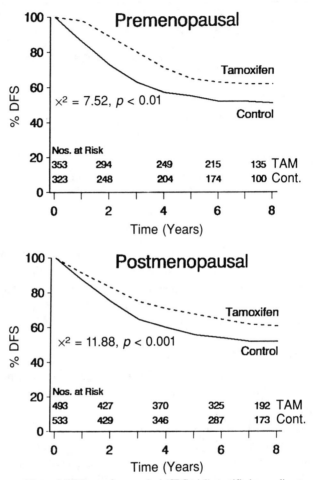

Figure 5.6. Disease-free survival (CRC trial) stratified according to menopausal status.

VI. *Discussion*

The data from both these trials of adjuvant tamoxifen again demonstrate the unequivocal beneficial effect of 2 years of tamoxifen on disease-free survival amongst patients with early breast cancer. As with the world overview, the results seem to improve with time, and there is as yet no suggestion of a rebound (NATO 1983). There is no significant improvement in overall sur-

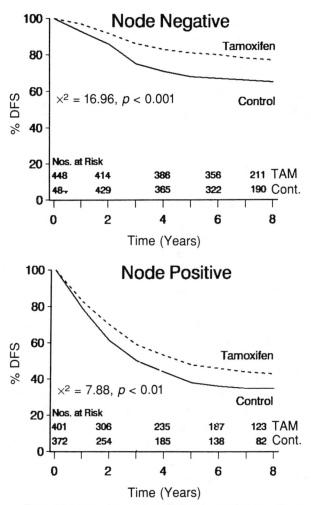

Figure 5.7. Disease-free survival (CRC trial) stratified according to pathological node status at randomization.

vival in the CRC trial, which appears to be inconsistent with the results from the NATO trial. This showed a much earlier and more promising improvement in the overall survival rates in the tamoxifen-treated group (Baum et al. 1983). If, however, the results are expressed as relative risk reduction, the 95% confidence intervals for the two survival results overlap in a manner that fails to suggest a genuine heterogeneity (Fig. 5.10).

Table 5.6. Incidence of contralateral breast cancer

	RR	χ^2	p	χ^2(int)	p
All patients	0.85 (0.48–1.52)	0.31	0.58		
Age					
<50	1.78 (0.64–4.91)	1.22	0.27		
≥50	0.60 (0.30–1.21)	2.04	0.15	3.00	0.08
Menstrual status					
Premenopausal	1.41 (0.60–3.32)	0.60	0.44		
Postmenopausal	0.49 (0.22–1.09)	3.04	0.08	3.08	0.08

RR = relative risk
χ^2(int) = χ^2 test for interaction.

The log hazard ratio analysis for events and survival from the NATO trial also provides an interesting pointer for the future, suggesting that the maintained long-term benefit of adjuvant tamoxifen is a result of the delay in recurrence amongst the patients whilst receiving the drug. This would indicate that tamoxifen for more than 2 years might produce an improved cumulative reduction in mortality. The implication from the recent world overview (Early Breast Cancer Trialists' Collaborative Group 1992a), both from indirect comparisons of duration of therapy and from the continued divergence in mortality beyond 5 years, which closely follows the prolonged disease-free survival, add weight to this hypothesis. Results from currently recruiting trials of duration of therapy will have to be awaited to provide reliable data.

Of great importance in the analysis of the CRC data is the demonstration that tamoxifen has a significant impact in reduction of the risk of relapse amongst premenopausal women which is identical with that for postmenopausal women. These data are counter to popular prejudice and appear to contradict the reported results of the world overview (Early Breast Cancer Trialists' Collaborative Group 1992a). It must be emphasized, however, that in the world overview, patients from trials where tamoxifen was added to chemotherapy were included together with trials where tamoxifen was compared with a control group. A more detailed and sophisticated reading of the world overview demonstrates consistency of the CRC result with that of other trials, where the tamoxifen effect in the premenopausal group was not confounded by the synchronous administration of long-term polychemotherapy (A'Hern et al. 1991; Early Breast Cancer Trialists' Collaborative Group 1992a,b).

Two years ago the National Cancer Institute issued a "Medi-alert" on the basis of the results from two American trials suggesting adjuvant systemic therapy might also be of value in node-negative patients, in addition to the conventional practice for node-positive patients. It is ironic that no such

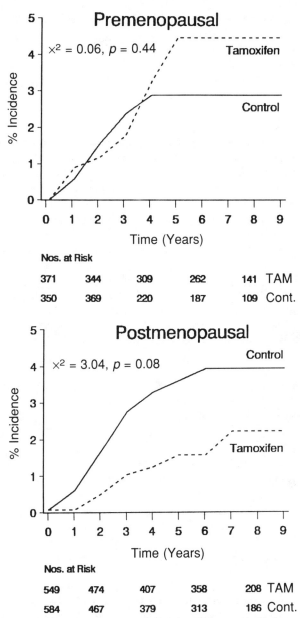

Figure 5.8. Incidence of new contralateral disease stratified according to menopausal status at randomization to the CRC trial.
(NB: Numbers at risk are not identical to Figs. 5.6 and 5.7, because
patients of unknown menopausal status but under the age of 45
have been included in the premenopausal group and those over 55
in the postmenopausal group.)

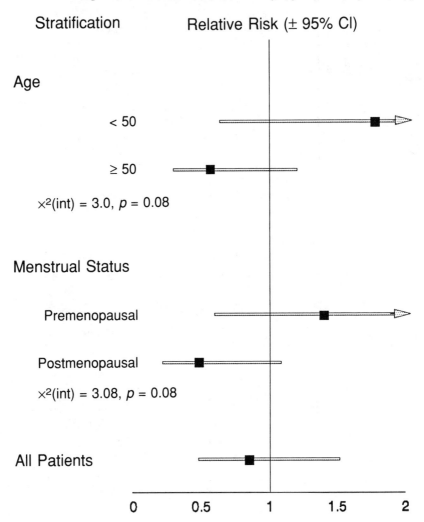

Stratification   Relative Risk (± 95% CI)

Age

< 50

≥ 50

x^2(int) = 3.0, *p* = 0.08

Menstrual Status

Premenopausal

Postmenopausal

x^2(int) = 3.08, *p* = 0.08

All Patients

0   0.5   1   1.5   2

Figure 5.9. Illustration of relative risks of developing contralateral breast cancer.

clinical alert appeared after the first description of the CRC trial 3 years before that, when we had demonstrated the value of adjuvant tamoxifen in node-negative patients. This new analysis reinforces this result and furthermore suggests a trend where the relative risk reduction is somewhat greater in the node-negative patients. Bearing in mind that node-positive patients relapse at a faster rate, it is likely that the absolute benefits for adjuvant tamoxifen might be similar in these two subgroups. If this is the case, then

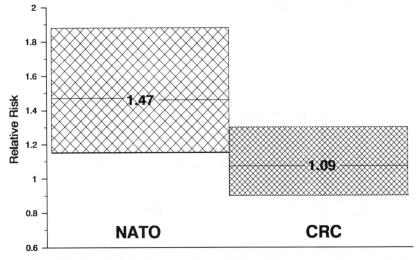

Figure 5.10. Overall relative risk estimation and 95% confidence intervals for survival in the NATO and CRC trials.

adjuvant tamoxifen could be ethically and logically prescribed for all patients with early breast cancer irrespective of nodal and menopausal status.

The CRC trial did not include an analysis of estrogen receptor status of the primary breast cancer. The NATO trial data still suggest that the estrogen receptor status of the primary tumor does not predict the likelihood of response to adjuvant tamoxifen. Once again this appears to contradict the analysis of ER within the world overview (Early Breast Cancer Trialists' Collaborative Group 1992a). It has been suggested already that the measurement of ER in a multicenter trial with inter- and intralaboratory variation will produce many false negative results. This may indeed be the case, but if ER assay fails to discriminate within the constraints of a well-conducted trial, then the role of ER assay to determine therapy within routine clinical practice (with variable levels of quality control) must be questioned.

An alternative explanation that we favor involves the confounding effect within the overview mechanism because of a putative negative interaction between chemotherapy and the non-receptor-mediated effect of adjuvant tamoxifen. For example, the assay of ER in the NATO study has indicated something of biological relevance about the primary cancer, because there is a powerful correlation between the ER status and prognosis and between ER status and histological grade, irrespective of adjuvant therapy (NATO 1985). Rather than ignore these data, it would be more fruitful to try to incorporate them within a modified hypothesis. There is little doubt that the major pathway mediating the antitumor effect of tamoxifen in advanced breast cancer is via the estradiol receptor; but the observations from the NATO trial raise the question whether tamoxifen exerts some of its effect on microscopic foci of the disease by another pathway. This is supported by recent observations in our laboratory demonstrating the induction of transforming growth factor (TGF)-ß from stromal fibroblasts exposed to tamoxifen (Colletta et al. 1990).

Antiestrogens might be better thought of as modulators of growth factors and their receptors, which are an expression of oncogene amplification. The environment of a metastasis is as important a determinant of "hormone" responsiveness as the malignant cells themselves. For example, locoregional disease without an intact stromal response mechanism might respond immediately to antiestrogens through mechanisms intrinsic to the tumor cells, whereas micrometastases might depend on interactions with the surrounding stroma, which are not reflected by the ER content of the primary tumor.

The most interesting aspect of the new analysis of the CRC data concerns the incidence of contralateral breast cancer. We recognize that there is a potential for the misdiagnosis of this event, particularly in patients who have already relapsed at other sites. However, on most occasions when the trial center was notified of new contralateral disease, the trial coordinators contacted the surgeon and pathologist involved and ascribed the new event as either a new primary in the opposite breast or a component of widespread metastatic disease which was not eligible for the analysis for contralateral breast cancer.

It is interesting to note that the initial effect of tamoxifen on contralateral breast cancer, originally described by Cuzick and Baum (1985), has disappeared. This is in keeping with animal models described by Jordan and his colleagues. These suggest breast cancer may remain suppressed at a subclinical level for as long as the subject was exposed to tamoxifen, but on withdrawing the drug the occult malignancy could reemerge (Jordan 1983). Such a simplistic interpretation of the data can be challenged by looking at the subgroups divided according to menopausal status. A striking difference emerges between the pre- and postmenopausal women which just fails to reach conventional levels of significance using the chi-squared test for interaction. A sustained reduction in contralateral breast cancer appears in the postmenopausal women with a relative risk of 0.49 (0.22–1.09), whereas the premenopausal women demonstrated a relative risk of 1.41 (0.60–3.32). A plausible biological explanation can be proposed if this is a true effect. Premenopausal women on long-term tamoxifen develop a sustained elevation of estradiol. This is not coupled with an associated increase in the sex hormone–binding globulin (Jordan et al. 1991). The breast epithelial cells are, therefore, exposed to high levels of free estradiol, as long as the patient is receiving the drug, and these high levels compete with tamoxifen for the estrogen receptor. Clearly this trend has to be compared with the overview data for the nonconfounded trials of tamoxifen versus control in premeno-pausal women. As well as biological significance, these data might have an effect on the planned recruitment of high-risk premenopausal women to trials of the chemoprophylaxis of breast cancer with tamoxifen.

VII. *Summary*

Over 3000 patients with early breast cancer were recruited into two trials (the Nolvadex Adjuvant Trial Organisation and the Cancer Research Campaign Adjuvant Trial) between 1977 and 1985. These trials were to investigate the benefit of tamoxifen at 20 mg daily for 2 years (the CRC trial also included a short course of perioperative cyclophosphamide). At the tenth year of follow-up in the CRC trial and longer for the NATO study, adjuvant tamoxifen-treated patients demonstrate a significant improvement in disease-free sur-vival, which increases with time during the follow-up period. The NATO trial also shows a survival advantage but, although a similar trend is obvious in the CRC trial, this does not reach conventional statistical significance. These results are in keeping with the world overview of trials of adjuvant tamoxifen.

The CRC study is unique, having a large number of node-negative patients and over 500 premenopausal women in a comparison of tamoxifen with control. The relative risk reductions for node-negative patients for disease-free survival are greater than for node-positive patients. This might suggest that the absolute benefit for adjuvant tamoxifen is similar in both groups of patients, bearing in mind the increased risk of relapse for node-positive patients. No trend for interaction emerges when data are stratified according to age or menopausal status, suggesting an identical benefit for the younger and older women. Of particular interest is the effect of tamoxifen on the development of contralateral breast cancer. The beneficial effect which emerged at the third year of follow-up now ceases to be apparent, but sub-group analysis according to menopausal status suggests a trend for interac-tion, with a reduction in the risk of contralateral breast cancer in post-menopausal women but an increased risk in premenopausal women. Plausible biological mechanisms exist to explain this difference in outcome. At a time when the chemoprophylaxis of breast cancer is being considered, these data need to be checked against other large trials of adjuvant tamoxifen before including high-risk premenopausal women in such trials.

Members of the CRC Breast Cancer Trials Group

Prof. M. Baum, Mr. D. Berstock, Dr. J. Dobbs., Dr. J. Haybittle, Ms. J. Houghton, Dr. I. Jackson, Mr. J. MacIntyre, Mr. A. McKinna, Prof. K. McPherson, Dr. T. Powles, Dr. G. Rees, Ms. D. Riley, Prof. R. Rubens, Mr. J. R. C. Sainsbury, Dr. T. Wheeler, Mr. A. Wilson.

Acknowledgments

We gratefully acknowledge the working parties and participants of the NATO and CRC clinical trial groups, without whose active support all this would have been impossible. We also acknowledge with gratitude the hard work of the clinical trials center staff, and thank the Cancer Research Campaign for generous financial support.

References

A'Hern, R. P., M. Baum, and M. Dowsett. 1991. How does tamoxifen interact with chemotherapy? *Lancet* 337:439–440.

Baum, M., D. M. Brinkley, J. A. Dossett, K. McPherson, J. S. Patterson, R. D. Rubens, F. G. Smiddy, B. A. Stoll, A. Wilson, J. C. Lea, D. Richards, and S. H. Ellis. 1983. Improved survival among patients with adjuvant tamoxifen after mastectomy for early breast cancer. *Lancet* 2:450.

CRC Adjuvant Breast Trial Working Party. 1988. Cyclophosphamide and tamoxifen as adjuvant therapies in the management of breast cancer. *British Journal of Cancer* 57:604–607.

Colleta, A. A., L. M. Wakefield, F. V. Howell, K. E. van Roozendaal, D. Danielpour, S. R. Ebbs, M. B. Spain, and M. Baum. 1990. Antioestrogens induce the secretion of active transforming growth factor beta from human fetal fibroblasts. *British Journal of Cancer* 62:405–409.

Cuzick, J., and M. Baum. 1985. Tamoxifen and contralateral breast cancer. *Lancet* 2:282.

Early Breast Cancer Trialists' Collaborative Group. 1992a. Systemic treatment of early breast cancer by hormonal, cytotoxic or immune therapy. 133 randomised trials involving 31,000 recurrences and 24,000 deaths among 75,000 women. *Lancet* 339:1–15.

Early Breast Cancer Trialists' Collaborative Group. 1992b. Systemic treatment of early breast cancer by hormonal, cytotoxic or immune therapy. 133 randomised trials involving 31,000 recurrences and 24,000 deaths among 75,000 women. *Lancet* 339:71–85.

Houghton, J., M. Baum, R. Nissen-Meyer, D. Riley, and R. A'Hern. 1989. Is there a role for perioperative adjuvant cytotoxic therapy in the treatment of early breast cancer? *Recent Results in Cancer Research* 115:54–61.

Jordan, V. C. 1976. Effect of tamoxifen (ICI 46,474) on initiation and growth of DMBA-induced rat mammary carcinoma. *European Journal of Cancer* 12:419–424.

Jordan, V. C. 1983. Laboratory studies to develop general principles for the adjuvant treatment of breast cancer with antiestrogens: problems and potential for future clinical applications. *Breast Cancer Research and Treatment* 3(Supplement)12:419–424.

Jordan, V. C., N. F. Fritz, S. M. Langan-Fahey, M. Thompson, and D. C. Tormey. 1991. Alteration of endocrine parameters in premenopausal women with breast cancer during long-term adjuvant monotherapy. *Journal of the National Cancer Institute* 83:1488–1491.

Nissen-Meyer, R., K. Kjellgren, and B. Mansson. 1971. Preliminary report from the Scandinavian Adjuvant Chemotherapy Study Group. *Cancer Chemotherapy Reports* 55:561–566.

Nolvadex Adjuvant Trial Organisation (NATO). 1983. Controlled trial of tamoxifen as adjuvant agent in the management of early breast cancer. Interim analysis at four years. *Lancet* 1:257–261.

Nolvadex Adjuvant Trial Organisation (NATO). 1985. Six year results of a controlled trial of tamoxifen as a single adjuvant agent in management of early breast cancer. *World Journal of Surgery* 258:3173.

Nolvadex Adjuvant Trial Organisation (NATO). 1988. Controlled trial of tamoxifen as a single adjuvant agent in the management of early breast cancer. Analysis at eight years. *British Journal of Cancer* 57:608–611.

Wilson, A. J., M. Baum, D. M. Brinkley, J. A. Dossett, K. McPherson, J. S. Patterson, R. D. Rubens, F. G. Smiddy, B. A. Stoll, D. Richards, and other NATO members. 1985. Six-year results of a controlled trial of tamoxifen as a single adjuvant agent in the management of early breast cancer. *World Journal of Surgery* 9:756–764.

6

The Stockholm Adjuvant Tamoxifen Trial

LARS E. RUTQVIST

I.	INTRODUCTION	116
II.	STUDY DESIGN	116
III.	NUMBER OF PATIENTS AND FOLLOW-UP	117
IV.	TAMOXIFEN EFFECTS ON RFS AND OS	117
V.	NEGATIVE INTERACTION BETWEEN TAMOXIFEN AND CHEMOTHERAPY?	119
VI.	TREATMENT EFFECT BY HORMONE RECEPTOR STATUS	121
VII.	ESTROGENIC EFFECTS OF TAMOXIFEN	123
VIII.	NEW PRIMARY MALIGNANCIES	124
IX.	TAMOXIFEN AND CONTRALATERAL BREAST CANCER	125
X.	TAMOXIFEN AND CARDIOVASCULAR DISEASE	128
XI.	CONCLUSIONS	128
XII.	SUMMARY	130
	REFERENCES	131

I. Introduction

THE Stockholm Adjuvant Tamoxifen Trial was initiated more than 15 years ago. It was originally designed to evaluate the effect of adjuvant tamoxifen in early breast cancer only on recurrence-free survival (RFS) and overall survival (OS). The trial included both low-risk, node-negative patients and high-risk, node-positive patients. In the latter group tamoxifen was given as an addition to either postoperative radiation therapy or adjuvant CMF chemotherapy. These features of the design have permitted an evaluation of putative interactions between the effect of tamoxifen and tumor stage as well as the effect of combined chemo-endocrine treatment.

Several Swedish, population-based registers—such as the National Cause-of-Death Registry and the National Cancer Registry—rely on a personal identification number to identify all registered individuals uniquely. This number has permitted computerized record linkages to study effects of tamoxifen on events that were not originally included as end points in the study protocol—such as second cancers and deaths due to intercurrent disease.

This chapter presents a summarized description of the main findings from the trials at a median follow-up of 7 years.

II. Study Design

The design—including the main inclusion criteria—is summarized in Figure 6.1. Note that all patients were postmenopausal; that is, more than 6 months should have elapsed since the last menstrual period. Randomization was between tamoxifen given postoperatively at a dose of 40 mg daily for 2 years or no adjuvant endocrine therapy. The selected daily dose was based on overviews of studies of advanced breast cancer done in the early 1970s suggesting higher objective response rates with 40 mg compared with lower doses (Mouridsen et al. 1978). In both the tamoxifen and control group, all patients treated with breast-conserving surgery received postoperative radiation therapy to the breast parenchyma (50 Gy/5 weeks).

Patients at high risk of disease recurrence—defined as those having involved axillary nodes or a tumor size greater than 30 mm—were entered in

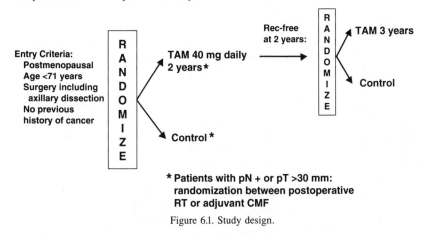

* Patients with pN + or pT >30 mm:
randomization between postoperative
RT or adjuvant CMF

Figure 6.1. Study design.

a concurrent randomized comparison of postoperative radiation therapy to the chest wall and regional nodes (46 Gy/5 weeks) or adjuvant CMF chemotherapy. Patients randomized to adjuvant chemotherapy and tamoxifen received the two treatments concurrently.

Tamoxifen patients who were disease-free at 2 years were randomly allocated to discontinue tamoxifen or to continue for 3 more years, i.e., a total treatment period of 5 years. This study is part of a multicenter, Swedish trial with a sample size of 5000 patients, so results relative to the 2-year versus 5-year comparison will not be presented in this chapter.

III. *Number of Patients and Follow-Up*

This chapter is mainly based on patients entered in the trial during 1976–1987. During this period a total of 2135 patients were randomized, of whom 788 (37%) had high-risk tumors. The follow-up ranges from 2 to 13 years with a mean of 7 years. All follow-up was by clinical examination alone, supplemented with yearly, routine mammogram. Accrual of patients did not stop until the 10-year data from the international overview of adjuvant tamoxifen trials became available in 1990, so the total number of patients in the trial now exceeds 2700.

IV. *Tamoxifen Effects on RFS and OS*

Figure 6.2 shows the RFS for all patients by allocated treatment. The relative hazard (tamoxifen versus control group) indicated a 23% reduction of treat-

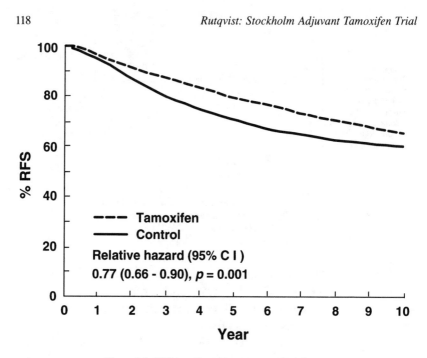

Figure 6.2. RFS by allocated treatment, all patients.

ment failures with tamoxifen ($p < 0.001$). There was a continued benefit during the entire follow-up; that is, there was no evidence to suggest that the initial benefit was lost or diminished after cessation of treatment. Table 6.1 presents a more detailed analysis of events: the most pronounced effect of tamoxifen was seen for locoregional recurrences, which were prevented to a greater extent than distant metastases and deaths. Figure 6.3 shows the overall survival rates. The estimated relative hazard suggested a 12% reduction of deaths in the tamoxifen group, but this result was not statistically significant ($p = 0.17$). However, because of the wide confidence interval the result is fully compatible with the result of the international overview of

Table 6.1. Analysis of total number of events, by allocated treatment

Type of event	TAM, % (n = 1074)	Control, % (n = 1061)	Relative hazard (TAM vs control)	p
Locoregional recurrences	9	13	0.66	<0.001
Distant metastases	18	21	0.81	<0.05
Death	20	22	0.88	0.17

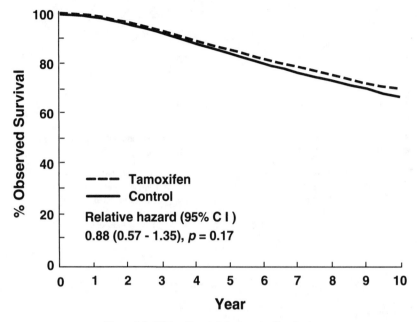

Figure 6.3. OS by allocated treatment, all patients.

adjuvant tamoxifen trials, which showed a reduction of about one-fifth in the odds of death with tamoxifen (Early Breast Cancer Trialists' Collaborative Group 1990).

As in many other adjuvant tamoxifen trials there was no significant inter-action between the effect of tamoxifen and tumor stage. The relative hazard in the analysis of RFS was 0.70 for the node-negative low-risk patients compared with 0.73 for the high-risk patients (Fig. 6.4). For overall survival, if anything, the effect of tamoxifen appeared to be better among the low-risk patients (relative hazard: 0.78) compared with the high-risk group (relative hazard: 0.97), but this numerical difference was not statistically significant.

V. *Negative Interaction between Tamoxifen and Chemotherapy?*

In recent years there has been a concern that tamoxifen therapy might interact negatively with concurrent adjuvant chemotherapy. One putative mechanism for such an interaction is that tamoxifen causes cell cycle arrest, which may make the tumor cells less sensitive to cytotoxic agents. In this trial the study design for high-risk patients permitted an unconfounded evaluation of the

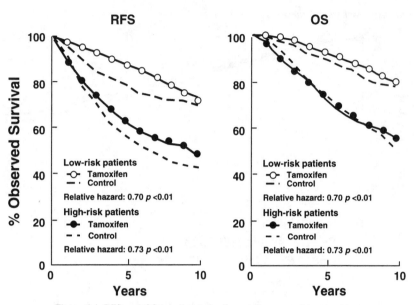

Figure 6.4. RFS and OS by allocated adjuvant therapy and tumor stage.

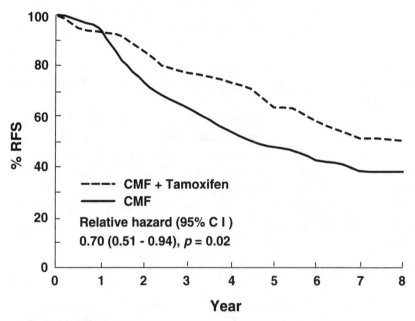

Figure 6.5. RFS by allocated adjuvant therapy among high-risk patients treated with concurrent chemotherapy.

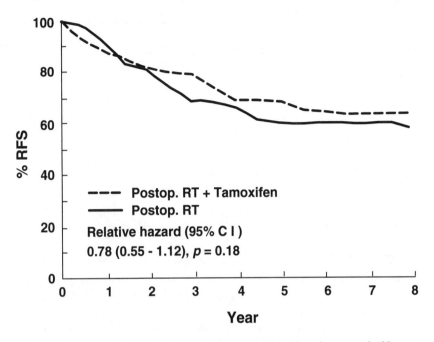

Figure 6.6. RFS by allocated adjuvant therapy among high-risk patients treated with post-operative radiation therapy.

effect of tamoxifen combined with concurrent CMF chemotherapy compared with tamoxifen without other systemic treatment.

Figure 6.5 shows the RFS for the tamoxifen and control patients who received concurrent CMF, and Figure 6.6 shows similar results for those treated with postoperative radiation therapy. The relative hazard (tamoxifen versus control group) was, if anything, slightly lower for those who were allocated to concurrent CMF (0.70) compared with radiation therapy (0.78), but this difference was not statistically significant. So, in this trial there was no evidence of a negative interaction between tamoxifen and chemotherapy. In fact, CMF plus tamoxifen was significantly better than CMF alone ($p = 0.02$).

VI. *Treatment Effect by Hormone Receptor Status*

Data on estrogen receptor (ER) content of the primary tumor were not required in the protocol but were available in 1847 patients (87%). Progesterone receptor (PgR) data were available in 1413 patients (66%). All assays were done in one laboratory using isoelectric focusing as previously described (Wrange et al. 1978). A rigorously low cutoff level of 0.05 fmol/μg

Table 6.2. Analysis of treatment failures, by ER or PgR level

Receptor level	Tamoxifen[a]	Control[a]	Relative hazard (95% CI)
ER–	73/198 (37)	67/202 (33)	1.16 (0.83–1.61)
ER+	89/377 (24)	128/394 (32)	0.68 (0.52–0.89)
ER++	89/345 (26)	117/331 (35)	0.64 (0.49–0.84)
PgR–	108/406 (27)	131/417 (31)	0.87 (0.68–1.13)
PgR+	28/144 (19)	52/169 (31)	0.58 (0.37–0.89)
PgR++	22/143 (15)	29/134 (22)	0.61 (0.35–1.07)

[a]Data are arranged as: number of failures/number of subjects in group (% of failures).

DNA was used to distinguish between receptor-positive and receptor-negative cases. This corresponds to about 2–5 fmol/mg of tissue protein. With this cutoff level, only about 20% of the patients were defined as ER-negative, which is lower than in many other trials.

Table 6.2 shows an analysis of treatment failures by ER and PgR levels separately. Treatment failure—that is, the end point in the calculations of RFS—was defined as a locoregional recurrence, distant metastasis, or death without a reported recurrence. In the ER-negative subgroup there was no evidence of any treatment benefit with tamoxifen, as evidenced by the relative hazard (tamoxifen versus control group) of 1.16, whereas there were highly significant benefits among patients with intermediate and high ER levels. Similarly, patients with intermediate and high PgR levels showed a greater benefit with tamoxifen than those who were PgR negative. However, as suggested by the relative hazard of 0.87, there was some evidence of benefit also among the PgR negatives, although the 95% confidence interval of the relative hazard was wide (0.68–1.13).

Table 6.3 shows an analysis of RFS in subgroups according to both ER and PgR levels. As expected, the greatest benefit was observed among those who were both ER and PgR positive. The relative hazard in this subgroup suggested a 43% reduction of treatment failures with tamoxifen. Among those who were negative for both receptors the relative hazard was 1.42, so, if anything, there was some evidence—although not statistically significant— of a detrimental effect of tamoxifen. A more detailed analysis of the results for this subgroup has revealed that the difference between the tamoxifen group and the control group was mainly the result of a higher frequency of

Table 6.3. Analysis of treatment failures, by hormone receptor status

Receptor level	Tamoxifen[a]	Control[a]	Relative hazard (95% CI)
ER–, PgR–	56/145 (37)	44/142 (33)	1.42 (0.96–2.11)
ER–, PgR+	2/10 (24)	26/6 (32)	0.88 (0.19–4.15)
ER+, PgR–	52/261 (26)	87/275 (35)	0.62 (0.45–0.87)
ER+, PgR+	48/277 (26)	75/277 (35)	0.57 (0.49–0.81)

[a]Data are arranged as: number of failures/number of subjects in group (% of failures).

breast cancer recurrences in the former group, whereas the mortality due to intercurrent diseases was similar (data not shown). However, whether tamoxifen can, in fact, stimulate the growth of tamoxifen-resistant tumors remains to be established. At any rate, the lower limit of the 95% confidence interval—that is, 0.96—clearly indicates that the result is incompatible with claims of any clinically worthwhile treatment benefit in this particular subgroup of patients.

VII. *Estrogenic Effects of Tamoxifen*

Tamoxifen has a complex mechanism of action in that it is both a partial estrogenic agonist and antagonist. The balance between agonism and antagonism is both species- and organ-specific. In postmenopausal women, tamoxifen acts as an estrogen in many tissues, such as the pituitary, liver, bone, and genital tract (Fornander et al. 1993; Ferazzi et al. 1977). An estrogenic effect can be demonstrated irrespective of whether the daily dose is 40 mg—as in this trial—or 20 mg, as in many other adjuvant trials (Boccardo et al. 1981). The effect of tamoxifen on normal breast tissue, however, remains unclear. The tamoxifen-induced changes in some markers of estrogenic activity suggest that the drug might be described as a weak estrogen, whereas the changes in other markers are more compatible with those of relatively potent estrogen. In 1984, Rössner and Wallgren showed tamoxifen-induced estrogen-like effects on serum lipoproteins with, for instance, a 20% decrease in low-density lipoprotein (LDL) cholesterol after 2 months of treatment (Rössner and Wallgren 1984). These observations raise questions about the potential effect of tamoxifen on the incidence of second cancers and cardiovascular disease. Estrogen therapy has been linked with an increased frequency of liver and endometrial cancer as well as thromboembolic events, but also with a decreased incidence of cardiac morbidity and mortality.

VIII. *New Primary Malignancies*

Tamoxifen induces liver tumors in laboratory animals (Fentiman and Powles 1987). *In vivo,* tamoxifen has been shown to stimulate the growth of endometrial cancer cells (Satyaswaroop et al. 1984). Previously we reported a significant increase of endometrial cancer among the tamoxifen patients in this trial (Fornander et al. 1989). That increase was most pronounced for those allocated to 5 years of tamoxifen, but there was some increase also among those treated for 2 years. Table 6.4 summarizes the current incidence of new primary malignancies in the trial. The data are based on a computerized record linkage with the Swedish National Cancer Registry. There was a continued significant difference between the tamoxifen group and the control group in terms of endometrial cancer, with 18 versus 2 cases ($p < 0.01$). There were two cases of liver cancer, both among patients in the tamoxifen group. The expected incidence of liver cancer in the tamoxifen group—based on general population incidence rates during the period of follow-up—was 0.5, so the estimate of the relative risk for the tamoxifen patients was about 4. However, this estimate is, of course, far from statistical significance because of the small number of cases.

There has been some controversy over the fact that an increase of endometrial and liver cancer has not been reported from other adjuvant tamoxifen trials. However, few such studies have included a prospective collection of data on second primaries other than contralateral breast cancers. Nor have such data been available from population-based cancer registries— except for studies done in the Scandinavian countries. Therefore, there is probably a considerable under-reporting of second primaries and corresponding lack of statistical power to detect a difference between the treated and the control groups in many of the currently available trials of more long-term adjuvant tamoxifen. Table 6.5 summarizes results from the three Scandinavian studies of adjuvant tamoxifen that have so far reported endometrial cancer incidence rates based on information obtained from population-based cancer registers. The treatment time (1 year) was shorter and the daily dose of tamoxifen (30 mg) was lower in both the Danish and the South Swedish trials than in the current trial (Andersson et al. 1991; Ryden et al. 1992), to confirm

Table 6.4. Number of new primary malignancies, by allocated treatment

Site	TAM	Control	Log rank p
Contralateral breast	33	52	<0.05
Corpus uteri			
Endometrium	18	2	<0.01
Other	—	3	NS
Liver	2	0	NS
Miscellaneous	47	47	NS
Total	100	104	NS

Table 6.5. Summarized description of three Scandinavian randomized trials of adjuvant tamoxifen in early breast cancer for which data are available on the relative risk of endometrial cancer (tamoxifen versus control group)

Study	Number of patients	Tamoxifen schedule	Median follow-up	RR of endometrial cancer[a] (95% CI)
Current trial	1846	40 mg 2–5 years	5 years	6.4 (1.4–28)
Danish Breast Cancer Group (CI, 11)	1710	30 mg 1 year	8 years	3.3 (0.6–32)
South Swedish Breast Group (CI, 12)	719	30 mg 1 year	9 years	2.2[b]

[a]Information in all three trials was obtained from population-based registers.
[b]Confidence interval not published.

our observations in showing increased relative risks for endometrial cancer with tamoxifen, although the increases were not as great as in our trial.

IX. *Tamoxifen and Contralateral Breast Cancer*

Estrogens are considered to act as promotors of initiated breast cells in the development of breast cancer. This suggests that the risk of the disease may be reduced by the prophylactic use of tamoxifen, provided that the drug actually has predominantly antagonistic estrogenic effect on breast epithelium. At present there are no data on the ability of tamoxifen to decrease breast cancer incidence in previously healthy women. Breast cancer patients compared with the general population have an increased risk of developing a second primary breast cancer. The annual risk is about 0.5–1%, giving a cumulative life-time risk of 2–15%, depending on the age of the patient at primary diagnosis.

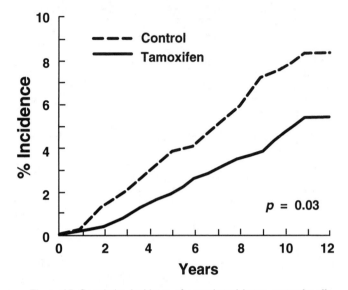

Figure 6.7. Cumulative incidence of contralateral breast cancer by allocated adjuvant therapy.

In this trial there were 29 cases of new primary, contralateral breast cancers in the tamoxifen group compared with 47 among the controls. The relative hazard (tamoxifen versus control group) was 0.60, which suggested a 40% reduction with tamoxifen (95% confidence interval: 6–62%, $p = 0.03$). Figure 6.7 shows cumulative incidence rates. At 10 years the estimated incidence was 5% for the tamoxifen group compared with 8% among the controls. Table 6.6 shows a comparison of clinical characteristics of the first and second, contralateral breast cancers in the tamoxifen and the control groups. In both groups the second tumors were most often small and node-negative. However, ER-negative second tumors were more frequent in the tamoxifen group than in the control group, indicating, as expected, that the tamoxifen

Table 6.6. Clinical characteristics of the first and contralateral breast cancers, by allocated
treatment

Characteristic	Tamoxifen			Control		
	1st (%)	2nd (%)	p^{a}	1st (%)	2nd (%)	p^{a}
pT1	67	96	<0.01	68	94	<0.01
pN0	67	83	0.11	69	79	0.18
ER-positive	79	53[b]	<0.05	79	88	0.35
PgR-positive	40	45	0.96	41	40	0.90

[a]Comparison between the first and second cancer in each group.
[b]Comparison between the second cancers in the tamoxifen and control group: $p < 0.05$.

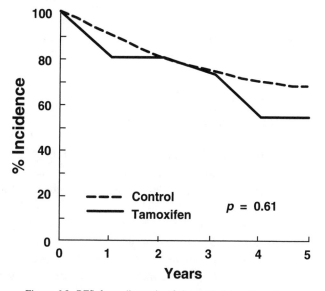

Figure 6.8. RFS from diagnosis of the contralateral breast cancer according to allocated initial adjuvant therapy.

treatment mainly prevented the occurrence of hormone-responsive, ER-positive tumors. This observation was explained only in part by spuriously low receptor values in tumors detected during treatment in which tamoxifen may have interfered with the receptor assay (data not shown). Despite this observation there was no significant difference between the second tumors in the tamoxifen group and the control group in terms of RFS (Fig. 6.8). This apparent inconsistency is probably explained by the fact that there were no differences between the groups in terms of tumor size or nodal status, which are both more important prognostic factors than ER status.

It might be argued that some of the contralateral cancers included in this analysis represented recurrences from the patient's first cancer rather than new, primary malignancies. However, the Swedish National Cancer Registry includes only cancers that are considered to be new primary malignancies according to both the responsible clinician and the pathologist. Moreover, the cumulative incidence of second breast cancer at 10 years in the control group was 8%, which is entirely as expected in an untreated group of breast cancer patients. The recurrence-free survival after the diagnosis of contralateral breast cancer was also about the same for the tamoxifen and the control patients. These circumstances all contradict the hypothesis that the excess of contralateral breast cancer in the control group was due to patients with recurrent disease. Nevertheless, until a decreased incidence of breast cancer with tamoxifen is demonstrated in a controlled trial including previously healthy women, the chemopreventive ability of the drug should be regarded as only tentative.

X. *Tamoxifen and Cardiovascular Disease*

In a previous report we published data on intercurrent morbidity according to allocated treatment (Fornander et al. 1991). The data were based on a record linkage to a computerized register of hospital admissions in Stockholm County. In that analysis, there was no significant benefit with tamoxifen in terms of cardiovascular disease. Numerically, there were slightly fewer admissions because of cardiac disease in the tamoxifen group. On the other hand, there were also slightly more admissions because of thromboembolic events in that group. Table 6.7 summarizes our latest update of cause-specific mortality in the trial. The total number of deaths was 456, out of which 91 (20%) were officially recorded as being due to causes other than breast cancer. There was no difference between the tamoxifen and the control group in terms of intercurrent mortality. In particular, there was no evidence of a decreased cardiovascular mortality with tamoxifen. However, the 95% confidence interval of the relative hazard was wide.

Table 6.7. Cause-specific mortality, by allocated treatment

Recorded underlying cause of death	Tamoxifen	Control	Relative hazard (95% CI) (tamoxifen vs control)	*p*
Breast cancer	172	193	0.86 (0.70–1.06)	0.17
Intercurrent diseases[a]	48	43	1.08 (0.72–1.64)	0.70
Other cancer	18	16	1.10 (0.56–2.16)	0.78
Heart disease	17	18	0.92 (0.48–1.79)	0.81

[a]Results for miscellaneous intercurrent diseases not given.

XI. *Conclusions*

Like several other adjuvant tamoxifen studies, this trial showed a significant improvement of RFS and a trend toward improved overall survival with tamoxifen. The benefit was similar irrespective of tumor stage. Moreover, the treatment benefit was sustained even during long-term follow-up; that is, there was no evidence of an increased rate of recurrence in the tamoxifen group after cessation of treatment. However, the benefit of a treatment longer than 2 years remains controversial.

In contrast with the NATO and Scottish trials there was no benefit among patients classified as ER-negative. In fact, among patients classified as both ER- and PgR-negative there was some evidence of a detrimental effect of tamoxifen. This observation supports the mentioned theories suggesting that tamoxifen may stimulate the growth of tamoxifen-resistant breast cancers.

In the first report of the international overview of adjuvant tamoxifen studies there was no significant interaction between the effect of tamoxifen and ER status (Early Breast Cancer Trialists' Collaborative Group 1990). However, when the trials in the overview are grouped according to the proportion of patients classified as ER-negative in each individual study, there is little if any benefit among the ER negatives in the studies with fewer than 25% ER-negative cases (Table 6.8). In contrast, the greatest benefit among ER negatives is observed in studies in which that subgroup constitutes more than 35% of all cases. This observation suggests that misclassification of patients in regard to ER status may help to explain the mentioned lack of interaction between treatment and ER. The ER protein is sensitive and may become undetectable if the tumor specimen is not rapidly chilled after excision. Moreover, if the assays are done in several laboratories, there might be a considerable interlaboratory variation. In the current trial, all assays were done in one laboratory, and a rigorously low cutoff point was used to distinguish reliably between ER-negative and ER-positive cases.

One argument for the use of tamoxifen also among ER negatives is that, although the benefit in terms of a reduced incidence of recurrences from the patient's first cancer may be small, there might be a benefit in terms of a reduced incidence of contralateral breast cancer and cardiovascular disease. Such benefits should theoretically not be dependent on the ER status of the primary tumor. In this trial there was, in fact, a reduced incidence of contralateral cancers with tamoxifen but no evidence of a reduced cardiovascular mortality. On the other hand, there was an increased incidence of endometrial cancer. In the adjuvant setting, the benefit of 2 years of tamoxifen in terms of improvement of recurrence-free and overall survival in ER-positive cases probably outweighs any increase of endometrial cancer, which in most cases is a disease with good prognosis. Studies evaluating the benefit of extending the treatment period beyond 2 years are currently under way in Europe.

Table 6.8. Summary of treatment results in terms of RFS among patients classified as ER-negative in the international overview of adjuvant tamoxifen studies, by proportion of patients who were classified as ER-
negative in the trial

% ER-negative in the trial	Relative hazard (95% CI)[a]
<25	0.95 (0.61–1.48)
25–35	0.77 (0.55–1.08)
>35	0.61 (0.40–0.76)

From data presented in Early Breast Cancer Trialists' Collaborative Group 1990.
[a]Tamoxifen versus control group, test for trend in the relative hazards: $p = 0.06$.

XII. *Summary*

The chapter summarizes the main findings of the 1991 update of the Stockholm Adjuvant Tamoxifen Trial. The study included more than 2100 postmenopausal patients with early breast cancer during 1976–1987, who were
randomly allocated to tamoxifen at 40 mg daily for 2 or 5 years, or to no
adjuvant endocrine therapy. The results concerning RFS and overall survival
confirmed and extended previous reports of the trial. There was a sustained
benefit in terms of RFS up to at least 10 years with adjuvant tamoxifen. There
was also an overall survival difference in favor of the tamoxifen patients,
which, however, was not significant. There was no negative interaction
between tamoxifen and CMF chemotherapy among high-risk patients who
received the two treatments concurrently. In this subgroup, those who
received tamoxifen plus CMF fared significantly better in terms of RFS than
those treated with CMF alone. Estrogen receptor–negative patients did not
appear to benefit from tamoxifen. This observation was probably related to
the use of a rigorously low definition of receptor negativity. Among patients
classified as negative for both estrogen and progesterone receptors there was
even some evidence of a detrimental effect of tamoxifen. Current theories
suggesting that tamoxifen can stimulate growth of hormone-resistant tumors
may possibly help to explain this observation. In the tamoxifen group there
was a significant reduction of contralateral breast cancers which were more
frequently estrogen receptor–negative than the contralateral cancers in the
control group. There was also a continued significant excess of endometrial
cancers in the tamoxifen group, a result that was recently confirmed in two
other Scandinavian, randomized trials of adjuvant tamoxifen.

Acknowledgments

This study was supported by the King Gustaf V Jubilee Fund and the Swedish Cancer Society.

References

Andersson, M., H. H. Storm, and H. T. Mouridsen. 1991. Incidence of new primary cancers after adjuvant tamoxifen therapy and radiotherapy for early breast cancer. *Journal of the National Cancer Institute* 83:1013–1017.

Boccardo, F., P. Bruzzi, A. Rubagotti, G. U. Nicolo, and R. Rosso. 1981. Estrogen-like action of tamoxifen on vaginal epithelium in breast cancer patients. *Oncology* 38:281–285.

Early Breast Cancer Trialists' Collaborative Group. 1990. Treatment of early breast cancer: worldwide evidence in 1985–1990. A systematic overview of all available randomized trials in early breast cancer of adjuvant endocrine and cytotoxic therapy. In *Treatment of Early Breast Cancer,* vol. 1. Oxford: Oxford University Press.

Fentiman, I. S., and T. J. Powles. 1987. Tamoxifen and benign breast problems. *Lancet* 2:1070–1072.

Ferazzi, E., G. Cartei, R. Mattarazzo, and M. Fiorentino. 1977. Oestrogen-like effect of tamoxifen on vaginal epithelium. *British Medical Journal* 1:1351–1352.

Fornander, T., L. E. Rutqvist, N. Wilking, K. Carlström, and B. von Schoultz. 1993. Oestrogenic effects of adjuvant tamoxifen in postmenopausal breast cancer. *European Journal of Cancer* 29A:497–500.

Fornander, T., L. E. Rutqvist, B. Cedermark, U. Glas, A. Mattsson, C. Silfversward, L. Skoog, A. Somell, T. Theve, N. Wilking, J. Askergren, and M. L. Hjalmer. 1989. Adjuvant tamoxifen in early breast cancer: occurrence of new primary cancers. *Lancet* 1:117–120.

Fornander, T., L. E. Rutqvist, B. Cedermark, U. Glas, A. Mattsson, L. Skoog, A. Somell, T. Theve, N. Wilking, J. Askergren, S. Rotstein, M. L. Hjalmar, and L. Perbeck. 1991. Adjuvant tamoxifen in early-stage breast cancer: effects on intercurrent morbidity and mortality. *Journal of Clinical Oncology* 9:1740–1748.

Mouridsen, H., T. Palshof, J. Patterson, and L. Battersby. 1978. Tamoxifen in advanced breast cancer. *Cancer Treatment Reviews* 5:131–141.

Rössner, S., and A. Wallgren. 1984. Serum lipoproteins and proteins after breast cancer surgery and effects of tamoxifen. *Atherosclerosis* 52:339–346.

Rydén, S., M. Fernö, T. Moller, K. Aspergren, L. Bergljung, D. Killander, and T. Landberg. 1992. Long-term effects of adjuvant tamoxifen and/or radiotherapy. The South Swedish Trial. *Acta Oncologica* (in press).

Satyaswaroop, P. G., R. J. Zaino, and R. Mortel. 1984. Estrogen-like effects of tamoxifen on human endometrial carcinoma transplanted into nude mice. *Cancer Research* 44:4006–4010.

Wrange, O., B. Nordenskjold, and J. A. Gustafsson. 1978. Cytosol estradiol receptor in human mammary carcinoma: an assay based on isoelectric focusing in polyacrylamide gel. *Analytical Biochemistry* 85:461–475.

7

Maintenance Tamoxifen after Induction Postoperative Chemotherapy in Node-Positive Breast Cancer Patients: The Eastern Cooperative Oncology Group Trials (ECOG)

D. C. TORMEY, R. GRAY, H. C. FALKSON
K. GILCHRIST, M. D. ABELOFF, G. FALKSON,
AND PARTICIPATING INVESTIGATORS

I.	INTRODUCTION	135
II.	MATERIALS AND METHODS	136
	A. PATIENT ELIGIBILITY	136
	B. RANDOMIZATION	137
	C. TREATMENT REGIMENS	137
	D. DRUG DOSAGE MODIFICATIONS	138
	E. PATIENT EVALUATION	139
	F. PATIENT EVALUABILITY	139
	G. STATISTICAL METHODS	139

III. RESULTS   140
      A. PATIENT CHARACTERISTICS   140
      B. TIME-TO-RELAPSE TREATMENT COMPARISONS   141
      C. SURVIVAL TREATMENT COMPARISONS   144
      D. EFFECT OF PROGNOSTIC FACTORS   144
      E. SITES OF FIRST RELAPSE AND CAUSES OF DEATH   145
      F. SIDE EFFECTS DURING TREATMENT   145
      G. DRUG DOSING DURING TREATMENT   148
IV.   DISCUSSION   149
V.   SUMMARY   151
      ACKNOWLEDGMENTS   153
      REFERENCES   153

134

I. Introduction

T_{HE} treatment of breast carcinoma in postoperative, ipsilateral, axillary node–positive women with 1 or more years of systemic chemotherapy was begun in 1972 and 1973. The early results in the premenopausal patients from these initial trials suggested an advantage for L-phenylalanine mustard (L-PAM) in patients with from one to three involved axillary nodes (Fisher et al. 1975) and for a cyclophosphamide, methotrexate, 5-fluorouracil (CMF) combination in patients with four or fewer involved axillary nodes (Bonadonna et al. 1976). During this period the Eastern Cooperative Oncology Group (ECOG) demonstrated the superiority of a CMF regimen over L-PAM (Canellos et al. 1976), and of CMF plus prednisone (CMFP) over CMF (Tormey, Gelman, et al. 1982) in patients with metastatic disease. Simultaneously the antiestrogen tamoxifen (TAM) became accepted as an active hormonal treatment for disseminated disease (Cole et al. 1971; Ward 1973; Tormey et al. 1976). The addition of tamoxifen to an advanced disease chemotherapy regimen in patients previously treated with chemotherapy was found to be beneficial (Tormey, Falkson, et al. 1982). On the basis of early data from these trials the ECOG in 1978 initiated adjuvant therapy trials in axillary node-positive women that compared the therapeutic effectiveness of 1 year of CMFP and CMFP plus tamoxifen (CMFPT). The results from these trials showed no significant difference with the addition of either prednisone or prednisone and tamoxifen for 1 year (Tormey et al. 1990). However, early analyses suggested there was an advantage with the CMFPT regimen in both pre- and postmenopausal patients. This program was thereby chosen as the control regimen for the subsequent trials.

The premenopausal trial was designed to test CMFPT to a regimen consisting of CMFPT plus halotestin (H) in the odd-numbered cycles and an adriamycin-containing regimen with the addition of tamoxifen in the even-numbered cycles. This latter regimen was the vinblastine, adriamycin, thio-TEPA, H regimen (VATH) reported by Hart et al. (1981) to be a very effective second-line therapy in advanced disease and verified in a concomitant ECOG trial (Skeel et al. 1989). The addition of this regimen in the premenopausal trial's alternating program also provided a test of partly non-cross-resistant drugs in concordance with the hypotheses of Goldie et al. (1982).

135

The postmenopausal trial was designed to test the 12 months of the CMFPT regimen to a shorter 4 months of chemotherapy. This design was an extension of two previous trials that directly tested chemotherapy duration. Early results had suggested that 12 months was equivalent to 24 months of treatment (Jungi et al. 1984), and that 6 months was equivalent to 12 months (Bonadonna et al. 1985).

Finally, both trials reported herein were also designed to test the concept of tamoxifen maintenance therapy beyond 2 years. This concept had its inception in the preclinical *in vivo* work of Jordan et al. (1979) and the subsequent *in vitro* reports from Green et al. (1981) and Osborne et al. (1983). Their results strongly suggested that tamoxifen was a cytostatic agent which provided a G_0/G_1 block which would be reversed when the drug was discontinued. The initial laboratory results from Jordan et al. (1979) led to a long-term toxicity trial, which showed the pharmacological feasibility and possible clinical benefit of up to 10 years or more of postchemotherapy tamoxifen maintenance therapy in the postoperative setting (Tormey and Jordan 1984; Tormey et al. 1987; Langan-Fahey et al. 1990). These data led ECOG in 1982 to test the concept of long-term tamoxifen maintenance.

The induction and maintenance results from these two ECOG adjuvant trials are updated herein.

II. *Materials and Methods*

A. PATIENT ELIGIBILITY

Women with infiltrating breast carcinomas pathologically ≤5 cm and a radical or modified radical mastectomy, one or more histopathologically involved ipsilateral axillary lymph nodes, and a biochemical estrogen receptor (ER) assay result were considered for entry. At least three axillary lymph nodes had to be pathologically examined. Premenopausal status was defined as one or more menses in the 12 months preceding the diagnosis; or, under age 52 and no menopausal symptoms in patients with a prior hysterectomy. Patients with a prior bilateral oophorectomy were considered postmenopausal if at least 12 months had elapsed before the diagnosis of breast cancer. At presentation the patients had no tumor fixation, nodal fixation, arm edema, ulceration or infiltration of the skin of more than 2 cm, peau d'orange involving more than one-third of the breast, clinical or pathological evidence of inflammatory cancer, satellite nodules or parasternal nodes, or other evidence of disseminated disease to clinical examination. Other eligibility criteria included: normal bone scan; or, if abnormal, skeletal X-rays had to demonstrate a nonmalignant cause of the abnormality or biopsy proof of absence of metastatic disease at the site of abnormality; diagnostic biopsy within 4 weeks of definitive surgery; randomization within 6 weeks of definitive surgery; WBC, ≥4000/mm^3; platelets, ≥100,000/mm^3; creatinine, ≤1.5 mg%; bilirubin, ≤1.5 mg%, and SGOT and alkaline phosphatase, ≤1½×normal; fasting glucose, <9.7 mmol/l (<175 mg%); no previous or concomitant malignancy (except curatively treated skin or cervix carcinoma); no contralateral breast malignancy; no prior treatment for breast carcinoma; no medical conditions precluding the treatment options (e.g., insulin-requiring diabetes mellitus, active peptic ulcer, recent myocardial infarction, drug-requiring psychiatric illnesses or pregnancy); and informed consent per the Department of Health, Education and Welfare, state, and institutional guidelines. Central pathological and clinical review of eligibility was performed prospectively by the study chairman and cochairmen when each patient entered the studies.

B. Randomization

Randomized treatment assignments in both trials for North American patients were by telephone to a central office for some and via sealed envelope for others. North American patients were stratified for induction by 1–3 versus 4–9 versus ≥10 histologically positive axillary nodes and by ER-negative (<10 fmol/mg protein) versus ER-positive (≥10 fmol/mg protein) status. The patients were additionally stratified by induction regimen in the premenopausal patients for the second and third randomizations at years 1 and 5. The randomization method used was permuted blocks within strata with a block size of two (Zelen 1974). Treatment balance within institutions was ensured using a dynamic randomization method (Zelen 1974).

C. Treatment Regimens

Each of the induction-treatment regimens consisted of cycles of therapy beginning 1–6 weeks after mastectomy. Drug dosages (Table 7.1) were based on each patient's body surface area, which was calculated from the patient's ideal or actual body weight, whichever was the lesser. Premenopausal patients received 12 cycles of induction therapy. Each 28-day cycle of the CMFPT regimen consisted of cyclophosphamide (100 mg/m^2 PO, days 1 through 14), methotrexate (40 mg/m^2 IV, days 1 and 8), 5-fluorouracil (600 mg/m^2 IV, days 1 and 8), prednisone (40 mg/m^2 PO, days 1 through 14), and tamoxifen (10 mg PO BID). Methotrexate was given immediately before fluorouracil. The alter-

Table 7.1. Drug doses

	CMFPTH regimen	VATH regimen
cyclophosphamide	100 mg/m^2 PO d1–14	vinblastine 4.5 mg/m^2 IV d1
methotrexate	40 mg/m^2 IV d1 and d8	adriamycin 45 mg/m^2 IV d1
5-fluorouracil	600 mg/m^2 IV d1 and d8	thioTEPA 12 mg/m^2 IV d1
prednisone	40 mg/m^2 PO d1–14	
tamoxifen	10 mg PO BID	
halotestin	10 mg PO BID	halotestin 10 mg PO BID

nating regimen (ALTER) consisted of the 28-day CMFPT regimen with the addition of halotestin (H) 10 mg PO BID in cycles 1, 3, 5, 7, 9, and 11. The prednisone was omitted after cycle 3. The even-numbered cycles consisted of 22-day courses of vinblastine (4.5 mg/m^2 IV, day 1), adriamycin (45 mg/m^2 IV, day 1), thioTEPA (12 mg/m^2 IV, day 1), halotestin, and tamoxifen (VATHT). After 12 cycles of induction therapy, patients were randomized to continue tamoxifen or to observation (Obs) for 4 additional years. In post-menopausal patients treatment consisted of the CMFPT regimen delivered for 4 or 12 cycles, or 12 cycles followed by tamoxifen for 4 additional years. In patients older than 60 years, the methotrexate dose was modified if the creatinine clearance was abnormal. For creatinine clearances of more than 70 ml/minute, 40 mg/m^2 was administered; for clearances 50–69, 30 mg/m^2; for 30–49, 20 mg/m^2; and for less than 30, 10 mg/m^2. Patients disease-free on tamoxifen 5 years after initial randomization in both studies were again randomized to continue tamoxifen or to observation. The data from this latter randomization are still too recent to have been decoded.

D. Drug Dosage Modifications

The CMF and VAT doses in subsequent cycles were to be reduced 25% if the nadir WBC was <2000/mm^3 or the nadir platelet was <75,000/mm^3, and increased by 25% if the nadir WBC was >3500/mm^3 and the nadir platelet was >125,000/mm^3. Treatment delays of up to 2 weeks were allowed prior to each cycle to allow for recovery from hematological toxicity. On days 1 and 8 of each cycle CMF and VAT doses were to be reduced to 50% if the WBC was ≤4000/mm^3 or platelets were ≤100,000/mm^3, and omitted if the WBC was <2500/mm^3 or platelets were <75,000/mm^3.

Cyclophosphamide was to be replaced by 1-phenylalanine mustard at 4 mg/m^2 PO days 1 through 5 in the event of hemorrhagic cystitis. Dosage modification guidelines for gastrointestinal, renal, hepatic, and neurological toxicity were also specified but seldom required. If steroid-related toxicity occurred the prednisone was reduced.

Table 7.2. Patient accrual and evaluability

	E5181				E4181		
	Induction		Maintenance				
	ALTER	CMFPT	TAM	Obs	×12→T	×12	×4
Randomized	330	328	238	239	320	319	323
Exclusions							
Inadequate data	5	7	3	4	5	1	4
Treatment refusal	2	0	0[a]	0	3	4	6
Ineligible induction	53	59	34[a]	39[a]	40	45	50
maintenance	—	—	0	1[b]	—	—	—
Analyzed	270	262	201	195	272	269	263

[a]From induction randomization.
[b]Patient had bilateral oophorectomy during induction.

E. PATIENT EVALUATION

During the first year follow-up was to include a history and physical examination, blood counts, BUN, or creatinine and glucose prior to day 1 of each cycle; blood counts prior to day 8 of each cycle; bilirubin, alkaline phosphatase, SGOT, serum calcium, and chest X-ray every 3 months; a bone scan every 6 months; and a mammogram after 12 months. Thereafter, the patients were scheduled to obtain a clinic visit with blood studies every 3 months, a chest X-ray every 6 months, and a bone scan and mammography every 12 months.

F. PATIENT EVALUABILITY

There were 658 patients randomized to the premenopausal trial and 962 women randomized to the postmenopausal trial. Patients were excluded from the primary analyses because of inadequate data, refusal of all treatment, and ineligible characteristics (Table 7.2). The majority of those excluded involved abnormal prestudy bloods or counts not done, tumors >5 cm or with muscle or dermal lymphatic invasion, or abnormal prestudy scans or X-rays or neither done. The 532 analyzed premenopausal cases were distributed with 262 randomized to CMFPT, 270 to ALTER, and subsequently 201 to continue TAM and 195 to Obs. The median follow-up for this report is 5.6 years for the induction regimens and 4.6 years for the maintenance TAM and Obs randomization. There were 804 analyzed postmenopausal cases with 263 receiving CMFPT×4, 269 CMFPT×12, and 272 CMFPT×12T; and a median follow-up of 5.9 years.

G. STATISTICAL METHODS

The analyses measured both time to relapse (TTR) and survival from the time of randomization to relapse or death, respectively. The date of relapse

Table 7.3. Percentage distribution of treatment regimens, by patient characteristics

| | Premenopausal trial | | | | Postmenopausal trial | | |
| | Induction | | Maintenance | | | | |
Characteristic	ALTER	CMFPT	TAM	Obs	$\times 12 \to T$	$\times 12$	$\times 4$
Axillary N+ >3	47	46	46	46	52	50	51
ER+	63	63	67	64	70	68	71
PgR+	57	52	55	59	43	43	39
PgR–	31	33	30	28	39	40	44
T_p <3.0 cm	52	52	57	50	58	59	62
Age (medians)	44	42	44	42	60	60	61

was taken as the first evidence of subsequently documented relapse as judged by previously published guidelines (Tormey et al. 1977). Separate TTR and survival treatment comparisons were also performed by analyzing all randomized entries and, again, by counting disease-unrelated deaths as failures. The results from these analyses were similar to those obtained from the major analyses. Comparison of the distribution of prognostic factors between treatments used exact tests (Mehta and Patel 1983) for categorical factors and Wilcoxon rank sum tests (Hajek 1969) for continuous valued factors. The method of Kaplan and Meier (1958) was used to estimate TTR and survival curves. The marginal relationships of treatment or patient characteristics with TTR and survival were analyzed using the log rank test (Peto and Peto 1972). The proportional hazards model (Cox 1972) was used to analyze these relationships while adjusting simultaneously for multiple patient characteristics. The association of amenorrhea with TTR and survival was evaluated using a landmark analysis (Anderson et al. 1983). Amenorrhea was defined as 6 or more months without menstrual activity. The associations of site of relapse with treatment were evaluated using exact tests (Mehta and Patel 1983). The toxicity analyses were based upon all analyzed entries for each toxicity type and used the Wilcoxon midrank test (Lehmann 1975). All *p* values are from two-sided tests, and the term "significant" refers to two-sided *p* values ≤ 0.05.

III. *Results*

A. Patient Characteristics

The treatment regimens were well-balanced with respect to major patient characteristics (Table 7.3). These and other characteristics were controlled for in the treatment comparison analyses where appropriate.

Table 7.4. Five-year relapse-free survival, by premenopausal treatment group

Group	n	ALTER (%)	CMFPT (%)	log rank p value	n	TAM (%)	Obs (%)	log rank p value
Overall	532	70	63	0.04	396	72	63	0.05
ER+	334	78	68	0.06	258	78	68	0.02
ER–	198	57	54	0.29	138	60	55	0.53
N+								
1–3	284	77	73	0.17	214	81	69	0.03
>3	248	63	52	0.12	182	64	56	0.30

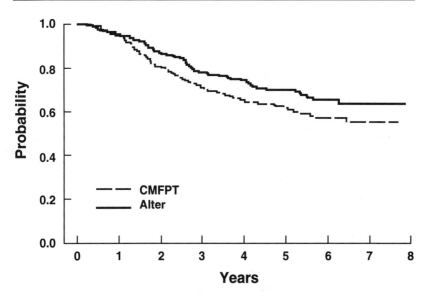

Figure 7.1 Time to relapse with the CMFPT and ALTER regimens for all analyzed premeno-pausal patients. The log rank *p* value is 0.04.

B. TIME-TO-RELAPSE TREATMENT COMPARISONS

The estimated proportion of premenopausal patients free of disease at 5 years was 70% among those receiving ALTER therapy, as compared with 63% in the CMFPT group ($p = 0.04$, Table 7.4, Fig. 7.1). Among the stratified subgroups the strongest trend favored ALTER therapy among the ER+ patients (78% vs 68% for CMFPT, $p = 0.06$).

During maintenance in the premenopausal trial those patients randomized to continue tamoxifen had an estimated 5-year relapse-free survival of 72% compared with 63% for those randomized to observation ($p = 0.05$, Table 7.4, Fig. 7.2). This difference was significant in the ER+ strata (78% vs 68%, $p = 0.02$, Fig. 7.3) and in the CMFPT strata (73% vs 60%, $p = 0.05$). Among the

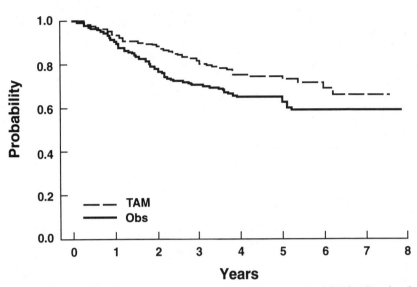

Figure 7.2. Time to relapse with the maintenance regimens of TAM and Obs for all analyzed premenopausal patients. The log rank *p* value is 0.05.

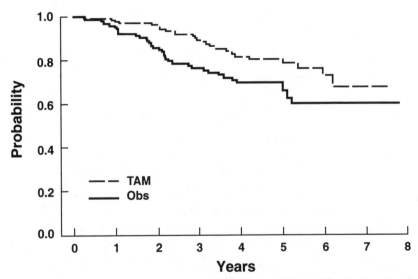

Figure 7.3. Time to relapse with the maintenance regimens of TAM and Obs for the analyzed ER+ premenopausal patients. The log rank *p* value is 0.02.

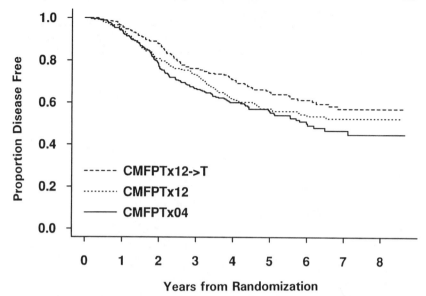

Figure 7.4. Time to relapse with the induction regimens for all analyzed postmenopausal patients. The log rank *p* value is 0.02.

Table 7.5. Five-year relapse-free survival, by postmenopausal treatment group

Group	n	×12→T (%)	×12 (%)	×4 (%)	*p* value
Overall	804	65	57	56	0.02
ER+	561	68	60	57	0.02
ER−	243	58	52	53	0.56
N+					
1–3	393	84	70	65	0.003
>3	411	48	45	47	0.60

patients from the ALTER strata the proportions of those relapse-free at 5 years randomized to TAM or Obs were, respectively, 73% and 67% (*p* = 0.24).

The estimated time to relapse (TTR) in the postmenopausal trial's analyzed patients (Fig. 7.4) is longer for patients on CMFPT×12 plus continuous TAM than for CMFPT×4 (*p* = 0.005) or CMFPT×12 (*p* = 0.08). The difference between 4 or 12 cycles of CMFPT is not significant. Relapse-free rates at 5 years are 65% for CMFPT×12 plus continuous TAM, 57% for CMFPT×12, and 56% for CMFPT×4 (Table 7.5).

Table 7.6. Five-year survival rates (%), by treatment group

Group	Premenopausal trial				Postmenopausal trial		
	ALTER	CMFPT	TAM	Obs	×12→T	×12	×4
Overall	79	76	82	78	71	73	72
ER+	88	84	90	85	76	79	75
ER–	65	62	66	66	60	58	63
N+							
1–3	85	84	87	83	83	82	79
>3	73	66	76	72	59	64	65

C. SURVIVAL TREATMENT COMPARISONS

The 5-year overall survival rate in the premenopausal trial was 79% for the ALTER group, as compared with 76% for the CMFPT group ($p = 0.56$, Table 7.6). The 5-year overall survival rate was 82% for the TAM-maintained group, as compared with 78% for the Obs group ($p = 0.75$, Table 7.6). The differences between the various induction and maintenance strata are also not significant at this time. The survival results in the postmenopausal trial were similar in that there are currently no significant differences in survival between the three regimens (Table 7.6).

D. EFFECT OF PROGNOSTIC FACTORS

The effects of the common pretreatment characteristics upon TTR were analyzed unadjusted by the log rank procedure and then by a proportional hazards multivariate model (Cox 1972). Those on-study factors found to be associated with a shorter TTR in the premenopausal trial were increasing nodal involvement ($p < 0.001$), negative ER status ($p < 0.001$), decreasing age ($p = 0.001$), induction CMFPT ($p = 0.04$), and negative PgR status ($p = 0.09$). It was observed that patients developing amenorrhea during therapy had a longer TTR (log rank, $p = 0.04$), with the effect being qualitatively similar in both ER+ and ER– patients. The proportions disease free at 5 years with amenorrhea versus no amenorrhea, respectively, were: overall, 74% vs 63%; ER+, 79% vs 69%; and ER-, 64% vs 52%. Shorter survivals in a proportional hazards multivariate model (Cox 1972) were associated with increasing nodal status ($p < 0.001$), negative ER assay ($p = 0.006$), negative PgR assay ($p = 0.007$), and increasing primary tumor size ($p = 0.02$). It was also observed that patients developing amenorrhea during therapy had a better survival (log rank, $p = 0.04$), with qualitatively similar effects in both ER+ and ER– patients. The proportions alive at 5 years with amenorrhea versus no amenor-

Table 7.7. Rates (%) of first relapse, by site and treatment received

	Premenopausal trial				Postmenopausal trial		
Site of relapse	ALTER (n = 270)	CMFPT (n = 263)	TAM (n = 201)	Obs (n = 195)	×12→T (n = 272)	×12 (n = 269)	×4 (n = 263)
Locoregional only	6	9	4	11	7	14	11
Distant only	18	23	16	21	24	24	26
Distant soft only	2	2	2	<1	2	2	4
Bone only	6	9	5	10	7	9	10
Visceral only	5	6	5	5	11	7	6
Distant + loco- regional	4	5	6	4	5	4	8
Any recurrence	29	37	25	36	36	42	46

rhea, respectively, were: overall, 86% vs 78%; ER+, 94% vs 87%; and ER–, 71% vs 63%.

The association of hormone receptor status and number of involved nodes with TTR and with survival is also highly significant in the postmenopausal trial. A shorter TTR and survival were associated with increasing nodal status ($p < 0.0001$ for both), negative ER status ($p < 0.0004$ and 0.0003, respectively), and negative PgR status ($p < 0.02$ and 0.0001, respectively). Because the use of long-term tamoxifen was part of the initial randomization, this variable was also analyzed and was associated with an improved TTR ($p = 0.03$).

E. Sites of First Relapse and Causes of Death

Table 7.7 displays the sites of first relapse with each regimen categorized as locoregional or distant. There were no statistical differences in the relapse patterns between the premenopausal induction regimens, although the ALTER regimen tended to have fewer locoregional and distant only recurrences. The tamoxifen maintenance regimen in premenopausal patients was associated with fewer locoregional relapses (4.0%) than the observation group (11.0%, $p = 0.02$). In the postmenopausal patients there was also a trend toward fewer locoregional relapses with maintenance tamoxifen (7%) than with observation (14% and 11%).

The major cause of death in all groups in both trials was breast cancer (336 patients). Only 49 patients died from other causes.

F. Side Effects during Treatment

The major side effects encountered during the induction treatments are shown in Table 7.8. In the premenopausal patients a significantly higher

Table 7.8. Rates (%) of major side effects occurring during induction treatment, by regimen

| | Premenopausal trial | | Postmenopausal trial | |
| | E5181 | | E4181 | |
Side effect[a]	ALTER	CMFPT	CMFPT×12	CMFPT×4
WBC				
<2000/mm^3	40	37	38	31
<1000/mm^3	3	7	8	7
Platelets <75,000/mm^3	4	8	19	5
Hemoglobin below normal	20	30	35	19
Sepsis: clinical/documented	2/0	3/0	6/1	4/1
Persistent nausea or emesis	5	2	20	0
Oral ulcerations requiring therapy	3	1	2	3
Epigastric pain	17	19	15	10
Cushingoid changes	10	19	15	7
Edema: mild–moderate/worse	32/1	35/1	44/1	18/1
Insomnia	20	29	22	17
Psychiatric requiring dose decrease	4	5	6	2
Elevated blood sugar	26	30	44	35
Weight gain >10%	7	20	24	10
Skin	38	20	19	12
Alopecia	74	61	60	49
Deep vein thromboses	4	7	11	7
Amenorrhea >6 months	66	67		
Hot flashes	59	66	31	22

[a]Based on ECOG grades ordering from 0 (no toxicity) to 5 (lethal), per Oken et al. 1982.

incidence of the following side effects was observed with the ALTER regimen: acne/skin, allergic, nausea/emesis, alopecia, hirsutism, peripheral nervous system symptoms, and joint pains. The CMFPT regimen was associated with a significantly higher incidence of anemia, thrombocytopenia, infection, Cushingoid changes, insomnia, weight gain, and eye complaints. Various mild or moderate toxic events were observed in 40% of the CMFPT group and 40% of the ALTER group, whereas severe or life-threatening events occurred in, respectively, 60% and 58%. There was one death on CMFPT associated with a WBC = 900/mm^3 and a mesenteric venous occlusion occurring in cycle 3. The ALTER regimen was associated with three deaths due to cerebral vascular accidents in cycles 1, 1, and 7, and one death in cycle 3 associated with a bilateral brainstem infarction. The percentage of patients not completing induction therapy for reasons other than relapse was 21% for CMFPT and 18% for ALTER therapy.

The use of maintenance tamoxifen in the premenopausal trial was associated with more hot flashes (67% vs 53%, $p = 0.008$), but less bone pain (6% vs 12%, $p = 0.05$). There were two patients with life-threatening events during maintenance, one cardiac on tamoxifen and one CNS symptom in observation. Severe toxicities on tamoxifen included leukopenia (1), infection (1), CNS symptom (1), deep vein thrombosis (1), pruritus (1), weight gain (2), and weight loss (2). In observation severe toxicities were CNS symptom (1) and weight gain (3). Other side effects recorded with tamoxifen and observation were: epigastric distress (4% and 3%, respectively), peripheral edema (11% and 8%), insomnia (2% and 1%), hyperglycemia (6% and 7%), vaginal discharge (2% and 1%), and vaginal bleeding (6% and 4%). There were three patients that developed amenorrhea during maintenance tamoxifen and five in observation; however, of the patients developing amenorrhea during induction or maintenance, 15% of the observation and 18% of the tamoxifen patients resumed menstruation.

Seven second nonbreast cancers have been reported in the premenopausal trial. There is one each of endometrial carcinoma, sarcoma, colorectal carcinoma, left conjunctival squamous cell carcinoma *in situ,* melanoma, basal cell carcinoma, and leukemia in patients receiving, respectively, CMFPT/ TAM, ALTER/Obs, CMFPT/TAM, ALTER/TAM, CMFPT/Obs, CMFPT/ TAM, and ALTER/off study.

The most commonly encountered side effects in the postmenopausal trial were hematological problems, nausea and vomiting, and alopecia. Table 7.8 shows the severity of toxicity according to whether the patient received 4 or 12 cycles of CMFPT. In general, there were fewer side effects among those patients receiving 4 courses of CMFPT than those receiving 12. In addition, 31% of the patients receiving 12 cycles and 22% of the patients receiving 4 cycles had hot flashes. There were 77 cases reported with life-threatening toxicity and 7 with lethal toxicities. In three of the patients, death was attributed to a thromboembolic event, three other patients died with severe hematopoietic depression and septicemia, and one patient died of acute pancreatitis. Worth noting is that 10.6% of patients receiving 12 cycles and 6.9% of patients receiving 4 cycles experienced severe or worse clotting problems. Side effects reported for patients on continuous tamoxifen after 12 months were qualitatively similiar to those reported in the observation groups.

There were 24 cases of second primaries other than breast cancer reported in the postmenopausal trial with 9 on CMFPT×4, 7 on CMFPT×12, and 8 on CMFPT×12→T. In the CMFPT×4 and ×12 programs these have been colorectal (5), head and neck (1), leukemia (1), melanoma (1), skin (4), cervical (2), uterine (1), endometrium (1), and kidney (1). The second cancers on the CMFPT×12→T regimen are pancreas (1), colorectal (1), skin (3), uterine (1), endometrium (1), and kidney (1).

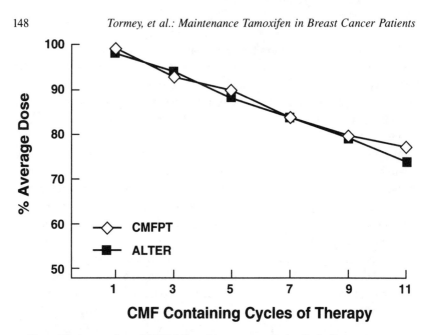

Figure 7.5. Average dose of CMF delivered in premenopausal patients. Dose averages were calculated by dividing the actual dose of C + M + F received by the 100% projected dose of C + M + F for each cycle. Patients who relapsed during a cycle or were lost to follow-up were censored at that time. Patients who did not receive a drug in any cycle without relapse were assigned doses of zero. The time to complete each of the first 11 cycles of therapy among these 392 patients ranged from 306 to 476 days for CMFPT, and from 255 to 401 days for ALTER. For each regimen the number of observations in cycle 1 and 12 were, respectively, 190 and 140 for CMFPT, and 202 and 156 for ALTER.

G. Drug Dosing during Treatment

Drug dosing was evaluated in random order for 392 of the 533 eligible premenopausal patients. There were at least 6 cycles of induction therapy delivered to 88% on ALTER and 89% on CMFPT. Twelve cycles were delivered to 78% on ALTER and 74% on CMFPT. The average dose of CMF delivered during the odd cycles in each of the induction regimens is displayed in Figure 7.5. There was a similar drug delivery in both regimens (Wilcoxon rank sum test; Hajek 1969). In cycles 1 and 3 the average dose of prednisone was 95.1% and 80.9% in CMFPT, and 97.1% and 83.0% with ALTER therapy. These analyses indexed all analyzable patients whether or not they received therapy so long as they had not relapsed. Treatment interruption due to relapse led to censoring of the subsequent data. The percentage of ideal dose was 100 times the actual dose divided by the protocol ideal dose, where the protocol ideal did not take into account dose modifications. For CMF these were calculated separately for each drug and averaged.

The proportion of premenopausal patients discontinuing tamoxifen for reasons other than relapse during induction was 14%, most because of stopping all therapy (see above). The proportion discontinuing tamoxifen during the first 5 years of maintenance was 9%, and during years 1 to 5 after the maintenance randomization the proportions were, respectively, 1.6%, 3.2%, 0.6%, 0.7%, and 2.1%.

For postmenopausal patients randomized to receive 4 cycles, 10.7% were given 1 to 3 cycles, 87% were given 4 cycles, and 2.3% were given more than 4 cycles. For patients randomized to receive 12 cycles, 10.3% were given 1 to 4 cycles, 16.8% were given 5 to 11 cycles, and 72% were given the full 12 cycles. Disease-free survival and survival analyses were based on patients as randomized, not as drugs received.

The proportion of postmenopausal patients discontinuing tamoxifen for reasons other than relapse during induction was 14%, most because of stopping all therapy (see above). The proportions discontinuing tamoxifen during years 1 to 5 after the maintenance randomization were, respectively, 3.3%, 0.7%, 1.5%, 2.9%, and 5.9%.

IV. *Discussion*

The present trials have demonstrated an overall therapeutic impact in premenopausal women by the addition of an adriamycin-based rotating induction regimen compared with a CMF-based regimen, and the continuation of a tamoxifen maintenance for at least 5 years compared with observation in both premenopausal and postmenopausal patients. In addition there is no evidence that treatment of postmenopausal women with 12 courses of CMFPT is superior to 4 courses. The results with the adriamycin-containing regimen are similar to multiple advanced disease trials wherein the use of adriamycin-containing regimens were superior to nonadriamycin regimens (Bull et al. 1978; Tormey et al. 1984; Smalley et al. 1977; Tormey, Gelman, and Falkson 1983). They have also provided additional evidence that such regimens are superior to non-adriamycin-containing regimens in postoperative patients (Misset et al. 1984; Fisher et al. 1989). The tamoxifen maintenance results verify the preclinical experiments (Jordan et al. 1979) as well as the early clinical suggestions of its effectiveness (Tormey and Jordan 1984; Tormey et al. 1987). The relative reduction of locoregional relapses in the tamoxifen-maintained patients also suggests a role for the drug in the prevention of second breast cancers or of breast cancer in high-risk cohorts of women.

Unlike the clear rationale for an expected benefit of tamoxifen in ER+ patients, the rationale for the advantage of the alternating adriamycin program is not clear. However, it is of interest that adriamycin-containing regimens in the treatment of metastatic disease have been reported to be most effective in older patients (Tormey et al. 1984). This may be an indication that the drug is more effective in the same patient cohort that is responsive to tamoxifen. Alternatively, the partial cross-resistance of the two regimens in the ALTER regimen may have provided an advantage in concert with a special case hypothesis of Goldie et al. (1982). In contrast with this is the observation that the adriamycin regimen tends to be superior to CMF-based regimens (see above), and that the rotation of two disparately active regimens yields results similar to those which would be obtained with use of only the more active regimen (Tormey, Gelman, and Falkson 1983). On this basis it would appear that the key factor providing for the improved results with the ALTER regimen is the VATH component.

Several trials (Jungi et al. 1984; Bonadonna et al. 1985; Henderson et al. 1986; Rivkin et al. 1984; Velez-Garcia et al. 1984) addressing the issue of duration of adjuvant therapy have not shown an advantage for a longer duration of chemotherapy. However, one study from Ontario showed a significant survival advantage for patients randomized to 36 weeks of CMFVP compared with those given 12 weeks of CMFVP followed by single-agent doxorubicin (Levine et al. 1988). Results reported here show that neither the TTR nor the survival was significantly different for 4 or 12 cycles of CMFPT in postmenopausal patients.

The results from the present trials further support reports of the prognostic importance of the number of nodes involved, estrogen receptor status, and size of the primary tumor (Tormey, Weinberg, et al. 1983; Tancini et al. 1983; Glucksberg et al. 1982; Hubay et al. 1981; Fisher et al. 1969). Contrary to a previous report (Bonadonna et al. 1981), but in keeping with our previous data (Tormey et al. 1990), we have observed a greater therapeutic effect among premenopausal patients developing amenorrhea. This implies that the induction of an ovarian ablation contributes to the therapeutic effect of adjuvant therapy in premenopausal patients. Further trials are needed to assess this observation directly.

Side effects with the various regimens were as expected from previous ECOG trials, including the nonsignificant reduction of side effects with 4 courses of therapy as compared with 12 courses.

There was a suggestive difference in the locoregional recurrence rate among patients treated with the tamoxifen maintenance. As in other reported trials (Tormey, Weinberg, et al. 1983; Tancini et al. 1983; Glucksberg et al. 1982) the overall incidence of locoregional recurrences was similar to historical postoperative radiotherapy data. Despite these observations it would appear that the major therapeutic problem continues to be inadequate systemic therapy, as judged by the incidence of distant recurrences. Although more prolonged therapy may eliminate some of these, it is our view, on the basis of other data sets (Falkson et al. 1990; Tormey and Gelman 1981; Tormey 1991), that more aggressive shorter-term therapy is needed.

On the basis of the results of these and other trials, the ECOG is currently participating in trials to evaluate further the role of maintenance hormone therapy in both node-negative and node-positive pre- and postmenopausal patients (Figs. 7.6–7.8). The node-negative trial also includes an evaluation of CMF versus CAF. In ER– node-positive patients an "aggressive" chemotherapy regimen is compared with a standard CAF regimen (Fig. 7.9).

These trials provide evidence that the incorporation of an adriamycin-containing regimen in the induction chemotherapy program facilitates an improvement in the therapeutic effect for premenopausal patients. They also provide strong evidence for incorporating a maintenance program of long-term tamoxifen therapy in both premenopausal and postmenopausal patients. This latter benefit appears to be most pronounced in ER+ patients. The prognostic value of nodal status, ER results, and tumor size were reaffirmed. The retrospective reaffirmation of a beneficial effect of amenorrhea in premenopausal patients suggests that strategies which promote amenorrhea may be important and should be explored prospectively.

V. *Summary*

Prospective randomized trials were undertaken to evaluate the therapeutic effect of long-term administration of postchemotherapy tamoxifen maintenance in postoperative ipsilateral axillary node-positive patients with breast carcinoma. The premenopausal trial also evaluated an adriamycin-containing induction regimen, and the postmenopausal trial also evaluated 4 months versus 12 months of induction chemotherapy. Women in both trials were postoperatively stratified by degree of nodal involvement and estrogen receptor status prior to randomization. Premenopausal patients received 1 year of induction treatment with 12 28-day cycles of cyclophosphamide (100 mg/m^2

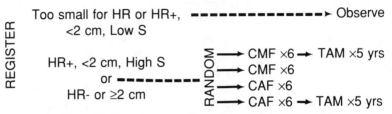

Figure 7.6. Current postoperative node-negative intergroup trial.

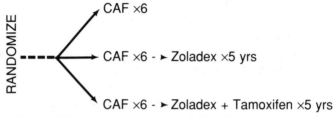

Figure 7.7. Current postoperative node-positive ER+ premenopausal trial.

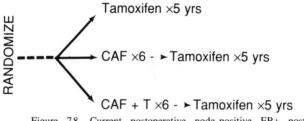
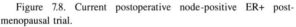

Figure 7.8. Current postoperative node-positive ER+ post-menopausal trial.

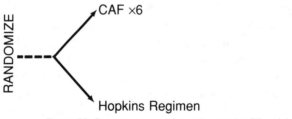

Figure 7.9. Current postoperative node-negative ER– trial.

PO, days 1 through 14), methotrexate (40 mg/m^2 IV, days 1 and 8), 5-fluo-rouracil (600 mg/m^2 IV, days 1 and 8), prednisone (40 mg/m^2 PO, days 1 through 14), and tamoxifen (10 mg PO BID) (CMFPT), or the same regimen plus halotestin (10 mg PO BID) (CMFPTH) alternating with 22-day cycles of vinblastine (4.5 mg/m^2 IV, day 1), adriamycin (45 mg/m^2 IV, day 1), thioTEPA (12 mg/m^2 IV, day 1), halotestin, and tamoxifen (VATHT). In the alternating regimen (ALTER) the prednisone was stopped after the second CMFPTH cycle. After 12 cycles of therapy, disease-free patients were again randomized to continue or stop tamoxifen. Postmenopausal patients were randomized to receive CMFPT×4 months, ×12 months, or ×12 months with tamoxifen continued to 5 years. A third randomization to continue or stop tamoxifen was performed in both protocols after 5 years of therapy among those disease-free patients continuing tamoxifen. In the premenopausal trial there were 532 analyzed induction cases and 396 analyzed maintenance cases. There were 804 analyzed postmenopausal entries. Treatment arms in both studies were balanced with respect to pretherapy characteristics. The median follow-up time for the premenopausal study is 5.6 years for induction and 4.6 years for maintenance; and for the postmenopausal study the median follow-up time is 5.9 years. Among the premenopausal patients the overall time to relapse (TTR) was superior for ALTER ($p = 0.04$) and for the maintenance continuation of tamoxifen ($p = 0.03$). Among the postmenopausal patients the overall TTR was greater for CMFPT×12T ($p = 0.02$), whereas CMFPT×12 and CMFPT×4 were equivalent. Overall survival comparisons between the regimens in each trial are not significantly different at this time. The results of the present analyses suggest significant overall TTR therapeutic benefits for an adriamycin-containing induction regimen in premenopausal patients and for continuing maintenance tamoxifen for at least 5 years in both pre- and postmenopausal patients.

Acknowledgments

The authors gratefully acknowledge the participation of all the involved investigators and patients, as well as the data management and analytical help provided by Ms. Rochelle Aro, Mrs. Lorraine Danforth, Ms. Grace Mellin, and Ms. Wendy Fischer.

References

Anderson, J. R., K. C. Cain, and R. D. Gelber. 1983. Analysis of survival by tumor response. *Journal of Clinical Oncology* 1:710–719.

Bonadonna G., P. Valagussa, A. Rossi, G. Tancini, C. Brambilla, M. Zambetti, and U. Veronesi. 1985. Ten-year experience with CMF-based adjuvant chemotherapy in resectable breast cancer. *Breast Cancer Research and Treatment* 5:95–115.

Bonadonna, G., A. Rossi, G. Tancini, E. Bajetta, S. Marchini, C. Brambilla, J. D. Tesoro Tess, P. Valagussa, A. Banfi, and U. Veronesi. 1981. Adjuvant combination chemotherapy for operable breast cancer. Trials in progress at the Instituto Nazionale Tumori of Milan. *Cancer Treatment Reports* 65(Supplement)1:61–65.

Bonadonna, G., E. Brusamolino, P. Valagussa, A. Rossi, L. Brugnatelli, C. Brambilla, M. De Lena, G. Tancini, E. Bajetta, R. Musumeci, and U. Veronesi. 1976. Combination chemotherapy as an adjuvant treatment in operable breast cancer. *New England Journal of Medicine* 294:405–410.

Bull, J. M., D. C. Tormey, S. H. Li, P. P. Carbone, G. Falkson, J. Blom, E. Perlin, and R. Simon. 1978. A randomized comparative trial of adriamycin versus methotrexate in combination drug therapy. *Cancer* 41:1649–1657.

Canellos, G. P., S. J. Pocock, S. G. Taylor III, M. E. Sears, D. J. Klaasen, and P. R. Band. 1976. Combination chemotherapy for metastatic breast carcinoma. Prospective comparison of multiple drug therapy with L-phenylalanine mustard. *Cancer* 38:1882–1886.

Cole, M. P., C. T. Jones, and I. D. Todd. 1971. The treatment of advanced carcinoma of the breast with the antioestrogenic agent tamoxifen (ICI 46,474)—a series of 96 patients. In *Advances in antimicrobial and antineoplastic chemotherapy,* ed. M. Hejzlar, M. Semonsky, and S. Masak, 529–531. *Proceedings of the 7th International Congress of Chemotherapy,* Prague. Baltimore: University Park Press.

Cox, D. R. 1972. Regression models and life tables. *Journal of Royal Statistical Society* (Series B) 34:187–198.

Falkson, H. C., R. Gray, W. H. Wolberg, K. W. Gilchrist, J. E. Harris, D. C. Tormey, and G. Falkson. 1990. Adjuvant trial of 12 cycles of CMFPT followed by observation or continuous tamoxifen versus four cycles of CMFPT in postmenopausal women with breast cancer: an Eastern Cooperative Oncology Group phase III study. *Journal of Clinical Oncology* 8:599–607.

Fisher, B., N. H. Slack, and I. D. Bross. 1969. Cancer of the breast: size of neoplasm and prognosis. *Cancer* 24:1071–1080.

Fisher, B., P. P. Carbone, S. G. Economou, R. Frelick, A. Glass, H. Lerner, C. Redmond, M. Zelen, P. Band, D. L. Katrych, N. Wolmark, and E. R. Fisher. 1975. L-phenylalanine mustard (L-PAM) in the management of primary breast cancer. A report of early findings. *New England Journal of Medicine* 292:117–122.

Fisher, B., C. Redmond, D. L. Wickerham, D. Bowman, H. Schipper, N. Wolmark, R. Sass, E. R. Fisher, P. Jochimsen, S. Legault-Poisson, N. Dimitrov, J. Wolter, R. Bornstein, E. G. Elias, N. Licalzi, C. M. Sutherland, and A. H. G. Paterson. 1989. Doxorubicin-containing regimens for the treatment of stage II breast cancer: the National Surgical Adjuvant Breast and Bowel Project experience. *Journal of Clinical Oncology* 7:572–582.

Glucksberg, H., S. E. Rivkin, S. Rasmussen, B. Tranum, N. Gad-el-Mawla, J. Costanzi, B. Hoogstraten, J. Athens, T. Maloney, J. McCracken, and C. Vaughn. 1982. Combination chemotherapy (CMFVP) versus L-phenylalanine mustard (L-PAM) for operable breast cancer with positive axillary nodes: a Southwest Oncology Group study. *Cancer* 50:423–434.

Goldie, J. H., A. J. Coldman, and G. A. Gudauskas. 1982. Rationale for the use of alternating non-cross-resistant chemotherapy. *Cancer Treatment Reports* 66:439–449.

Green, M. D., A. M. Whybourne, I. W. Taylor, and R. L. Sutherland. 1981. Effects of anti-oestrogens on the growth and cell cycle kinetics of cultured human mammary carcinoma cells. In *Nonsteroidal antioestrogens: molecular pharmacology and antitumour activity,* ed. R. L. Sutherland and V. C. Jordan, 397–412. Sydney: Academic Press.

Hajek, J. 1969. *A course in nonparametric statistics.* San Francisco: Holden Day.

Hart, R. D., M. Perloff, and J. F. Holland. 1981. One-day VATH (vinblastine, adriamycin, thiotepa, and halotestin) therapy for advanced breast cancer refractory to chemotherapy. *Cancer* 48:1522–1527.

Henderson, I. C., R. S. Gelman, J. R. Harris, and G. P. Canellos. 1986. Duration of therapy in adjuvant chemotherapy trials. *NCI Monographs* 1:95–98.

Hubay, C. A., O. H. Pearson, J. S. Marshall, T. A. Stellato, R. S. Rhodes, S. M. DeBanne, J. Rosenblatt, E. G. Mansour, R. E. Hermann, J. C. Jones, W. J. Flynn, C. Eckert, and W. L. McGuire. 1981. Adjuvant therapy of stage II breast cancer: 48-month follow-up of a prospective randomized clinical trial. *Breast Cancer Research and Treatment* 1:77–82.

Jordan, V. C., C. J. Dix, and K. E. Allen. 1979. The effectiveness of long-term tamoxifen treatment in a laboratory model for adjuvant hormone therapy of breast cancer. In *Adjuvant therapy of cancer,* vol. 2, ed. S. E. Salmon and S. E. Jones, 19–26. New York: Grune and Stratton.

Jungi, W. F., P. Alberto, K. W. Brunner, B. Mermillod, L. Barrelet, and F. Cavalli. 1984. Short- or long-term chemotherapy for node-positive breast cancer: LMF 6 versus 18 cycles. SAKK study, 27/76. *Recent Results in Cancer Research* 96:175–177.

Kaplan, E. L., and P. Meier. 1958. Nonparametric estimation from incomplete observations. *Journal of the American Statistical Association* 53:457–481.

Langan-Fahey, S. M., D. C. Tormey, and V. C. Jordan. 1990. Tamoxifen metabolites in patients on long-term adjuvant therapy for breast cancer. *European Journal of Cancer* 26:883–888.

Lehmann, E. L. 1975. *Nonparametrics: statistical methods based on ranks.* San Francisco: Holden Day.

Levine, M., H. Bush, and W. Gent. 1988. A randomized controlled trial comparing 12 weeks with 36 weeks of adjuvant chemotherapy in stage II breast cancer. *Proceedings of the American Society of Clinical Oncology* 7:8.

Mehta, C. R., and N. R. Patel. 1983. A network algorithm for performing Fisher's exact test in rxc contingency tables. *Journal of American Statistical Associates* 78:427–434.

Misset, J. L., F. De Vassal, and C. Jasmis. 1984. Five-year results of the French adjuvant trial for breast cancer comparing CMF to a combination of adriamycin (ADM), vincristine (VCR), cyclophosphamide (CPM), and 5-fluorouracil (5-FU). In *Adjuvant therapy of cancer IV,* ed. S. E. Salmon and S. E. Jones, 243–251. Orlando: Grune and Stratton.

Oken, M. M., R. H. Creech, D. C. Tormey, J. Horton, T. E. Davis, E. T. McFadden, and P. P. Carbone. 1982. Toxicity and response criteria of the Eastern Cooperative Oncology Group. *American Journal of Clinical Oncology* 5:649–655.

Osborne, C. K., D. H. Boldt, G. M. Clark, and J. M. Trent. 1983. Effects of tamoxifen on human breast cancer cell cycle kinetics: accumulation of cells in early G1 phase. *Cancer Research* 43:3583–3585.

Peto, R., and J. Peto. 1972. Asymptotically efficient rank invariant test procedures. *Journal of the Royal Statistical Society* (Series A) 135:185–198.

Rivkin, S. E., W. A. Knight, and A. Cruz. 1984. Adjuvant chemotherapy and hormonal therapy for operable breast cancer with positive axillary nodes. *Proceedings of the American Association for Cancer Research* 25:181.

Skeel, R. T., J. W. Andersen, D. C. Tormey, A. B. Benson III, R. F. Asbury, and G. Falkson. 1989. Combination chemotherapy of advanced breast cancer. Comparison of dibromodulcitol, doxorubicin, vincristine, and halotestin to thiotepa, adriamycin, vinblastine, and halotestin. An Eastern Cooperative Oncology Group study. *Cancer* 64:1393–1399.

Smalley, R. V., J. Carpenter, A. Bartolucci, C. Vogel, and S. Krauss. 1977. A comparison of cyclophosphamide, adriamycin, 5-fluorouracil (CAF) and cyclophosphamide, methotrexate, 5-fluorouracil, vincristine, prednisone (CMFVP) in patients with metastatic breast cancer: a Southeastern Cancer Study Group project. *Cancer* 40:625–632.

Tancini, G., G. Bonadonna, P. Valagussa, S. Marchini, and U. Veronesi. 1983. Adjuvant CMF in breast cancer: comparative 5-year results of 12 versus 6 cycles. *Journal of Clinical Oncology* 1:2–10.

Tormey, D. C. 1991. Intensive treatment considerations in breast cancer. In *High risk breast cancer—therapy*, ed. J. Ragaz and I. Ariel, 285–294. New York: Springer-Verlag.

Tormey, D. C., and R. S. Gelman. 1981. Relationship between time to treatment failure and survival and between time to response and response duration in metastatic breast cancer. Implications for treatment. *Cancer Clinical Trials* 4:355–362.

Tormey, D. C., and V. C. Jordan. 1984. Long-term tamoxifen adjuvant therapy in node-positive breast cancer: a metabolic and pilot clinical study. *Breast Cancer Research and Treatment* 4:297–302.

Tormey, D. C., R. S. Gelman, and G. Falkson. 1983. Prospective evaluation of rotating chemotherapy in advanced breast cancer. An Eastern Cooperative Oncology Group trial. *American Journal of Clinical Oncology* 6:1–18.

Tormey, D. C., P. Rasmussen, and V. C. Jordan. 1987. Long-term adjuvant tamoxifen study: clinical update (Letter). *Breast Cancer Research and Treatment* 9:157–158.

Tormey, D. C., R. M. Simon, M. E. Lippman, J. M. Bull, and C. E. Myers. 1976. Evaluation of tamoxifen dose in advanced breast cancer: a progress report. *Cancer Treatment Reports* 60:1451–1459.

Tormey, D. C., G. Falkson, J. Crowley, H. C. Falkson, J. Voelkel, and T. E. Davis. 1982. Dibromodulcitol and adriamycin ± tamoxifen in advanced breast cancer. *American Journal of Clinical Oncology* 5:33–39.

Tormey, D. C., R. Gelman, P. R. Band, M. Sears, S. N. Rosenthal, W. DeWys, C. Perlia, and M. A. Rice. 1982. Comparison of induction chemotherapies for metastatic breast cancer. An Eastern Cooperative Oncology Group trial. *Cancer* 50:1235–1244.

Tormey, D. C., R. Gray, K. Gilchrist, T. Grage, P. P. Carbone, J. Wolter, J. E. Woll, and F. J. Cummings. 1990. Adjuvant chemohormonal therapy with cyclophosphamide, methotrexate, 5-fluorouracil, and prednisone (CMFP) or CMFP plus tamoxifen compared with CMF for premenopausal breast cancer patients. An Eastern Cooperative Oncology Group trial. *Cancer* 65:200–206.

Tormey, D., B. Fisher, G. Bonadonna, S. Carter, H. Davis, O. Glidewell, R. G. Hahn, S. Payne, M. Zelen, and M. E. Sears. 1977. Proposed guidelines—report from the Combined Modality Trials Working Group in breast cancer: suggested protocol guidelines for combination chemotherapy trials and for combined modality trials. In *DHEW Publication No. NIH 77-11924*, ed. P. P. Carbone and M. E. Sears, 20–35. Washington, D.C.

Tormey, D. C., V. E. Weinberg, L. A. Leone, O. J. Glidewell, M. Perloff, B. J. Kennedy, E. Cortes, R. T. Silver, R. B. Weiss, J. Aisner, and J. F. Holland. 1984. A comparison of intermittent versus continuous and of adriamycin versus methotrexate 5-drug chemotherapy for advanced breast cancer. A Cancer and Leukemia Group B study. *American Journal of Clinical Oncology* 7:231–239.

Tormey, D. C., V. E. Weinberg, J. F. Holland, R. B. Weiss, O. J. Glidewell, M. Perloff, G. Falkson, H. C. Falkson, P. H. Henry, L. A. Leone, S. Rafla, S. J. Ginsberg, R. T. Silver, J. Blom, R. W. Carey, P. S. Schein, and G. J. Lesnick. 1983. A randomized trial of five and three drug chemotherapy and chemoimmunotherapy in women with operable node positive breast cancer. *Journal of Clinical Oncology* 1:138–145.

Velez-Garcia, E., M. Moore, C. L. Vogel, V. Marcial, A. Ketcham, M. Raney, and R. Smalley. 1984. Post-surgical adjuvant chemotherapy in women with breast cancer and positive axillary nodes. The Southeastern Cancer Study Group experience. In *Adjuvant therapy of cancer,* vol. 4, ed. S. E. Salmon and S. E. Jones, 273–282, Orlando: Grune and Stratton.

Ward, H. W. C. 1973. Antioestrogen therapy for breast cancer: a trial of tamoxifen at two dose levels. *British Medical Journal* 1:13–14.

Zelen, M. 1974. The randomization and stratification of patients to clinical trials. *Journal of Chronic Diseases* 27:365–375.

8

Prolonged Tamoxifen Treatment of Early Breast Cancer: The Experience of the Italian Cooperative Group for Chemohormonal Therapy of Early Breast Cancer

GRUPPO RICERCA ORMONO CHEMI
TERAPIA ADIUVANTE (GROCTA)
FRANCESCO BOCCARDO, DOMENICO AMOROSO,
ALESSANDRA RUBAGOTTI, MARIO CAPPELLINI,
PAOLO PACINI, LUIGI CASTAGNETTA, ADELE
TRAINA, ANTONIO FARRIS, STEFANO IACOBELLI,
GIORGIO MUSTACCHI, ITALO NENCI, ADRIANO
PIFFANELLI, PIERO SISMONDI, CORRADO
DE SANCTIS, MARIO MESITI, LUIGI GALLO,
EUGENIO VILLA, GIUSEPPE SCHIEPPATI, AND
OTHER PARTICIPANTS IN THE GROCTA STUDIES
(SEE APPENDIX)

159

I.	Background	161
II.	GROCTA I Trial: Patients and Methods	162
	A. Clinical Outcome	162
	B. Drug-related Toxicity	164
	C. Clinical Outcome and Menstrual Status	167
	D. Clinical Outcome and the Other Prognostic Factors	167
III.	General Comments and New Generation GROCTA Trials	169
IV.	Conclusions	174
V.	Summary	175
	Appendix	176
	References	177

I. *Background*

Iɴ 1983, a prospective nationwide study was initiated in Italy to establish whether prolonged tamoxifen treatment might represent an alternative to adjuvant chemotherapy in patients with early breast cancer and with estrogen receptor (ER)-positive tumors. At that time, chemotherapy was the chosen treatment for all patients with node-positive tumors (Henderson and Canellos 1980), although some concern about its possible role in postmenopausal women also arose in our country (Bonadonna et al. 1982). In fact, the benefit achieved by this treatment modality appeared to be limited to premenopausal patients—in particular, to those at a lower risk of relapse (Bonadonna et al. 1982). Why chemotherapy was effective in younger women only was not clear, although most investigators believed that the benefit achieved in this group of patients was strictly related to the ovarian suppression chemotherapy induces in 50–80% of them (Pourquier 1981).

Meanwhile, the early results of the first tamoxifen trials provided evidence that tamoxifen might represent a safe alternative to chemotherapy, especially in postmenopausal women (NATO 1983; Baum et al. 1983; Rose et al. 1983), in whom it was found not only to prolong time to recurrence but also to improve patient survival.

Such considerations provided us with the rationale to plan a prospective comparison between chemotherapy and tamoxifen treatment. Patients with ER-positive tumors appeared to be specifically suited for such a comparison, even from an ethical point of view, for several reasons: (1) they are the patients who can benefit most from endocrine therapy; (2) in metastatic disease, the benefit obtained in these patients from hormonal therapy is at least as great as that attainable with chemotherapy (Patterson 1982); (3) the fallout from biological and clinical trials suggests that estrogen receptor–positive patients might have a more indolent disease and, therefore, a better prognosis (Silvestrini et al. 1979). Moreover, because some synergistic or at least subadditive effects between chemotherapy and endocrine therapy have emerged from *in vitro* and *in vivo* studies (Stoll 1981; Boccardo 1984), a third arm based on the combination of tamoxifen and chemotherapy was also added, with the aim to investigate the ameliorative potential of a combined therapy with respect to both tamoxifen and chemotherapy alone.

II. GROCTA I Trial: Patients and Methods

Details on patient eligibility, treatment of primary tumor, allocated treatments after surgery, hormonal receptor assay, method of randomization, statistical procedures, and follow-up studies have been described elsewhere (Boccardo et al. 1990). In brief, 504 evaluable patients aged 35–65 years with node-positive, estrogen receptor–positive (≥10 fmol/mg protein) tumors were entered in the trial. Within 6 weeks from surgery, patients were randomized to receive: tamoxifen, 30 mg daily for 5 years (group T); 6 cycles of CMF (cyclophosphamide, 500 mg/sm, methotrexate 40 mg/sm, and 5-fluorouracil, 600 mg/sm) followed by 4 cycles of epidoxorubicin (75 mg/sm) (group CT); or the combination of both treatments (group CTT). All cytotoxic drugs were administered intravenously on day 1 every 3 weeks.

Prolonged tamoxifen treatment (i.e., 5 years) was selected on the basis of its suppressive action on tumor cell proliferation (Furr and Jordan 1984) and of the pioneering work by some leading investigators on animal models (Jordan 1978) and in humans (Tormey and Jordan 1984), indicating the feasibility and the superiority of prolonged or indefinite treatment with the antiestrogen. The cytotoxic schema was derived from a similar chemotherapeutic regimen developed at the Tumor Institute in Milan (Bonadonna et al. 1982). Epidoxorubicin was utilized instead of adriamycin in view of the equivalent activity shown in advanced disease and its lower cardiotoxicity (Jain et al. 1985), which rendered its use more appropriate in the adjuvant setting. Vincristine was deleted from the original Milan regimen because of its limited value in contributing to adriamycin efficacy as demonstrated in metastatic disease (Minton et al. 1980).

Main patient characteristics have been described in detail elsewhere (Boccardo et al. 1990; Boccardo et al. 1992) and are summarized in Table 8.1.

A. Clinical Outcome

Treatment results, at a median follow-up in excess of 60 months (range 42–92 months), are summarized in Tables 8.2 and 8.3. Overall, the best results have been obtained in patients receiving combined therapy, and the worst in those treated with chemotherapy alone. However, in no patient subset was the combined treatment significantly superior to tamoxifen alone. This was particularly true in postmenopausal women, especially when the duration of overall survival was the end point considered for statistical analysis. The concurrent use of tamoxifen and chemotherapy yielded an additional

Table 8.1. Distribution of study patients, by main characteristics and treatment

	T		CT		CTT	
	n	%	n	%	n	%
Total evaluable	168		165		171	
Menopausal status						
Premenopausal	79	47.1	81	49.1	77	45.1
Postmenopausal	89	52.9	84	50.9	94	54.9
Treatment of primary						
Surgery	140	83.3	134	81.2	139	81.3
Surgery + radiotherapy	28	16.7	31	18.8	32	18.7
Tumor size						
pT1	60	35.7	61	36.9	63	36.8
pT2	97	57.7	92	55.8	101	59.1
pT3	8	4.8	9	5.5	6	3.5
pT4	3	1.8	2	1.2	1	0.6
unknown	—	—	1	0.6	—	—
Nodal status						
≤3	96	57.1	88	53.3	106	61.9
>3	72	42.9	77	46.7	65	38.1
ER status						
10–29 fmol/mg prot.	49	29.1	49	29.7	47	27.5
30–100 fmol/mg prot.	73	43.5	57	34.5	69	40.4
>100 fmol/mg prot.	46	27.4	59	35.8	55	32.1

T = tamoxifen; CT = chemotherapy; CTT = chemotherapy plus tamoxifen

benefit with respect to tamoxifen alone in prolonging time to recurrence. However, as is shown in Table 8.4, such benefit was related to the major effectiveness of combined treatment in preventing locoregional relapses. This effect was evident both in pre- and postmenopausal women (data not shown). Although the number of events to have occurred so far is still limited, some interesting findings emerged from the analysis of the annual odds of recurrence or death of tamoxifen-treated patients and of those receiving combined treatment (Fig. 8.1).

The protective effect of tamoxifen with respect to death increased with time in both pre- and postmenopausal patients. In this regard, the concurrent use of chemotherapy provided some additional benefit only in the first 2–3 years after surgery. The analysis of the odds of recurrence disclosed some differences in the protective effect of tamoxifen in postmenopausal and in premenopausal patients. In fact, in older women, the protective effect of the antiestrogen on the annual risk of relapse was similar to that exerted on the risk of death. By contrast, premenopausal patients treated with tamoxifen alone appeared to show an excess of recurrences in the first year, although the

Table 8.2. Analysis of all events, overall and by menopausal and nodal status

	Number of patients	Number of events	Ratio of observed to expected events	p	Pairwise p
All patients					
T	168	63	0.89		0.002[a]
CT	165	90	1.49	0.000	0.23[b]
CTT	171	57	0.72		0.000[c]
Premenopausal					
T	79	30	0.96		0.31[a]
CT	81	39	1.25	0.19	0.5[b]
CTT	77	26	0.79		0.07[c]
Postmenopausal					
T	89	33	0.84		0.0006[a]
CT	84	51	1.8	0.000	0.27[b]
CTT	94	31	0.65		0.000[c]
Nodes ≤3					
T	96	23	0.84		0.015[a]
CT	88	35	1.58	0.0058	0.71[b]
CTT	106	25	0.76		0.0037[c]
Nodes >3					
T	72	40	0.92		0.0068[a]
CT	77	55	1.36	0.015	0.36[b]
CTT	65	32	0.74		0.0046[c]

T = tamoxifen; CT = chemotherapy; CTT = chemotherapy plus tamoxifen
[a]T vs CT
[b]T vs CTT
[c]CT vs CTT

absolute relapse rate was very low (three recurring patients in the tamoxifen arm versus no patients in the chemotherapy arm). Furthermore, a second peak of risk was observed in the third year of treatment. It is interesting to note that the concurrent use of chemotherapy appeared to decrease both peaks of risk.

B. Drug-Related Toxicity

Toxic effects induced by prolonged tamoxifen treatment were extremely mild, as was expected. About 20% of patients experienced a transient nausea of some degree during the first weeks of treatment, and another 20% suffered from weight increase. The more disturbing symptoms were hot flashes and spotting, which developed in 40% and 24% of patients, respectively. These symptoms, however, did not require any treatment discontinuation. Overall, tamoxifen-induced side effects were strikingly fewer and less serious than

Table 8.3. Analysis of all deaths, overall and by menopausal and nodal status

	Number	Number	Ratio of observed to expected	p	Pairwise
All patients					
T	168	40	0.81		0.0008[a]
CT	165	67	1.57	0.000	0.56[b]
CTT	171	37	0.71		0.000[c]
Premenopausal					
T	79	19	0.93		0.21[a]
CT	81	27	1.35	0.11	0.42[b]
CTT	77	14	0.71		0.045[c]
Postmenopausal					
T	89	21	0.72		0.0004[a]
CT	84	40	1.82	0.000	0.96[b]
CTT	94	23	0.71		0.0001[c]
Nodes ≤3					
T	96	11	0.64		0.012[a]
CT	88	22	1.59	0.026	0.42[b]
CTT	106	17	0.88		0.07[c]
Nodes >3					
T	72	29	0.88		0.028[a]
CT	77	45	1.48	0.0037	0.31[b]
CTT	65	20	0.65		0.0015[c]

T = tamoxifen; CT = chemotherapy; CTT = chemotherapy plus tamoxifen
[a]T vs CT
[b]T vs CTT
[c]CT vs CTT

those produced by chemotherapy, particularly with respect to gastrointestinal and myeloid toxicity.

It is noteworthy that 66% of premenopausal patients developed persistent amenorrhea during tamoxifen treatment as compared with 64% and 66%, respectively, of those receiving chemotherapy or concurrent chemotherapy-tamoxifen treatment. However, this did not prevent the development of gynecological disease, including uterine fibroids, the incidence being significantly higher than in premenopausal patients treated with tamoxifen alone (Table 8.5). This and the fact that the occurrence of gynecological diseases was instead prevented by the concurrent use of chemotherapy stress the different mechanisms involved in the development of amenorrhea in patients receiving chemotherapy or tamoxifen. As Table 8.5 shows, no extra increase in the incidence of endometrial carcinoma has occurred so far in postmenopausal women receiving tamoxifen or concurrent tamoxifen-chemotherapy treatment.

Table 8.4. Number of patients with recurrence according to sites of relapse

	Treatment arm		
Site of relapse	T	CT	CTT
Second malignancy	1	2	2
Contralateral breast	—	4	1
Locoregional[a]	20	22	8
Distant[b]	34	49	37
Locoregional and distant[b]	7	8	7
Dead without cancer	1	5	2
Total	63	90	57

T = tamoxifen; CT = chemotherapy; CTT = chemotherapy plus tamoxifen
[a]T vs CT: $p = 0.82$; T vs CTT: $p = 0.026$; CT vs CTT: $p = 0.0095$
[b]T vs CT: $p = 0.056$; T vs CTT: $p = 0.87$; CT vs CTT: $p = 0.1$

Postmenopausal

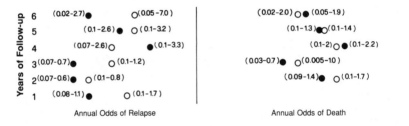

Premenopausal

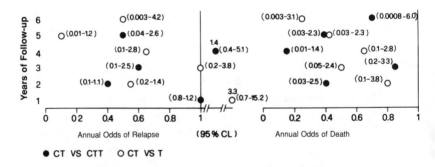

● CT VS CTT   ○ CT VS T

Figure 8.1. Annual odds of relapse and death according to menopausal status.

Table 8.5. Incidence of gynecological disease, by menopausal status and allocated treatment

	T (n = 168)	CT (n = 165)	CTT (n = 171)
Premenopausal patients			
Uterine fibroids[a]	14/79	2/81	1/77
Ovarian cysts[a]	3/79	—	—
Endometrial hyperplasia	1/79	1/81	—
Postmenopausal patients			
Uterine fibroids	1/89	1/84	3/94
Ovarian cysts	—	—	—
Endometrial hyperplasia	—	—	1/94
Endometrial cancer	—	—	1/94

Note: Data are arranged as: number of events/number of patients.
T = tamoxifen; CT = chemotherapy; CTT = chemotherapy plus tamoxifen
[a]T vs CT vs CTT: $p = 0.0000$

C. Clinical Outcome and Menstrual Status

Table 8.6 shows that actual menstrual status, as defined on the basis of the time elapsed since the last menstrual cycle both at the beginning of the study and during the treatment, was not able to affect the response to tamoxifen. By contrast, actual menstrual status was shown to influence the responsiveness to chemotherapy of our patients. The details of this analysis have been previously reported (Rubagotti et al. 1990). It is interesting to note also how, in patients receiving chemotherapy alone, the longer the time elapsed since the last menstrual period, the worse the results obtained with chemotherapy.

D. Clinical Outcome and the Other Prognostic Factors

In addition to menstrual status, other variables have been included in a multivariate analysis to investigate the predictive value of any single factor, both overall and within each treatment arm.

In particular, the purpose was to assess whether progesterone receptor (PgR) assay might be of additional value in predicting the response to adjuvant tamoxifen treatment. This could be expected on the basis of a biological premise, because PgR synthesis occurs in tumors with "functioning" estrogen receptors only. Table 8.7 clearly shows that overall PgR concentration was a strong predictor of clinical outcome. However, it was not predictive of response to tamoxifen treatment, and surprisingly it did predict the response to chemotherapy or combined chemotamoxifen treatment.

Table 8.6. Distribution of events (relapses and/or death), by treatment and menstrual status

Menstrual status	Number of patients	Number of events	Expected number of events	Ratio of observed to expected events	p
T treatment arm					
PM	89	21	22.0	0.95	
AM	25	5	6.7	0.75	0.50
PA	48	15	12.3	1.22	
CT treatment arm					
PM	84	41	22.9	1.37	
AM	20	4	9.6	0.42	0.012
PA	56	19	24.5	0.77	
CTT treatment arm					
PM	94	20	19.8	1.01	
AM	18	2	2.7	0.73	0.89
PA	56	12	11.5	1.05	

T = tamoxifen; CT ≐ chemotherapy; CTT = chemotherapy plus tamoxifen
PM = postmenopausal patients; AM = actively menstruating patients; PA = patients with persistent drug-induced amenorrhea

Table 8.7. Results achieved, by multivariate analysis in each treatment arm

Variable	T		CT		CTT	
	RR (95% CI)	p	RR (95% CI)	p	RR (95% CI)	p
Menopausal status		0.97		0.78		0.69
Pre	1		1		1	
Post	1.2 (0.7–2.3)		1.4 (0.8–2.3)		1.1 (0.5–2.1)	
Nodal status		0.001		0.000		0.004
1–3	1		1		1	
>3	3.5 (2.1–6.1)		2.3 (1.5–3.7)		3.4 (1.8–6.6)	
PgR		0.11		0.015		0.019
≤30 fmol/mg	1		1		1	
>30 fmol/mg	1.1 (0.6–2.0)		0.5 (0.3–1.2)		0.7 (0.4–1.3)	
ER		0.10		0.17		0.99
≤100 fmol/mg	1		1		1	
>100 fmol/mg	0.6 (0.3–1.2)		1.3 (0.8–2.2)		1.1 (0.5–2.2)	

T = tamoxifen; CT = chemotherapy; CTT = chemotherapy plus tamoxifen
RR = relative risk

III. General Comments and New Generation GROCTA Trials

Specific comments to our findings have been previously reported in detail (Boccardo et al. 1990; Boccardo et al. 1992; Rubagotti et al. 1990). Here, we will discuss whether and how our findings do agree with those that emerged from two major events which have contributed to the present state of the art in adjuvant therapy for early breast cancer, i.e., the NIH Consensus Conference (Breast Cancer Chemotherapy Consensus Conference 1985) and the Early Breast Cancer Trialists' Collaborative Group (EBCTCG) metanalysis of adjuvant trials (Early Breast Cancer Trialists' Collaborative Group 1992). In addition, we will discuss how the conclusions from these overviews and our findings have contributed to generating new GROCTA trials.

The EBCTCG metanalysis has clearly shown that the effectiveness of chemotherapy was strictly related to patient age, although some benefit in elderly patients was apparent at the 10-year analysis. In particular, the benefit produced by chemotherapy in patients aged 50 or older was about half of that yielded by tamoxifen. Indeed, looking at the behaviors of control patients in chemotherapy and tamoxifen trials, it was clear that patients who were recruited in the former trials probably had a more aggressive disease. Therefore, the indirect comparison between the overall results achieved in chemotherapy and tamoxifen trials warrants caution. Nevertheless, 1985 Consensus Conference panelists identified tamoxifen as the therapy of choice for postmenopausal breast cancer patients with node-positive and ER-positive tumors. This mainly inductive conclusion seems now to be strengthened by the results of the GROCTA I study, in which the difference between tamoxifen treatment and chemotherapy in postmenopausal patients was strikingly in favor of women treated with tamoxifen, irrespective of the end point chosen for statistical analysis. The results, both from the 10-year metanalysis (Early Breast Cancer Trialists' Collaborative Group 1992) and from two recently published individual trials (Fisher et al. 1990; Pearson et al. 1989), seem to suggest that the addition of chemotherapy to tamoxifen can further improve the therapeutic potential of antiestrogenic therapy in postmenopausal women. These findings are in contrast with our own, because in the GROCTA I study no difference at all was evident between the survival of patients receiving concurrent tamoxifen-chemotherapy treatment and that of patients treated with tamoxifen alone. Our personal belief is that the GROCTA findings are probably more reliable in this regard, although they have been achieved in a relatively small number of patients. In fact, in our opinion, the conclusions of metanalysis on chemohormonal therapy trials are somewhat flawed by two important points: (1) the great majority of the studies included in the metanalysis had recruited women without taking into proper account the receptor status of the disease; (2) most women had received tamoxifen for 1 or 2 years only, i.e., probably for an inadequate period of time. A similar selection bias might have invalidated the results both of the National Surgical Breast and Bowel Project B16 (Fisher et al. 1990) and of the Case Western Reserve University trial (Pearson et al. 1989). In the former study, at least 20% of the patients arbitrarily defined as "tamoxifen-responsive" had ER-negative tumors, and therefore very little chance of benefiting from tamoxifen treatment. Moreover, the superiority of chemohormonal therapy was proved only for one of the three chemotherapeutic regimens initially scheduled. The small study by Pearson and co-workers (1989) again included a proportion of women scarcely responsive to tamoxifen, because these investigators adopted an inadequate cutoff to define ER assay positivity. Therefore, we believe that tamoxifen should remain the treatment of choice for postmenopausal women with ER-positive tumors, keeping in mind that this therapy might not represent the best one for all postmenopausal patients and that the use of chemotamoxifen therapy might be worthwhile in some subgroups.

In fact, our study has shown a trend favoring chemotamoxifen treatment in patients with four or more involved nodes. It also has shown that the combined treatment was more effective in preventing locoregional relapses. Therefore, the concurrent use of tamoxifen and chemotherapy might be considered for patients with more advanced disease (i.e., those with four or more involved nodes), or for women more prone to local relapse (i.e., patients with very large primaries or with skin infiltration), or, in any case, for patients with more aggressive disease. In fact, patients with poorly differentiated or highly proliferating tumors have shown to derive limited benefit from tamoxifen treatment alone (NATO 1988; Paradiso et al. 1990).

The addition of chemotherapy to tamoxifen, while probably being more suitable for patients at higher risk of relapse, cannot interfere with the development of tamoxifen-resistant clones. A growing amount of experimental evidence suggests that adaptation phenomena (King and Dabre 1989) do intervene in the first steps of tumor progression and that mutational events can enhance the intrinsic susceptibility of breast cancer cells to the estrogenic action of tamoxifen (Jiang and Jordan 1992). The "early" use (i.e., before the development of clinical failure) of a second-line hormonal therapy different from tamoxifen should therefore help in circumventing tamoxifen failure in a certain proportion of patients. This hypothesis is being prospectively tested in the GROCTA IV trial, whose design is shown in Table 8.8, in which all new generation GROCTA trials are summarized.

GROCTA IV is recruiting postmenopausal patients with ER-positive tumors and giving them tamoxifen for 3 years. Patients are then randomized either to continue on tamoxifen treatment for a further 2 years or to be alternatively switched to 2 years of low-dose aminoglutethimide. About 300 patients have so far been recruited in the trial.

The 1985 Consensus Conference has left unresolved the issue about the more appropriate management of postmenopausal patients with ER-negative tumors. Indeed, the metanalysis results and those retrospectively achieved in individual trials have shown that the therapeutic effectiveness of tamoxifen in this group of patients is not so closely related to the positivity of ER assay as might be expected (NATO 1988; Breast Cancer Trials Committee 1987).

In fact, *in vitro* studies suggest that tamoxifen should be regarded as a "growth factor modulator" rather than as an antiestrogen. However, the low activity of tamoxifen in ER-negative tumors does not imply that anti-estrogenic treatment should be preferred to chemotherapy in this subgroup of patients. This issue is still open, because so far no trial has prospectively compared the value of tamoxifen and chemotherapy in postmenopausal women with ER-negative tumors.

This issue is being addressed by the GROCTA V study (Table 8.8), in which patients are randomly allocated to receive either tamoxifen or tamoxifen plus chemotherapy. Unfortunately, it can be expected that the comparison between tamoxifen and chemotherapy plus tamoxifen in this subgroup of patients will probably represent a "poor man's war." However, the need for chemotherapy in this group of women is worth being prospectively investigated, considering that it will certainly produce more toxicity.

Metanalysis results have shown that the protective effect exerted by tamoxifen in premenopausal women is very low, if any. These results have probably forced NIH Consensus Conference panelists to exclude hormono-therapy from the therapeutic armamentarium in premenopausal women. However, it should be taken into account that metanalysis results might have been flawed by the methodology followed in putting trials together. In fact, metanalysis included both trials comparing the value of tamoxifen with nil (or placebo) and trials comparing the effectiveness of tamoxifen plus chemo-therapy with chemotherapy alone. Indeed, the trials of the latter type were the majority, and certainly the baseline use of chemotherapy might have diluted the benefit produced by tamoxifen. This interpretation is confirmed if we

Table 8.8. New generation GROCTA trials

GROCTA II trial

Pre-perimenopausal patients, with ER-positive, node-positive, or high-risk negative tumors

R
A ————————→ classic CMF (for 6 cycles)
N
D
O ————————→ tamoxifen (for 5 years) + goserelin depot
M

GROCTA III trial

Pre-perimenopausal patients, with ER-negative, node-positive, or high-risk negative tumors

R
A ————————→ classic CMF (for 6 cycles)
N
D
O ————————→ classic CMF (2 cycles) followed by epidoxorubicin + vincristine
M   (2 cycles) and mitomycin C + vindesin (2 cycles)

GROCTA IV trial

Postmenopausal patients, with ER-positive/unknown, node-positive, or high-risk negative tumors

REGISTRATION: tamoxifen for 3 years, then

R
A ————————→ tamoxifen for 2 years
N
D
O ————————→ "low dose" aminoglutethimide for 2 years
M

GROCTA V trial

Postmenopausal patients, with ER-negative, node-positive, or high-risk negative tumors

R
A ————————→ tamoxifen for 5 years
N
D
O ————————→ tamoxifen for 5 years + "classic" CMF (6 cycles)
M

observe the results achieved by metanalysis only in trials comparing tamoxifen with nil, or placebo: a protective effect of tamoxifen emerges in women aged less than 50 which is similar to that exerted by this drug in older women. These data are consistent with the results of individual trials, including the first GROCTA study, which have shown that the effectiveness of tamoxifen is not related to age or menopausal status (NATO 1988; Breast Cancer Trials Committee 1987; Fisher et al. 1989).

A few trials have prospectively compared the effectiveness of tamoxifen with that of chemotherapy in premenopausal breast cancer patients. The differences between these trials, which include the GROCTA I trial, have been previously discussed (Boccardo et al. 1990, 1992) and may probably account for the different conclusions they have achieved. GROCTA I trial conclusions do not prove or suggest that tamoxifen treatment should be used instead of chemotherapy in younger women, even if they had ER-positive tumors. However, our results indicate that tamoxifen might represent an alternative or useful complement to chemotherapy in this group of patients. Also, the results of the metanalysis of ovarian ablation trials enforce the concept that hormone therapy should have a role in the management of premenopausal women. Indeed, the preliminary results of a Scottish trial show the similar efficacy of oophorectomy and CMF treatment in premenopausal women (Early Breast Cancer Trialists' Collaborative Group 1992).

Therefore, when we speak of the more appropriate management of premenopausal women, we should not oppose chemotherapy for hormonotherapy, but rather try to identify patients who might be safely managed by hormonotherapy alone. In fact, if we look at the results of the first GROCTA trial, we can see that ER assay, or better yet the cutoff value which is commonly used to define ER-assay positivity, is not as appropriate and predictive of the response to hormonotherapy in premenopausal women as it seems to be in postmenopausal women. Although the overall response to tamoxifen was similar in pre- and postmenopausal women, two peaks of risk in premenopausal patients were evident when we analyzed the annual odds of relapse in younger women. This leads to speculation that a different proportion of premenopausal women with ER-positive tumors might have a more aggressive disease that is not controlled by tamoxifen as it is by chemotherapy. Indeed, the retrospective analysis of the clinical outcome of GROCTA I patients with respect to drug-induced amenorrhea, and, in particular, the fact that patients still actively menstruating have shown a significantly better outcome than postmenopausal women, has led us to hypothesize that a different kinetics of the disease might exist in pre- and postmenopausal women in relation to the modulatory effect of endogenous hormones over the proliferation of the ER-positive clones (Rubagotti et al. 1990). These differences might have also influenced the initial response to tamoxifen as a function of the hyper-estrogenic stimulation which is known to occur in premenopausal women during antiestrogenic treatment (Ravdin et al. 1988) and which is documented in our study by an extra-incidence of gynecological disease. Should this be true, the concurrent use of tamoxifen and oophorectomy could be safer than the use of tamoxifen alone in younger women.

This issue is being addressed by the GROCTA II trial, which is limited to premenopausal women with node-positive (or "high-risk" node-negative), ER-positive tumors. In this trial, women are randomly allocated to receive either chemotherapy or tamoxifen plus goserelin depot (Zoladex). The main goal of this study is to verify whether the use of a more appropriate hormonotherapy might reproduce the results achieved by the first GROCTA trial in a larger series of patients. The classic CMF regimen has been selected for this study in order to render its results more extrapolatory. In fact, the CMF regimen has been identified by Peto's metanalysis as the chemotherapeutic regimen of choice, in that the protective effect exerted by different regimens was no better than that provided by CMF (Early Breast Cancer Trialists' Collaborative Group 1988). In addition, no individual trial has proved so far that the addition or the incorporation of an anthracycline into the original regimen can achieve significantly better results than standard CMF (Armand et al. 1984; Moliterni et al. 1991). The GROCTA II study was initiated in 1990 and so far has recruited 158 patients. Preliminary blind results show that a similar number of events, six and five, respectively, have occurred in each treatment arm, thus confirming that, in this selected group of patients, chemotherapy and hormonotherapy are equivalent.

IV. *Conclusions*

Our findings confirm that prolonged tamoxifen therapy is a safe and effective treatment for patients with early breast cancer, irrespective of menopausal status.

Patients with ER-positive tumors are the best candidates for antiestrogenic treatment. However, the selection criteria to assign patients to hormonotherapy should probably be redefined. This could be achieved both through the adoption of a more appropriate threshold to define ER assay positivity (taking into account that the response to hormonotherapy in the adjuvant setting is not likely to be related to ER content in a linear fashion, as it appears to be in advanced disease) and the use of other discriminants, such as tumor differentiation or proliferative activity. In fact, PgR assay was of no help in predicting the response to hormonotherapy in our study, although this finding should be considered with caution, inasmuch as it comes from a retrospective analysis.

In hormone-responsive patients, the efficacy of tamoxifen might be further increased by the concurrent (or sequential?) use of chemotherapy. However, this approach has proved to be more toxic and should be reserved for patients with more advanced or more aggressive disease.

V. *Summary*

The introduction of adjuvant therapy for early breast cancer has modified the natural history of the disease. The use of adjuvant chemotherapy has prolonged both time to recurrence and survival of premenopausal patients, and tamoxifen has been shown to be the endocrine therapy of choice for postmenopausal women, prolonging both disease-free and overall survival of treated of patients.

These are the conclusions most consistent with the results deriving from the first generation of adjuvant individual studies. The recent findings of both 5- and 10-year metanalysis of adjuvant tamoxifen trials have confirmed that tamoxifen, administered for an appropriate duration (i.e., for 2 or more years), significantly reduces the likelihood of recurrence and death in patients aged 50 or older. However, only indirect comparisons have suggested that tamoxifen might be more effective than chemotherapy in older women and that possibly chemotherapy might be more effective than tamoxifen in younger ones. Unfortunately, very few trials have directly compared these two treatment modalities in each patient subset to draw firm conclusions.

The GROCTA I trial has tested the hypothesis that there could be an additive or synergistic effect of the combination of tamoxifen and chemotherapy, in order to improve patient outcome. The findings from the GROCTA I trial confirm that prolonged tamoxifen is an effective therapy for patients with estrogen receptor–positive tumors, irrespective of menopausal status, thus raising the question whether tamoxifen treatment could be an alternative to chemotherapy in selected premenopausal patients. This issue is under active investigation by the GROCTA II study.

Moreover, the prolonged use of tamoxifen (i.e., for 5 or more years) raises some concern about the development of tamoxifen-resistant clones. The GROCTA IV trial is addressing the question by randomizing postmenopausal patients to be switched to a second-line hormonotherapy other than tamoxifen before the appearance of clinical failure.

The optimal treatment of postmenopausal patients with ER-negative tumors has yet to be defined, but the GROCTA V study is evaluating the effectiveness of tamoxifen compared with tamoxifen plus combination chemotherapy.

The results from the GROCTA I study indicate that the use of concurrent (or sequential?) chemotherapy might benefit some subgroups of patients, such as those with more aggressive or advanced estrogen receptor–positive disease. However, the proper selection of patients who may benefit from combined treatment has yet to be fully defined.

Appendix

Institutions contributing to GROCTA I and new-generation GROCTA trials

INVESTIGATORS	CENTER
Dr. A. Giovaninetti, Dr. E. Piatto	Ospedale Civile, Bollate
Dr. C. Epifani, Dr. G. Scognamiglio	Ospedale S. Anna, Camerlata
Dr. I. Spinelli, Dr. S. Venturini	Ospedale Civile, Carrara
Prof. P. Malacarne, Dr. D. Donati	Arcispedale S. Anna, Ferrara
Prof. M. Cappellini, Dr. P. Pacini	Ospedale Careggi, Firenze
Dr. A. Piano	Casa Sollievo della Sofferenza, S. Giovanni Rotondo
Dr. L. Gallo	Ospedale Galliera, Genova
Dr. E. Rinaldi, Dr. R. Biasioli	Ospedale Civile, Magenta
Dr. F. Smerieri, Dr. M. Pini	Ospedale Civile, Mantova
Dr. V. Visca, Dr. F. Mensi	Ospedale Predabissi, Melegnano
Dr. R. Scappaticci, Dr. A. Silvani	Ospedale Civile, Melzo
Dr. G. P. Benetti, Dr. S. Banducci	Ospedale Civile, Merate
Dr. A. Scanni, Dr. M. Tomirotti	Ospedale Fatebene Fratelli, Milano
Dr. E. Villa, Dr. A. Bolognesi	Istituto Scientifico S. Raffaele, Milano
Prof. G. Palazzotto, Dr. A. DiCarlo, Dr. A. Traina	Ospedale Oncologico M. Ascoli, Palermo
Dr. R. Canaletti, Dr. C. Rodino	Ospedale Civile, Piacenza
Prof. P. Trompeo, Dr. L. Allara	Ospedale Civile, Pinerolo
Dr. M. Marangolo, Dr. G. Cruciani	Ospedale S. Maria delle Croci, Ravenna
Prof. F. Saccani, Dr. M. Sassi	Ospedale S. Maria Nuova, Reggio Emilia
Dr. A. Beni	Ospedale S. Giacomo, Roma
Dr. C. Gatti	Ospedale Civile, S. Remo
Dr. G. Schieppati, Dr. G. Burani	Ospedale Civile, Saronno

INVESTIGATORS	CENTER
Prof. A. Farris	Università Sassari
Dr. L. Galletto	Ospedale Civile, Savigliano
Prof. P. Sismondi, Dr. F. Genta,	Università di Torino
Dr. C. De Sanctis	
Dr. G. Mustacchi, Dr. F. De Lazzer	Centro Tumori, Trieste
Dr. B. Marsilio	Ospedale Civile, Udine
Dr. F. Buzzi, Dr. R. Bartolucci	Ospedale S. Maria, Terni
Prof. M. Mesiti, Dr. F. Delia	Istituto Oncologico, Messina
Dr. M. Svanosio, Dr. F. Rolfo,	Ospedale S. Croce, Moncalieri
Dr. B. Castagna	
Prof. F. D'Addato, Dr. Repinto	Ospedale S. Andrea, Vercelli
Prof. F. Crucitti, Dr. C. Lombardi	Università Cattolica, Roma

References

Armand, J. P., P. Hurteloup, and M. Hayat. 1984. Phase III chemotherapy comparing FAC versus FEC in advanced breast cancer. In *Proceedings of American Society of Clinical Oncology* 3:118.

Baum, M., D. M. Brinkley, J. A. Dossett, K. McPherson, J. S. Patterson, R. D. Rubens, F. G. Smiddy, B. A. Stoll, A. Wilson, J. C. Lea, D. Richards, and S. H. Ellis. 1983. Improved survival among patients treated with adjuvant tamoxifen after mastectomy for early breast cancer. (Letter.) *Lancet* 2:450–452.

Boccardo, F. 1984. Concurrent or sequential tamoxifen/chemotherapy treatment of advanced breast cancer? *Review on Endocrine-related Cancer* 19:23–26.

Boccardo, F., A. Rubagotti, P. Bruzzi, M. Cappellini, G. Isola, I. Nenci, A. Piffanelli, A. Scanni, P. Sismondi, L. Santi, F. Genta, F. Saccani, M. Sassi, P. Malacarne, D. Donati, A. Farris, L. Castagnetta, A. DiCarlo, A. Traina, L. Galletto, F. Smerieri, and F. Buzzi. 1990. Chemotherapy versus tamoxifen versus chemotherapy plus tamoxifen in node-positive, estrogen receptor–positive breast cancer patients: results of a multicentric Italian study. *Journal of Clinical Oncology* 8:1310–1320.

Boccardo, F., A. Rubagotti, D. Amoroso, P. Sismondi, F. Genta, I. Nenci, A. Piffanelli, A. Farris, L. Castagnetta, A. Traina, M. Cappellini, P. Pacini, M. Sassi, P. Malacarne, D. Donati, G. Mustacchi, L. Galletto, G. Schieppati, E. Villa, A. Bolognesi, and L. Gallo. 1992. Chemotherapy versus tamoxifen versus chemotherapy plus tamoxifen in node-positive, estrogen-receptor positive breast cancer patients. An update at 7 years of the first GRO-CTA (Breast Cancer Adjuvant Chemo-hormone Therapy Cooperative Group) trial. *European Journal of Cancer* 28:673–680.

Bonadonna, G., A. Rossi, G. Tancini, C. Brambilla, and P. Valagussa. 1984. Adjuvant chemotherapy trials in resectable breast cancer with positive axillary nodes. The experience of the Milan Cancer Institute. In *Adjuvant therapy of cancer IV*, ed. S. E. Salmon and S. E. Jones, 195–208. New York: Grune and Stratton.

Bonadonna, G., P. Valagussa, A. Rossi, G. Tancini, C. Brambilla, S. Marchini, and U. Veronesi. 1982. Multimodal therapy with CMF in resectable breast cancer with positive axillary nodes. The Milan Institute experience. *Recent Results in Cancer Research* 80:149–156.

Breast Cancer Trials Committee, Scottish Cancer Trials Office. 1987. Adjuvant tamoxifen in the management of operable breast cancer: the Scottish trial. *Lancet* 2:171–175.

Breast Cancer Chemotherapy Consensus Conference. 1985. Adjuvant chemotherapy for breast cancer. *Journal of the American Medical Association* 254:3451–3463.

Early Breast Cancer Trialists' Collaborative Group. 1988. Effects of adjuvant tamoxifen and of cytotoxic therapy on mortality in early breast cancer. An overview of 61 randomized trials among 28,896 women. *New England Journal of Medicine* 319:1681–1692.

Early Breast Cancer Trialists' Collaborative Group. 1992. Systemic treatment of early breast cancer by hormonal, cytotoxic, or immune therapy. 133 randomized trials involving 31,000 recurrences and 24,000 deaths among 75,000 women. *Lancet* 339:1–15 and 71–85.

Fisher, B., J. Costantino, C. Redmond, R. Poisson, D. Bowman, J. Couture, N. V. Dimitrov, N. Wolmark, D. L. Wickerham, E. R. Fisher, R. D. Margolese, C. Sutherland, A. Glass, R. Foster, and R. Caplan. 1989. A randomized clinical trial evaluating tamoxifen in the treatment of patients with node-negative breast cancer who have estrogen-receptor-positive tumors. *New England Journal of Medicine* 320:479–484.

Fisher, B., C. Redmond, S. Legault-Poisson, N. V. Dimitrov, A. M. Brown, D. L. Wickerham, N. Wolmark, R. G. Margolese, D. Bowman, A. G. Glass, C. G. Kardinal, A. Robidoux, P. Jochimsen, W. Cronin, M. Deutsch, E. R. Fisher, D. B. Myers, and J. L. Hoehn. 1990. Postoperative chemotherapy and tamoxifen compared with tamoxifen alone in the treatment of positive-node breast cancer patients aged 50 years and older with tumors responsive to tamoxifen: results from the National Surgical Adjuvant Breast and Bowel Project B-16. *Journal of Clinical Oncology* 8:1005–1018.

Furr, B. J., and V. C. Jordan. 1984. The pharmacology and clinical uses of tamoxifen. *Pharmacology and Therapeutics* 25:127–205.

Goldie, J. H., and A. J. Coldman. 1979. A mathematic model for relating the drug sensitivity of tumors to their spontaneous mutation rate. *Cancer Treatment Reports* 63:1727–1733.

Henderson, I. C., and G. P. Canellos. 1980. Cancer of the breast: the past decade. *New England Journal of Medicine* 302:17–30.

Jain, K. K., E. S. Casper, N. L. Geller, T. B. Hakes, R. J. Kaufman, V. Currie, W. Schwartz, C. Cassidy, G. R. Petroni, C. W. Young, and R. E. Wittes. 1985. A prospective randomized comparison of epirubicin and doxorubicin in patients with advanced breast cancer. *Journal of Clinical Oncology* 3:818–826.

Jordan, V. C. 1978. Use of the DMBA-induced rat mammary carcinoma system for the evaluation of tamoxifen treatment as a potential adjuvant therapy. *Reviews on Endocrine Related Cancer* (October Supplement):49–55.

Jaing, S. Y., and V. C. Jordan. 1992. A molecular strategy to control tamoxifen resistant breast cancer. In *Cancer surveys—Growth regulation of nuclear hormone receptors*, ed. M. G. Parker, 55–70. Long Island, N.Y.: Cold Spring Harbor Laboratory Press.

Jordan, V. C. 1991. Personal communication.

Minton, M. J., S. A. Sexton, B. M. Cantwell, G. E. Sparrow, R. K. Knight, and R. D. Rubens. 1980. Does vincristine contribute to adriamycin in the treatment of advanced breast cancer? In *Proceedings of the American Association for Cancer Research* 21:408.

Moliterni, A., G. Bonadonna, P. Valagussa, L. Ferrari, and M. Zambetti. 1991. Cyclophosphamide, methotrexate, and fluorouracil with and without doxorubicin in the adjuvant treatment of resectable breast cancer with one to three positive axillary nodes. *Journal of Clinical Oncology* 9:1124–1130.

Nolvadex Adjuvant Trial Organisation (NATO). 1983. Controlled trial of tamoxifen as adjuvant agent in the management of early breast cancer. Interim analysis at four years. *Lancet* 1:257–261.

Nolvadex Adjuvant Trial Organisation (NATO). 1988. Controlled trial of tamoxifen as a single adjuvant agent in the management of early breast cancer. Analysis at eight years. *British Journal of Cancer* 57:608–611.

Paradiso, A., S. Tommasi, A. Mangia, V. Lorusso, G. Simone, and M. De Lena. 1990. Tumor-proliferative activity, progesterone receptor status, estrogen receptor level, and clinical outcome of estrogen receptor positive advanced breast cancer. *Cancer Research* 50:2958–2962.

Patterson, J. S., L. A. Battersby, and D. G. Edwards. 1982. Review of the clinical pharmacology and international experience with tamoxifen in advanced breast cancer. In *The role of tamoxifen in breast cancer,* ed. S. Iacobelli, M. E. Lippman, and G. Robustelli Della Cuna, 17–33. New York: Raven Press.

King, R. J. B., and P. D. Dabre. 1989. Progression from steroid responsive to unresponsive state in breast cancer. In *Endocrine therapy of breast cancer,* vol. 3, ed. F. Cavalli, 4–15. Berlin: Springer-Verlag.

Pearson, O. H., C. A. Hubay, N. H. Gordon, J. S. Marshall, J. P. Crowe, B. M. Arafah, and W. McGuire. 1989. Endocrine versus endocrine plus five-drug chemotherapy in postmenopausal women with stage II estrogen receptor–positive breast cancer. *Cancer* 64:1819–1823.

Pourquier, H. 1981. The results of adjuvant chemotherapy are predominantly caused by the hormonal changes such therapy induces. In favor. In *Medical oncology controversies in cancer treatment,* ed. M. B. Van Scoy-Mosher, 83–99. Boston: G. K. Hall and Company.

Ravdin, P. M., N. F. Fritz, D. C. Tormey, and V. C. Jordan. 1988. Endocrine status of premeno-pausal node-positive breast cancer patients following adjuvant chemotherapy and long-term tamoxifen. *Cancer Research* 48:1026–1029.

Rose, C., S. M. Thorpe, H. T. Mouridsen, J. A. Andersen, H. Brincker, and K. W. Andersen. 1983. Antiestrogen treatment of postmenopausal women with primary high risk breast cancer. *Breast Cancer Research and Treatment* 3:77–84.

Rubagotti, A., F. Boccardo, P. Sismondi, F. Genta, M. Sassi, P. Malacarne, A. Farris, A. Traina, F. Buzzi, G. Mustacchi, and G. Schieppati for the Italian Cooperative Group for Adjuvant Chemohormono Therapy of Early Breast Cancer (GROCTA). 1990. Effect of menstrual status on response to adjuvant chemotherapy and/or endocrine therapy. In *Adjuvant therapy of cancer,* vol. 6, ed. S. E. Salmon, 349–356. Philadelphia: Saunders Company.

Silvestrini, R., M. G. Daidone, and G. Di Fronzo. 1979. Relationship between proliferative activity and estrogen receptors in breast cancer. *Cancer* 44:665–670.

Stewart, H. J., for the Scottish Cancer Trials and the Guy's (ICRF) Breast Groups. 1991. Oophorectomy versus chemotherapy (CMF) in premenopausal node positive breast cancer. Programme and Abstract Book, *5th EORTC Breast Cancer Working Conference,* September 3–6, Pauscollege Leuven, Belgium, A 116.

Stoll, B. A. 1981. Recent developments in the hormonal therapy of metastatic breast cancer. *Review in Endocrine-related cancer* 9:391–398.

Tormey, D. C., and V. C. Jordan. 1984. Long-term tamoxifen adjuvant therapy in node-positive breast cancer: a metabolic and pilot clinical study. *Breast Cancer Research and Treatment* 4:297–302.

9

Interactions of Tamoxifen with Cytotoxic Chemotherapy for Breast Cancer

C. K. OSBORNE

I. INTRODUCTION   182
II. CELLULAR EFFECTS OF TAMOXIFEN   182
III. INTERACTIONS OF TAMOXIFEN WITH SPECIFIC CYTOTOXIC DRUGS   184
    A. ALKYLATING AGENTS   184
    B. ANTIMETABOLITES   192
    C. DOXORUBICIN   193
IV. DISCUSSION   194
    REFERENCES   196

I. *Introduction*

Tamoxifen is the most widely used drug in breast cancer management today. It is taken by thousands of women worldwide to delay recurrence and prolong survival following local therapy of primary breast cancer, and for palliation of those with metastatic disease. Although the drug has a variety of effects on tumor cells, the dominant antitumor activity is mediated by competitive blockade of estrogen receptors (ER).

Used as a single agent, tamoxifen therapy results in a 20% proportional reduction in early mortality in the adjuvant setting (Early Breast Cancer Trialists' Collaborative Group 1992). The greatest benefit is in patients with ER-positive tumors. In metastatic receptor-positive breast cancer, about 50% of patients attain temporary remissions lasting 9–18 months (Saez and Osborne 1989). In an attempt to improve therapeutic results, tamoxifen has been combined with cytotoxic chemotherapy. Clinical trials of chemo-endocrine treatment, however, have been disappointing. With some exceptions, the addition of tamoxifen to combination chemotherapy regimens has resulted in little or no survival benefit compared with the sequential use of the two modalities either in patients with advanced breast cancer or in those with primary disease (Early Breast Cancer Trialists' Collaborative Group 1992; Lippman 1983). An adverse effect of the addition of tamoxifen to melphalan and 5-fluorouracil was seen in several patient subsets in a National Surgical Adjuvant Breast and Bowel Project (NSABP) trial (Fisher et al. 1986). These clinical studies suggest the possibility that tamoxifen could interact antagonistically with certain cytotoxic drugs. In this chapter biochemical mechanisms by which tamoxifen could interact with cytotoxic agents and preclinical data from experimental models demonstrating important drug interactions will be reviewed, focusing on data from our own laboratory.

II. *Cellular Effects of Tamoxifen*

A myriad of cellular effects that potentially could alter sensitivity to cytotoxic drugs are observed when tamoxifen is incubated with cultured breast cancer cells (Fig. 9.1). In cells containing ER, tamoxifen binds to the hormone-binding domain of the receptor, blocks the binding of estrogen, and inhibits

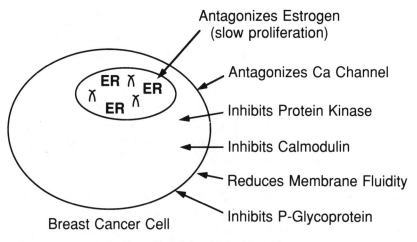

Figure 9.1. Cellular effects of tamoxifen.

cell proliferation. Cell cycle kinetic studies have shown that a major effect of tamoxifen is to slow cell cycle transit reversibly by delaying progression through the G_1 phase (Osborne et al. 1983; Osborne et al. 1984; Taylor et al. 1983). After several days of incubation with clinically relevant concentrations of tamoxifen (≤ 1 μM), cells accumulate in G_1 phase at the expense of S and $G_2 M$ phases, conceivably rendering them less vulnerable to S-phase specific cytotoxic agents. This "cytostatic" effect is reversible with estrogen replenishment, resulting in a synchronous wave of cells progressing through G_1 phase and entering S phase (Osborne et al. 1984).

Data from an *in vivo* model lend support to the idea that the predominant antitumor effect of tamoxifen is cytostatic rather than cytocidal. Tamoxifen treatment of castrated nude mice inhibits tumorigenesis of MCF-7 breast cancer cells inoculated subcutaneously. This effect is not lethal to all cells, however, because subsequent estrogen treatment given months later can induce the cells to proliferate and form tumors. Furthermore, tamoxifen treatment of mice with established tumors results in a stabilization or only slight reduction in tumor size but not in significant tumor regression (Osborne et al. 1985; Osborne et al. 1987). Tumors from treated mice appear viable histologically, but they do have a reduced mitotic rate. Clonogenicity of these tumor cells in soft agar is maintained, and tumor growth can be restored when mice are retreated with estrogen, indicating continued viability despite long-term tamoxifen treatment. Neither cultured breast cancer cells nor tumors from nude mice treated with tamoxifen show the "ladder" effect of sheared DNA in agarose gels that is observed with glucocorticoid treatment of lymphocytes (unpublished observation). Other studies have shown some evidence both *in vitro* and *in vivo* of a cytotoxic effect of tamoxifen (Barden et al. 1987; Brünner et al. 1989), but the cumulative data suggest that the dominant antitumor effect is a slowing of cell proliferation that could theoretically antagonize cell cycle–dependent drugs.

Tamoxifen has other biochemical effects on cells that could influence drug cytotoxicity. The drug inhibits calcium-dependent cellular processes. It antagonizes calmodulin- and phospholipid-activated protein kinase, and it is an effective calcium channel antagonist—effects that could alter drug uptake (Greenberg et al. 1987; Lam 1984; Su et al. 1985). Protein kinase C is inhibited by tamoxifen, albeit at suprapharmacological concentrations, in breast cancer as well as nonbreast cancer tissue, apparently via non-ER-mediated mechanisms (O'Brian et al. 1986). It has also been suggested that lipophilic tricyclic triparanol analogues including tamoxifen can interact with the cell membrane lipid domain, thereby altering packing density and, secondarily, diffusion rates of certain drugs (Ramu et al. 1984). High concentrations of tamoxifen have been shown to reduce fluidity of cell membranes derived from both ER-positive and ER-negative breast cancer cell lines (Clarke et al. 1990). Very high concentrations of tamoxifen (≥ 10 μM) can reverse the multidrug-resistant (MDR) phenotype presumably through an interaction with the membrane-associated P-glycoprotein efflux pump (Berman et al. 1991). Finally, tamoxifen has also been shown to be an inhibitor of the P-450 system, which could influence metabolism or activation of certain drugs (Reidy and Murray 1989)

III. *Interactions of Tamoxifen with Specific Cytotoxic Drugs*

A. ALKYLATING AGENTS

1. Melphalan

We have evaluated the effects of the coadministration of tamoxifen with the alkylating agent melphalan on the cytotoxicity of human breast cancer cells by examining dose-survival curves of these agents used alone or in combination in the ER-positive MCF-7 breast cancer cell line in a colony-forming assay (Osborne et al. 1989). In initial experiments, the effect of a 72-hour preincubation of tamoxifen on melphalan cytotoxicity was examined. We have previously shown that under these conditions, tamoxifen induces a G_1 block, resulting in a marked reduction in the percentage of S-phase cells (Osborne et al. 1983). Dose-survival curves for cells treated with melphalan

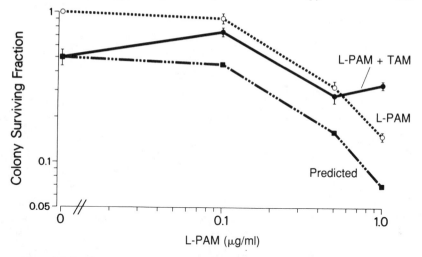

Figure 9.2. Dose-survival curves of melphalan (L-PAM) for 1 hr without or with tamoxifen (1 μM, 72-hr preincubation) in MCF-7 cells. (Reprinted from Osborne et al. 1989, with permission from W. B. Saunders Company.)

alone, or with melphalan and a clinically relevant tamoxifen concentration (1 μM), were compared with a theoretical predicted curve assuming an additive interaction (Fig. 9.2). Predicted values were obtained by finding the product of the actual colony surviving fractions (SFs) observed with each drug used alone ($SF_A \times SF_B$). A dose-response effect on colony survival of MCF-7 cells was evident with melphalan concentrations between 0.1 and 1.0 μg/ml. The colony surviving fraction of cells treated with tamoxifen alone was 0.5. Colony survival with melphalan plus tamoxifen was consistently greater than that predicted for an additive effect. At the highest melphalan concentration, more colonies survived treatment with the combination (SF = 0.33) than with melphalan alone (SF = 0.15). Thus, the addition of a clinically relevant concentration of tamoxifen to melphalan was significantly antagonistic in this model system.

Figure 9.3 shows a reciprocal experiment in which the effect of the tamoxifen concentration without or with a single dose of melphalan (0.5 μg/ml) was examined. The 72-hour preincubation with tamoxifen alone reduced the SF in a dose-response fashion with an SF of 0.21 observed at a concentration of 1 μM in this experiment. The SF observed with melphalan alone was 0.3. When the cells were treated with a combination of the two drugs, the dose-survival curve was consistently above that predicted for an additive effect, and more colonies actually survived with the drug combination than with

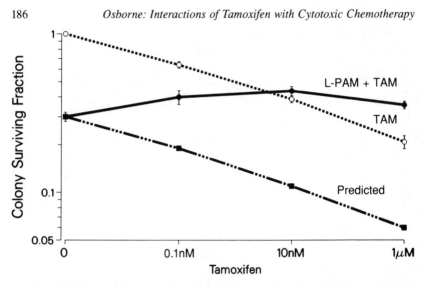

Figure 9.3. Dose-survival curves of tamoxifen (72 hrs) without or with melphalan (L-PAM, 0.5 μg/ml) in MCF-7 cells. (Reprinted from Osborne et al. 1989, with permission from W. B. Saunders Company.)

melphalan alone, again demonstrating an antagonistic interaction even with very low tamoxifen concentrations (0.1 nM). In all these experiments, the cells were first incubated with tamoxifen for 72 hours, and melphalan was added for the final hour, prior to plating in the cloning assay.

Other Antiestrogens

To determine whether the antagonism observed in the above experiments was specific for tamoxifen, we examined several other triphenylethylene antiestrogens (Osborne et al. 1989). The antagonistic interaction with melphalan was observed with all these antiestrogens (Table 9.1). Toremifene, LY 156758, and nafoxidine, as well as tamoxifen, significantly inhibited colony survival when used alone, although to a variable degree. However, when these antiestrogens were combined with melphalan, the observed SF in each case was greater than that predicted for an additive effect. Furthermore, the actual number of colonies surviving with the antiestrogen-melphalan combinations was greater than that seen with melphalan alone, a clearly antagonistic interaction.

Duration of Tamoxifen Treatment

We have previously shown that the 72-hour preincubation with tamoxifen used in the above experiments results in an accumulation of cells in the G_1 phase prior to melphalan treatment (Osborne et al. 1983). To assess whether this G_1 arrest is necessary for the antagonistic effect, MCF-7 cells were

Table 9.1. Effect of antiestrogens on melphalan cytotoxicity in MCF-7 cells

| Group[a] | Colony number ± SE | Surviving fraction | |
		Observed	Predicted
Controls	150 ± 4	—	—
L-PAM	66 ± 3	0.44	—
TAM	79 ± 2	0.52	—
+ L-PAM	106 ± 5	0.71	0.23
LY 156758	86 ± 4	0.57	—
+ L-PAM	101 ± 3	0.67	0.25
Toremifene	116 ± 3	0.77	—
+ L-PAM	125 ± 5	0.83	0.34
Nafoxidine	90 ± 7	0.60	—
+ L-PAM	76 ± 1	0.50	0.26

[a]Cells were incubated with vehicle alone (controls), antiestrogens alone
(0.5 μM for 72 hrs), melphalan alone (L-PAM for 1 hr), or the combination.

Table 9.2. Effect of tamoxifen pretreatment duration on melphalan cytotoxicity in
MCF-7 cells

| Group[a] | Colony number ± SE | Surviving fraction | |
		Observed	Predicted
Control	124 ± 6	—	—
L-PAM	22 ± 2	0.18	—
TAM 72 hrs	39 ± 14	0.31	—
+ L-PAM	39 ± 7	0.32	0.06
TAM 1 hr	156 ± 8	1.25	—
+ L-PAM	72 ± 3	0.58	0.22

[a]TAM (1 μM), melphalan (L-PAM, 0.5 μg/ml)

incubated with tamoxifen either for 72 hours or for only 1 hour prior to the
addition of melphalan (Table 9.2) (Osborne et al. 1989). A 1-hour preincubation was insufficient to cause a significant perturbation of cell-cycle phase
distributions (Osborne et al. 1983), and in this experiment it did not reduce
colony number. However, tamoxifen for only 1 hour did antagonize the effects
of melphalan as indicated by the comparison of the observed and predicted
SFs. Thus, the antagonistic interaction observed in these experiments cannot
be explained on a cell kinetic basis. Furthermore, the antagonism observed
does not require a prolonged exposure to the antiestrogen.

Effect of ER Status

To determine if the antagonistic interaction between tamoxifen and melphalan was mediated via the estrogen receptor, we examined the interaction
in a panel of cell lines, some ER-positive and some ER-negative (Table 9.3)
(Osborne et al. 1989). The ER-positive ZR75-1 cell line, like MCF-7, was
inhibited by tamoxifen and by melphalan alone. When tamoxifen was com-

Table 9.3. Effect of tamoxifen plus melphalan in breast cancer cell lines

	Surviving fraction for TAM + L-PAM	
Cell line	Observed	Predicted
ZR75-1	0.63	0.33
BT-20	0.81	0.69
MDA-231	0.79	0.38
BRL-3A	0.45	0.31

bined with melphalan, the observed SF (0.63) was nearly twice that predicted for an additive interaction for these agents (0.33), again indicating antagonism. As expected, tamoxifen by itself had no effect on the colony SF of two ER-negative human breast cancer cell lines, BT-20 and MDA-MB-231. Nevertheless, tamoxifen still antagonized melphalan cytotoxicity in each of these cell lines, because the observed SF with the combination was greater than that predicted for an additive effect. As shown in the table, antagonism was observed with tamoxifen and melphalan in the BRL-3A ER-negative rat liver cell line. Thus, the antagonistic effects of tamoxifen are not mediated via the estrogen receptor and are not even specific for breast cancer tissue.

Other hormones

To determine if melphalan antagonism was specific for the triphenyethylene antiestrogens, we examined the effects of pharmacological concentrations of several other agents used in breast cancer management (Osborne et al. 1989). Table 9.4 shows the effects of dexamethasone, 17ß-estradiol, and medroxyprogesterone acetate, all of which inhibited colony formation slightly when used alone. When the last two agents were combined with melphalan, the SF was actually less than that with melphalan alone, and the observed values were similar to those predicted, suggesting an additive effect. On the other hand, an antagonistic interaction was also observed with dexamethasone, an agent commonly used at high doses in breast cancer patients as an antiemetic at the time of chemotherapy administration. This observation requires additional study with other chemotherapeutic agents, but the cumulative data suggest that the routine use of other drugs at the time of chemotherapy may not be totally innocuous and has the potential for an antagonistic interaction.

The above studies do not provide a mechanism for the antagonistic interaction between tamoxifen and melphalan. They suggest that the interaction was not a consequence of the ability of tamoxifen to induce a cell cycle arrest, because antagonism was still observed under conditions in which tamoxifen had no antiproliferative or cell kinetic effects. Furthermore, tamoxifen was

Table 9.4. Effect of other hormones on melphalan cytotoxicity in MCF-7 cells

Group	Colony number ± SE	Surviving fraction	
		Observed	Predicted
Control	369 ± 13	—	—
L-PAM	70 ± 4	0.19	—
Dexamethasone	256 ± 7	0.69	—
+ L-PAM	92 ± 4	0.25	0.13
17β-estradiol	261 ± 14	0.71	—
+ L-PAM	35 ± 8	0.09	0.13
Medroxyprogesterone	325 ± 10	0.88	—
+ L-PAM	50 ± 4	0.14	0.17

antagonistic even in ER-negative breast cancer cells. Other studies by Goldenberg and Froese, who also found an antagonistic interaction between tamoxifen and melphalan, provide a possible mechanism for this effect (Goldenberg and Froese 1985). These investigators reported that tamoxifen reduced the cellular uptake of melphalan, perhaps resulting in a reduced cytotoxic effect. It is not clear, however, if this mechanism was operative in our studies, because these investigators used extraordinarily high concentrations of tamoxifen ranging from 5 to 25 μM, concentrations that are substantially higher than those used in our *in vitro* experiments and substantially higher than concentrations observed in patients on tamoxifen. These concentrations could have nonspecific and perhaps clinically irrelevant membrane effects. Whether the lower concentrations of tamoxifen used in our experiments also inhibit melphalan uptake into cells will require additional study.

2. Cyclophosphamide

The above studies indicate that tamoxifen antagonizes the effects of melphalan on cultured human breast cancer cells. An important question is whether this antagonism is specific for melphalan or is also observed with other alkylating agents. To examine this question, we investigated the effects of tamoxifen on the cytotoxicity of cyclophosphamide using 4-hydroxycyclophosphamide, the active metabolite. In contrast with melphalan, no antagonism was observed when tamoxifen was combined with 4-hydroxycyclophosphamide (Fig. 9.4). In fact, the colony SF when the drugs were combined overlapped the predicted curve, indicating an additive effect. It is interesting that 4-hydroxycyclophosphamide is transported into the cell by a carrier-mediated mechanism different from that of melphalan (Goldenberg 1975). This raises the possibility that the effects of tamoxifen are specific for certain amino acid, carrier-mediated, uptake mechanisms.

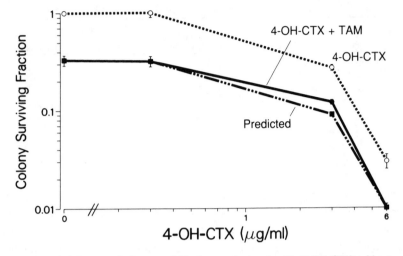

Figure 9.4. Dose-survival curves of 4-hydroxycyclophosphamide (4-OH-CTX) without or with tamoxifen in MCF-7 cells. (Reprinted from Osborne et al. 1989, with permission from W. B. Saunders Company.)

Although tamoxifen did not antagonize cyclophosphamide's *in vitro* activity, the *in vitro* metabolic pathways for these two drugs suggest another possible mechanism by which an important drug interaction could occur. Cyclophosphamide is somewhat distinct among alkylating agents, in that it must be metabolized to produce alkylating compounds by hepatic microsomal enzymes (Colvin 1982). Several individual P-450 enzymes are thought to be the major contributors to cyclophosphamide activation (LeBlanc and Waxman 1989). These include P-450IIC6, P-450IIB1, and P-450IIC11. Certain P-450 substrates, including hexobarbital, testosterone, and cortisol, inhibit cyclophosphamide activation presumably by competitive inhibition at the P-450 active site (LeBlanc and Waxman 1989). The parent drug is metabolized initially to 4-hydroxycyclophosphamide, then to aldophosphamide, and finally to phosphoramide mustard, all active alkylating agents. 4-Hydroxycyclophosphamide and aldophosphamide are also oxidized by soluble enzymes to inactive metabolites (Colvin 1982).

Tamoxifen has also been shown to undergo significant hepatic metabolism by microsomal enzymes. One such metabolite is the potent antiestrogen 4-hydroxytamoxifen. This suggests the possibility that tamoxifen could antagonize activation of cyclophosphamide and reduce its cytotoxic effects by competitive inhibition of microsomal enzymes. It has been reported that tamoxifen and several of its metabolites are inhibitors of certain P-450

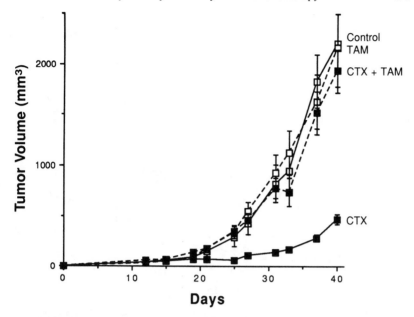

Figure 9.5. Effect of tamoxifen (□--□), cyclophosphamide (CTX, ■—■), or the combination (■--■), on growth of MDA-231 breast cancer cells (control, □—□) in athymic nude mice.

enzymes including IIC11 and IIB1, both of which are involved in cyclophosphamide activation (Reidy and Murray 1989).

To address this issue, in preliminary studies we have examined the effect of tamoxifen treatment on the cytotoxicity of cyclophosphamide using the estrogen receptor–negative MDA-MB-231 breast cancer cell line growing as a subcutaneous tumor in the athymic nude mouse model. This cell line was chosen for study because tamoxifen by itself has no effect on its growth *in vitro* or *in vivo*. Mice with established growing MDA-MB-231 tumors were treated with vehicle alone, tamoxifen alone, cyclophosphamide alone, or the combination of tamoxifen and cyclophosphamide (Fig. 9.5). Tamoxifen treatment, at doses resulting in blood concentrations similar to those observed in patients, had no effect on tumor growth in this model. Cyclophosphamide alone, however, significantly inhibited tumor growth. The addition of tamoxifen to cyclophosphamide nearly abolished the inhibitory effects of cyclophosphamide alone. To determine whether this antagonism might have been due to reduced activation of cyclophosphamide to its active metabolites, two other groups of mice were treated with the active metabolite 4-hydroxycyclophosphamide, either alone or combined with tamoxifen (Fig. 9.6).

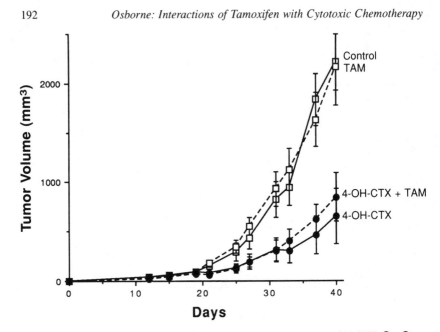

Figure 9.6. Effect of tamoxifen (□--□), 4-hydroxycyclophosphamide (4-OH-CTX, ●—●), or the combination (●--●), on growth of MDA-231 cells (control, □—□) in athymic nude mice.

4-Hydroxycyclophosphamide, like the parent drug, significantly inhibited tumor growth. However, in contrast with the effects observed when tamoxifen was combined with cyclophosphamide, tamoxifen had no antagonistic effect when combined with 4-hydroxycyclophosphamide. Although these data need to be confirmed and extended, they suggest another possible mechanism by which tamoxifen can interfere with cytotoxic chemotherapy by altering metabolic pathways in the liver.

B. Antimetabolites

The interaction of tamoxifen with certain antimetabolites has also been studied *in vitro* with cultured human breast cancer cell lines. When MCF-7 breast cancer cells were incubated for 72 hours with tamoxifen alone, for 1 hour with 5-FU alone, or with the combination of tamoxifen preincubation and 5-FU, an antagonistic interaction was observed (Fig. 9.7) (Osborne et al. 1989). At all concentrations tested, the colony SF with the combination of 5-FU and tamoxifen was well above that predicted for an additive effect.

An antagonistic interaction between tamoxifen and 5-fluorouracil has not been a universal finding. Another group reported a synergistic interaction between fluorouracil and high doses of tamoxifen in 47-DN human breast

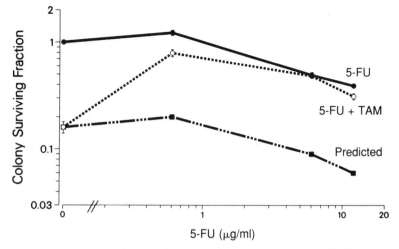

Figure 9.7. Dose-survival curves of 5-FU without or with tamoxifen in MCF-7 cells.

cancer cells (Benz, Santos, and Cadman 1983; Benz, Cadman, et al. 1983). The investigators hypothesized that this interaction may have been due to tamoxifen-enhanced RNA-mediated toxicity of 5-FU. On the other hand, another group reported antagonism between tamoxifen and fluorouracil in MCF-7 and MDA-468 breast cancer cells, data similar to our own (Hug et al. 1985). The discrepancies reported in different studies on the interaction of tamoxifen with fluorouracil cannot readily be explained. They could be related to differences in cultured cell lines, differences in experimental conditions, or differences in the drug doses and schedules employed. The mechanism by which tamoxifen alters cellular sensitivity to fluorouracil remains to be clarified.

C. DOXORUBICIN

Doxorubicin is the most highly active cytotoxic agent used in the management of breast cancer. Several studies have investigated the interaction between tamoxifen and doxorubicin. We reported that an additive or even synergistic interaction occurred when tamoxifen was combined with doxorubicin (Fig. 9.8) (Osborne et al. 1989). At all concentrations of doxorubicin tested, the colony surviving fraction with the combination of doxorubicin plus tamoxifen resulted in a lower surviving fraction than that predicted by an additive effect. A synergistic effect was even noted at a tamoxifen concentration that by itself had no effect on colony growth. These results, however, must still be considered controversial, because another group has reported

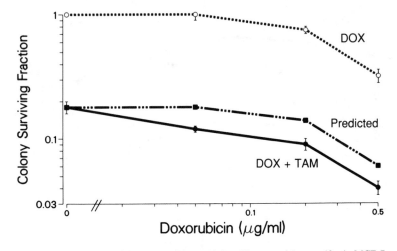

Figure 9.8. Dose-survival curves of doxorubicin without or with tamoxifen in MCF-7 cells.

an antagonistic interaction between tamoxifen and doxorubicin in cultured breast cancer cells (Hug et al. 1985). Still other reports suggest that tamoxifen can be used to enhance the sensitivity of doxorubicin in P388 leukemia cells resistant to the drug (Ramu et al. 1984). The mechanism for the increased sensitivity of cells to the combination of tamoxifen plus doxorubicin is not known, but it is interesting to speculate that it is related to the ability of tamoxifen to reverse the multi-drug-resistant phenotype resulting in increased intracellular accumulation of drug (Berman et al. 1991). Alternatively, tamoxifen's effects on membrane lipid packing density and membrane fluidity may also be involved (Ramu et al. 1984; Clarke et al. 1990).

IV. *Discussion*

The preclinical studies suggest the possibility that important drug interactions could occur when tamoxifen is given to patients simultaneously with chemotherapy. Whether this interaction is favorable or unfavorable may depend on the agents used as well as on their dose and schedule. From the data discussed above, melphalan, 5-FU, and cyclophosphamide are potential candidates for an antagonistic net interaction when combined with tamoxifen. On the other hand, the interaction of doxorubicin with tamoxifen may be more favorable, yielding an additive or synergistic interaction.

It is difficult to predict the net interaction when tamoxifen is added to drug combinations. However, antagonism might be expected when tamoxifen is added to the combination of melphalan plus 5-FU. A previously reported NSABP trial randomized pre- and postmenopausal node-positive patients to melphalan plus 5-FU alone or combined with tamoxifen (Fisher et al. 1986). Postmenopausal patients "benefited" from the addition of tamoxifen to chemotherapy. Unfortunately, a tamoxifen-alone arm was not included in this study, making full interpretation difficult. In this subset, tamoxifen could have inhibited any small disease-free or overall survival advantage provided by the chemotherapy, but the net effect was beneficial, because tamoxifen alone is very beneficial in such patients. Premenopausal patients failed to benefit from the addition of tamoxifen to chemotherapy in this study. In fact, a detrimental effect was observed, especially in ER-negative subsets. The detrimental effect could have resulted from an antagonistic interaction between tamoxifen and melphalan plus 5-FU in a group of patients in which the chemotherapy provides the greatest benefit and in which tamoxifen by itself has little activity.

In the majority of studies reported to date in the adjuvant setting or in advanced disease, tamoxifen has been added to chemotherapy regimens composed of cyclophosphamide (C), methotrexate (M), and 5-FU (F) (Early Breast Cancer Trialists' Collaborative Group 1992; Lippman 1983; Henderson 1987). In adjuvant therapy trials, although a disease-free survival advantage is evident in some studies, a significant survival advantage cannot be documented for combinations of CMF plus tamoxifen compared with CMF alone in premenopausal patients, or for CMF plus tamoxifen compared with tamoxifen alone in older patients. The Southwest Oncology Group recently completed a three-arm study in postmenopausal, ER-positive, node-positive patients, in which only 1 year of tamoxifen was equivalent to 1 year of CMFVP (CMF plus vincristine and prednisone) or to the combination of tamoxifen plus CMFVP in both disease-free and overall survival (Rivkin et al. 1990). Lack of benefit with the combination could be attributed to an antagonistic interaction. In advanced-disease trials, combinations of CMF plus tamoxifen do not result in higher response rates or longer survival compared with the sequential use of the agents alone (Lippman 1983).

The data from trials employing tamoxifen plus a doxorubicin-based combination are fewer and somewhat inconsistent. On the basis of the preclinical data, one might predict a significant benefit by adding tamoxifen to doxorubicin alone. Predicting the net effect of combining tamoxifen with regimens containing doxorubicin (A) plus cyclophosphamide ± 5-FU is more problematic. A trial of CAF alone versus CAF plus tamoxifen failed to show a higher response rate or longer survival with the combination compared with CAF alone (Perry et al. 1987). Similar results were observed in another trial comparing AC with AC plus tamoxifen (Australian and New Zealand Breast Cancer Trials Group 1986).

A recently reported NSABP trial, however, does show an advantage for the combination of AC plus tamoxifen (but not PAF plus tamoxifen) compared with tamoxifen alone (Fisher et al. 1990). The authors of this trial interpreted these data to suggest that combining chemotherapy with tamoxifen does not result in an antagonistic interaction. However, in the absence of a chemotherapy-alone arm or an arm in which the chemotherapy and tamoxifen were given sequentially, such conclusions are premature. In view of the preclinical data showing a synergistic or additive interaction between tamoxifen and doxorubicin, it is of interest that this is the only such trial that shows a survival benefit for the combination. It is even possible that tamoxifen antagonized the cyclophosphamide but synergized with the doxorubicin in this regimen to give the "net" modest beneficial effect observed in this trial.

In any event, it is clear that, although the preclinical studies of tamoxifen-chemotherapy interactions are interesting, they may not be directly extrapolated to the clinical setting in the absence of supporting clinical trial information. The question of whether tamoxifen should be given simultaneously with chemotherapy or sequentially when chemotherapy is completed is currently being addressed in an intergroup trial in postmenopausal, ER-positive, node-positive patients. This three-arm trial compares tamoxifen alone for 5 years versus CAF with tamoxifen for 6 cycles versus CAF followed by tamoxifen for 5 years. This trial will provide additional evidence for the role of chemotherapy in postmenopausal patients, and should provide important information on the optimal method of combining these two treatment modalities.

References

Australian and New Zealand Breast Cancer Trials Group, Clinical Oncological Society of Australia. 1986. A randomized trial in postmenopausal patients with advanced breast cancer comparing endocrine and cytotoxic therapy given sequentially or in combination. *Journal of Clinical Oncology* 4:186–193.

Bardon, S., F. Vignon, P. Montcourrier, and H. Rochefort. 1987. Steroid receptor–mediated cytotoxicity of an antiestrogen and an antiprogestin in breast cancer cells. *Cancer Research* 47:1441–1448.

Benz, C., G. Santos, and E. Cadman. 1983. Tamoxifen and 5-fluorouracil in breast cancer: modulation of cellular RNA. *Cancer Research* 43:5304–5308.

Benz, C., E. Cadman, and J. Gwin, T. Wu, J. Amara, A. Eisenfeld, and P. Dannies. 1983.

Tamoxifen and 5-fluorouracil in breast cancer: cytotoxic synergism in vitro. *Cancer Research* 43:5298–5303.

Berman, E., M. Adams, R. Duigou-Osterndorf, L. Godfrey, B. Clarkson, and M. Andreeff. 1991. Effect of tamoxifen on cell lines displaying the multidrug-resistant phenotype. *Blood* 77:818–825.

Brünner, N., D. Bronzert, L. L. Vindelov, K. Rygaard, M. Spang-Thomsen, and M. E. Lippman. 1989. Effect on growth and cell cycle kinetics of estradiol and tamoxifen on MCF-7 human breast cancer cells grown in vitro and in nude mice. *Cancer Research* 49:1515–1520.

Clarke, R., H. W. van den Berg, and R. F. Murphy. 1990. Reduction of the membrane fluidity of human breast cancer cells by tamoxifen and 17beta-estradiol. *Journal of the National Cancer Institute* 82:1702–1705.

Colvin, M. 1982. The alkylating agents. In *Pharmacologic principles of cancer treatment,* ed. B. Chabner, 276–308. Philadelphia: W. B. Saunders.

Early Breast Cancer Trialists' Collaborative Group. 1992. Systemic treatment of early breast cancer by hormonal, cytotoxic, or immune therapy. 133 randomised trials involving 31,000 recurrences and 24,000 deaths among 75,000 women. *Lancet* 339:1–15 and 71–85.

Fisher, B., C. Redmond, A. Brown, E. R. Fisher, N. Wolmark, D. Bowman, D. Plotkin, J. Wolter, R. Bornstein, S. Legault-Poisson, and E. A. Saffer. 1986. Adjuvant chemotherapy with and without tamoxifen in the treatment of primary breast cancer: five year results from the National Surgical Adjuvant Breast and Bowel Project trial. *Journal of Clinical Oncology* 4:459–471.

Fisher, B., C. Redmond, S. Legault-Poisson, N. V. Dimitrov, A. Brown, D. L. Wickerham, N. Wolmark, R. G. Margolese, D. Bowman, A. G. Glass, C. G. Kardinal, A. Robindoux, P. Jochimsen, W. Cronin, M. Deutsch, E. R. Fisher, D. B. Myers, and J. L. Hoehn. 1990. Postoperative chemotherapy and tamoxifen compared with tamoxifen alone in the treatment of positive-node breast cancer patients aged 50 years and older with tumors responsive to tamoxifen: results from the National Surgical Adjuvant Breast and Bowel Project B-16. *Journal of Clinical Oncology* 8:1005–1018.

Goldenberg, G. J. 1975. The role of drug transport in resistance to nitrogen mustard and other alkylating agents in L518Y lymphoblasts. *Cancer Research* 35:1687–1692.

Goldenberg, G. J., and E. K. Froese. 1985. Antagonism of the cytocidal activity and uptake of melphalan by tamoxifen in human breast cancer cells in vitro. *Biochemical Pharmacology* 34:763–770.

Greenberg, D. A., C. L. Carpenter, and R. O. Messing. 1987. Calcium channel antagonists properties of the antineoplastic antiestrogen tamoxifen in the PC12 neurosecretory cell line. *Cancer Research* 47:70–74.

Henderson, I. C. 1987. Adjuvant systemic therapy for early breast cancer. *Current Problems in Cancer* 11:125–207.

Hug, V., G. N. Hortobagyi, B. Drewinko, and M. Finders. 1985. Tamoxifen-citrate counteracts the antitumor effects of cytotoxic drugs in vitro. *Journal of Clinical Oncology* 3:1672–1677.

Lam, H. Y. 1984. Tamoxifen is a calmodulin antagonist in the activation of cAMP phosphodiesterase. *Biochemical and Biophysical Research Communication* 118:27–32.

LeBlanc, G. A., and D. J. Waxman. 1989. Interaction of anticancer drugs with hepatic monooxygenase enzymes. *Drug Metabolism Reviews* 20:395–439.

Lippman, M. E. 1983. Efforts to combine endocrine chemotherapy in the management of breast cancer: do two plus two equal three? *Breast Cancer Research and Treatment* 3:117–127.

O'Brian, C. A., R. M. Liskamp, D. H. Solomon, and I. B. Weinstein. 1986. Triphenylethylenes: a new class of protein kinase C inhibitors. *Journal of the National Cancer Institute* 76:1243–1246.

Osborne, C. K., D. H. Boldt, and P. Estrada. 1984. Human breast cancer cell cycle synchronization by estrogens and antiestrogens in culture. *Cancer Research* 44:1433–1439.

Osborne, C. K., E. B. Coronado, and J. P. Robinson. 1987. Human breast cancer in the athymic nude mouse: Cytostatic effects of long-term antiestrogen therapy. *European Journal of Cancer and Clinical Oncology* 23:1189–1196.

Osborne, C. K., K. Hobbs, and G. M. Clark. 1985. Effect of estrogens and antiestrogens on growth of human breast cancer cells in athymic nude mice. *Cancer Research* 45:584–590.

Osborne, C. K., L. Kitten, and C. L. Arteaga. 1989. Antagonism of chemotherapy-induced cytotoxicity for human breast cancer cells by antiestrogens. *Journal of Clinical Oncology* 7:710–717.

Osborne, C. K., D. H. Boldt, G. M. Clark, and J. M. Trent. 1983. Effects of tamoxifen on human breast cancer cell kinetics: accumulation of cells in early G_1 phase. *Cancer Research* 43:3583–3585.

Perry, M. C., C. G. Kardinal, A. H. Korzun, S. J. Ginsberg, P. C. Raich, J. F. Holland, R. R. Ellison, S. Kopel, A. Schilling, J. Aisner, P. Schulman, V. Weinberg, M. A. Rice, and W. Wood. 1987. Chemohormonal therapy in advanced carcinoma of the breast: cancer and leukemia group B protocol 8081. *Journal of Clinical Oncology* 5:1534–1545.

Ramu, A., D. Glaubiger, and Z. Fuks. 1984. Reversal of acquired resistance to doxorubicin in P388 murine leukemia cells by tamoxifen and other triparanol analogues. *Cancer Research* 44:4392–4395.

Reidy, G. F., and M. Murray. 1989. In vitro inhibition of hepatic steroid hydroxylation by tamoxifen, a series of tamoxifen analogues and related compounds. *Biochemical Pharmacology* 38:195–199.

Rivkin, S., S. Green, B. Metch, A. Cruz, R. McDivitt, W. Knight, J. Glick, and C. K. Osborne. 1990. Adjuvant combination chemotherapy (CMFVP) vs tamoxifen (TAM) vs CMFVP + TAM for postmenopausal women with ER+ operable breast cancer and positive axillary lymph nodes. *Proceedings of American Society of Clinical Oncology* 26:24.

Saez, R. A., and C. K. Osborne. 1989. Hormonal treatment of advanced breast cancer. In *Current clinical oncology*, ed. B. J. Kennedy, 163–172. New York: Alan R. Liss, Inc.

Su, H. D., G. J. Mazzei, W. R. Vogler, and J. F. Kuo. 1985. Effect of tamoxifen, a non-steroidal antiestrogen, on phospholipid/calcium-dependent protein kinase and phosphorylation of its endogenous substrate proteins from the rat brain and ovary. *Biochemical Pharmacology* 34:3649–3653.

Taylor, I. W., P. J. Hodson, M. D. Green, and R. L. Sutherland. 1983. Effects of tamoxifen on cell cycle progression of synchronous MCF-7 human mammary carcinoma cells. *Cancer Research* 43:4007–4010.

10

Tamoxifen-Resistant Growth

Douglas M. Wolf, Marco M. Gottardis,
and V. Craig Jordan

I.	Introduction	200
II.	Clinical Experience	200
	A. Tamoxifen in Advanced Disease	201
	B. Adjuvant Tamoxifen	202
III.	Models for Tamoxifen-Resistant Growth	203
	A. Tamoxifen Insensitivity	203
	B. Tamoxifen-Stimulated Growth	206
IV.	Conclusion and Future Prospects	213
	References	214

I. *Introduction*

Tamofixen is the most effective single-agent therapy currently available for the treatment of endocrine-responsive breast cancer. In the past 2 decades tamoxifen has moved from use as a palliative treatment for advanced breast cancer in elderly women to its current use as a treatment for both pre- and postmenopausal women with all stages of the disease. Most of the adverse effects of tamoxifen are fairly innocuous (see Fritsch and Wolf, Chapter 12 in this volume), especially in comparison with other chemotherapeutic agents commonly used to treat breast cancer.

However, the development of tamoxifen-resistant tumor growth is a concern that consistently arises with the application of tamoxifen treatment. Tamoxifen is considered to act primarily as a tumoristatic rather than a tumoricidal agent, and eventually a subset of tumor cells might be expected to overcome this growth inhibition and begin to grow even though the presence of tamoxifen is maintained. Most patients with advanced disease who initially respond to tamoxifen treatment will eventually fail therapy. In addition, many women treated with tamoxifen as an adjuvant also experience disease recurrence. The study of the mechanism or mechanisms by which endocrine-responsive breast tumors eventually overcome growth inhibition by tamoxifen is therefore of considerable importance. This chapter will discuss current laboratory models of tamoxifen failure and, in particular, will concentrate on the phenomenon of tamoxifen-stimulated tumor growth.

II. *Clinical Experience*

Tamoxifen was introduced into the clinic as a palliative treatment for advanced breast cancer (Cole et al. 1971), but its use has been broadened to cover all stages of the disease in both pre- and postmenopausal women. An overview analysis of the effectiveness of adjuvant tamoxifen, compiled from 40 trials with a total accrual of nearly 30,000 women, was published recently (Early Breast Cancer Trialists' Collaborative Group 1992). It has been suggested that tamoxifen may be effective against breast cancer even before the tumors are clinically detectable; a pilot study evaluating tamoxifen as a preventive has been completed in the United Kingdom (Powles et al. 1989,

1990). In the United States, the National Cancer Institute and the National Surgical Adjuvant Breast and Bowel Project (NSABP) have started a study intended to evaluate tamoxifen as a breast cancer preventive in 16,000 healthy volunteers. The application of tamoxifen to the prevention of breast cancer will be discussed in Chapter 13 (by Morrow and Jordan).

A. Tamoxifen in Advanced Disease

Tamoxifen treatment can be expected to produce a beneficial response in about one-third of patients with advanced breast cancer (Jordan et al. 1988). If a subset of patients with estrogen receptor (ER) and progesterone receptor (PgR) positive primary tumors is selected for tamoxifen therapy, it is possible to achieve a response rate as high as 80% (Jordan et al. 1988). These data are usually interpreted as an indication that tamoxifen administration will benefit only women with ER-positive primary tumors. However, when women with advanced, ER-negative disease are treated with tamoxifen, about 10% experience an objective response (Jordan et al. 1988). Several investigators have taken this as evidence that the action of tamoxifen is multimodal in nature, and that not all the effects of the drug are ER mediated.

For example, members of the transforming growth factor (TGF) ß family often act as inhibitors of epithelial cell growth. TGF-ß inhibits mammary epithelial cell growth (Sporn et al. 1986; Knabbe et al. 1987). Colletta and co-workers (1990) reported results that may be important in explaining the responsiveness of some ER-negative tumors to tamoxifen treatment. They showed that tamoxifen can induce the production of TGF-ß by fibroblasts, cells which do not usually contain estrogen receptors. They argue that, because mammary tumors are not a homogeneous mass of epithelial cells, but rather a mixture of stromal and epithelial cell types, the production of TGF-ß by tumor fibroblasts exposed to tamoxifen could lead to the control of some ER-negative tumors. Butta et al. (1992) recently presented clinical evidence that parallels these results. By analyzing pre- and posttamoxifen treatment biopsies from women with breast cancer, they have shown that tamoxifen treatment induces the production of TGF-ß by tumor fibroblasts from both ER-negative and ER-positive tumors. This evidence supports the argument that the action of tamoxifen may be multifaceted; women with ER-positive tumors could benefit on multiple levels, but even women with ER-negative tumors could benefit from what could be called the indirect action of tamoxifen.

There is another potential indirect action of tamoxifen as well. Insulin-like growth factors (IGFs), in particular IGF-I, have been shown to be stimulators of breast cancer cell growth *in vitro* (Karey and Sirbasku 1988; van der Burg et al. 1988; Arteaga and Osborne 1989). Huff et al. (1986) reported that ER-positive breast cancer cells produced IGFs in response to estrogen treatment, and that these IGFs might act as autocrine-growth stimuli. IGF production by breast cancer cells was later disputed by investigators using alternative, more sensitive assays (Karey and Sirbasku 1988; Yee et al. 1989; van der Burg et al. 1990). It remains clear, however, that IGFs can be growth effectors of breast cancer cells, possibly acting in a paracrine or endocrine (if not autocrine) fashion to stimulate breast cancer cell growth. There is evidence that tamoxifen can lower circulating IGF levels in breast cancer patients receiving the drug (Colletti et al. 1989; Pollack et al. 1990; Friedl et al., 1993). It is possible that part of the growth-inhibitory action of tamoxifen may be due to this effect, and that some of the ER-negative tumors that respond to treatment are IGF dependent.

Butta et al. (1992) and Jordan (1993) suggest, on the basis of the accumulated laboratory and clinical evidence, that all women with breast cancer could be offered the drug, especially since most side effects of treatment are relatively minor. Unfortunately, despite the fact that tamoxifen may act at sites other than ER to prevent tumor growth, tamoxifen therapy for advanced disease is not curative; almost all patients who initially respond will ultimately fail therapy and their disease will progress.

B. ADJUVANT TAMOXIFEN

It is difficult to make absolute statements about tamoxifen failure when the drug is used in the adjuvant setting. Most women who present clinically with stage II disease will experience disease recurrence at some time following their initial surgery, whether or not they receive tamoxifen. However, tamoxifen has been shown to confer significant increases in both disease-free and overall survival to this group (Early Breast Cancer Trialists' Collaborative Group 1992). The majority of women who are diagnosed as having stage I (node-negative) disease will be cured by removal of their primary tumor. Nevertheless, there will be some women in this group who will experience disease recurrence. Tamoxifen has been shown to increase both disease-free and absolute survival for these patients, although not to as great an extent as for stage II patients (Early Breast Cancer Trialists' Collaborative Group 1992).

Several important conclusions can be drawn from the overview analysis mentioned above (Early Breast Cancer Trialists' Collaborative Group 1992). The most obvious is that not all women benefit from adjuvant tamoxifen treatment. These women can be regarded as having *de novo* resistance to tamoxifen. Second, because tamoxifen confers both disease-free and overall survival benefits when compared with placebo, it can be concluded that the drug is interfering with the growth of micrometastases in a subset of patients. It is reasonable to assume that some women who experience disease recurrence during adjuvant tamoxifen treatment, especially after an extended treatment period, had an initial response to tamoxifen before metastatic tumor cells began to proliferate. The difference between this situation and that in advanced disease is that therapeutic response and subsequent development of tamoxifen resistance occurred entirely at a subclinical level.

All the above data and discussion must ultimately serve as a reminder that tamoxifen treatment failure is a complex phenomenon. A complete investigation must provide explanations for both tamoxifen-resistant relapse after initial therapeutic response and *de novo* tamoxifen resistance, especially in the case of patients with ER-positive tumors. Many investigators are currently addressing parts of these questions, and some of the more provocative results will be discussed in the following sections.

III. *Models for Tamoxifen Resistant Growth*

A. TAMOXIFEN INSENSITIVITY

Tamoxifen-resistant tumor growth could conceivably be achieved by a variety of mechanisms. Tumors could become hormone independent, circumventing the estrogen-response pathway so that occupation of ER by either agonist or antagonist ligands would have no effect on tumor growth. These tumors may or may not continue to maintain expression of ER. Estrogen receptor–positive but nonresponsive tumors of this type may account for many of the patients with ER-positive breast cancers that fail to respond to tamoxifen therapy.

The observation that not all patients with ER-positive breast tumors respond to tamoxifen led to the proposal that not all ER-positive tumors contain functional ER (Horwitz et al. 1975). Even if tumors were to contain an ER that bound estradiol, the hormone-receptor complex might fail to initiate the steps necessary to stimulate growth. Addition of the progesterone-receptor assay to the range of tests available for evaluation of the breast cancer patient has allowed the identification of a subset of patients with a very high likelihood of response to endocrine (tamoxifen) therapy (Jordan et al. 1988). However, there are patients with ER- and PgR-positive tumors who do not respond to endocrine therapy. The existence of such a patient population raises interesting questions. Have these patients' tumors adapted such that, even though they contain functional ERs, the growth control pathway regulated by estrogens is no longer affecting cell replication? Is the growth-arresting signal from tamoxifen being received and simply ignored? Or might something in the cell be interfering with the action of an otherwise normal ER?

It is possible that, in addition to wild-type ERs, tamoxifen-resistant tumors may also contain aberrant receptor forms that could either interfere with or circumvent normal receptor function. Several laboratories have demonstrated the presence of altered ER messenger RNAs (mRNAs) in breast tumor biopsies, breast cancer cell lines, and even in certain normal endometrial specimens. A detailed review of many of these variants has recently been published (McGuire et al. 1991).

Several of the variant estrogen receptors described to date contain deletions of some or all of the hormone-binding domain (Murphy and Dotzlaw 1989; Graham et al. 1990; Fuqua et al. 1991; Dotzlaw et al. 1992). Obviously, receptors lacking a functional hormone-binding domain could not be responsible for an ER-positive, tamoxifen-insensitive phenotype, because conventional hormone-binding assays would report these cells as ER negative. However, most of the hormone-binding-domain deficient ER mutants have been reported to be present against a background of varying concentrations of wild-type receptor. Although the function of wild-type ERs in these cells may be inhibited by tamoxifen, it is possible that mutant ERs with no hormone-binding domain could remain constitutively active in the presence of tamoxifen. The net effect would be antiestrogen resistance because of the action of the mutant receptors.

Fuqua et al. (1992) recently reported another potential action of receptors with truncated hormone-binding domains. They demonstrated that an ER variant lacking exon 7 is capable of interacting with and blocking the transcription-activation function of wild-type ERs. The exon 7 variant can act only in a negative fashion and does not exhibit transcription-activation activity when expressed alone. It is not clear what relevance a negatively acting receptor variant would have with respect to the development of tamoxifen resistance. It could be thought of as an antiestrogen which at one time may have been growth inhibitory, but to which the cells have become resistant. The ability to screen for receptor variants of this type may be useful in determining which patients might exhibit *de novo* resistance to tamoxifen, in which case alternative therapies could be suggested.

Not all truncated steroid receptors are completely transcriptionally inactive. Vegeto et al. (1992) recently reported that a progesterone receptor variant lacking a small portion of the carboxyl terminus does not bind and therefore cannot be induced to activate transcription by either progesterone or the synthetic progestin R5020. This truncated receptor does, however, still bind the antiprogestin RU 38486 with high affinity. Further, when the truncated progesterone receptor is occupied with RU 38486 it acts as a potent activator of progestin-mediated gene expression. Similar results have also been reported for the androgen receptor. The prostate carcinoma cell line LNCaP contains a mutant androgen receptor which is activated by both androgens and antiandrogens (Olea et al. 1990; Schuurmans et al. 1990; Veldscholte et al. 1990, Wilding et al. 1989), as well as by progestins and estrogens (Veldscholte et al. 1990).

In addition to the studies described above with deletion-containing receptors, there is evidence indicating that a single point mutation in the ligand-binding domain of the ER is sufficient to cause the receptor to respond to the tamoxifen metabolite 4-hydroxytamoxifen (4-OHT, normally a potent antiestrogen) as an agonist. Jiang, Langan-Fahey, et al. (1992) reported that, if ER-negative MDA-MB-231 breast cancer cells are transfected with the wild-type ER, E_2 inhibits their growth, and 4-OHT could block this effect, returning growth to non-E_2-treated levels. However, if MDA-MB-231 cells are transfected with an ER containing a valine for glycine substitution at position 400 in the hormone-binding domain, the resulting transfectants are growth inhibited by both E_2 and 4-OHT. Thus in cells containing the mutant ER, both E_2 and the antiestrogen 4-OHT act as ER agonists when compared with transfectants containing the wild-type ER. The results with both deletion- and point mutation–containing receptors may suggest an explanation for another type of tamoxifen resistance observed in the laboratory, i.e., tamoxifen-stimulated breast cancer cell growth. This concept will be addressed at length in the following section.

Finally, there is the possibility that a breast cancer cell may maintain expression of wild-type ER, not express any mutant ERs that interfere with the action of the wild-type receptor, and still be insensitive to tamoxifen. Recently our laboratory cloned an MCF-7 cell variant (clone 5C; Jiang, Wolf, et al. 1992) which expresses wild-type ER. No expression of a subset of mutant ERs was detectable in this line, yet these cells were neither growth stimulated by estrogens nor growth inhibited by tamoxifen. These cells expressed markedly reduced levels of PgR compared with the MCF-7 parental cells, and estrogen-stimulated reporter gene expression was also markedly reduced. These data suggest that processes downstream of ligand binding to the ER may act to circumvent the need for an E_2-occupied ER for growth stimulation. Further, changes of this nature appear to make it possible for the cell to ignore the growth inhibitory signal from a tamoxifen-occupied ER.

B. Tamoxifen-Stimulated Growth

As stated briefly above, an alternative mechanism that could lead to the failure of antiestrogen therapy is the occurrence of tamoxifen-stimulated tumor growth. Tamoxifen is not a pure ER antagonist; in many systems it has been shown to have partial agonist activity. In fact, many of the extramammary effects of tamoxifen in the clinic appear to be due primarily to agonist rather than antagonist effects (Wolf and Jordan 1992; Fritsch and Wolf, Chapter 12 in this volume). However, in human mammary tissue, tamoxifen appears to act primarily as an antiestrogen, at least initially (Walker et al. 1991).

Normally, if MCF-7 breast cancer cells or pieces of an established MCF-7 solid tumor are inoculated into the mammary fat pads of ovariectomized athymic mice, tumors will grow only if the mice are supplemented with estrogen (Shafie and Grantham 1981; Osborne et al. 1985; Gottardis, Robinson, and Jordan 1988). Tamoxifen administration will block the estradiol-stimulated growth of these tumors in a dose (i.e., serum concentration) dependent fashion (Iino et al. 1991).

In endometrial tissue tamoxifen seems to have a proliferative effect instead of the inhibitory effect seen on mammary tissue. There is clinical evidence that tamoxifen may be a weak promoter of endometrial carcinoma. An overall analysis of clinical trials to date indicates that patients treated with tamoxifen experience a 0.4% increased risk of developing endometrial carcinoma (Nayfield et al. 1991). In laboratory models, tamoxifen has been shown to be capable of stimulating endometrial tumor growth. The growth of EnCa 101 human endometrial tumors implanted into the flanks of athymic mice is stimulated rather than inhibited by tamoxifen (Satyaswaroop et al. 1984; Gottardis, Robinson, et al. 1988). If an EnCa 101 tumor is implanted into one flank of an athymic mouse and an MCF-7 tumor is implanted into the other, both tumors will grow if the animal is treated with estradiol. However, if the animal receives tamoxifen, only the EnCa 101 tumor will be stimulated to grow (Gottardis, Robinson, et al. 1988).

Breast tumors grown in athymic mice can develop a growth response similar to EnCa 101 tumors after chronic exposure to tamoxifen. If MCF-7

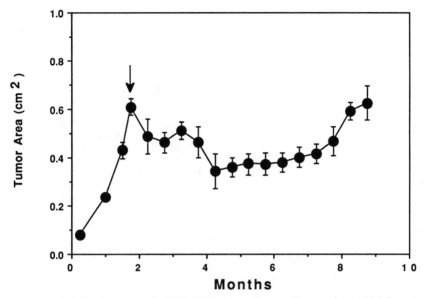

Figure 10.1. Development of the MCF-7 TAM tumor. Arrow indicates point at which E_2 was removed and replaced with TAM. (Adapted from Gottardis and Jordan 1988.)

tumors are allowed to grow for several weeks in estradiol-treated animals and then the estradiol is removed and replaced with tamoxifen, the tumors will regress partially and then their size will remain static for several weeks to months. Eventually some of the tumors will begin to grow again, although the presence of tamoxifen is maintained (Fig. 10.1; Osborne et al. 1987; Gottardis and Jordan 1988). When these tumors are removed and pieces of them are transplanted into new host animals, tumor growth can be stimulated over control growth rate by either estradiol or tamoxifen (Gottardis and Jordan 1988; Gottardis, Wagner, et al. 1989). A pure estrogen-receptor antagonist such as ICI 164,384 fails to stimulate the growth of these MCF-7 variant tumors (MCF-7 TAM). ICI 164,384 administered at sufficient doses is capable of blocking tamoxifen-stimulated growth in this model (Gottardis, Jiang, et al. 1989).

There are two principal hypotheses that have been suggested to explain the mechanism of tamoxifen-stimulated growth. The first suggests that tamoxifen-stimulated tumors have acquired the ability to modify tamoxifen or its metabolites in such a way that the resulting compounds act as potent estrogens. This hypothesis also suggests that tamoxifen-stimulated tumors are capable of actively lowering intracellular concentrations of tamoxifen and its antiestrogenic metabolites. The second hypothesis proposes that reproducible

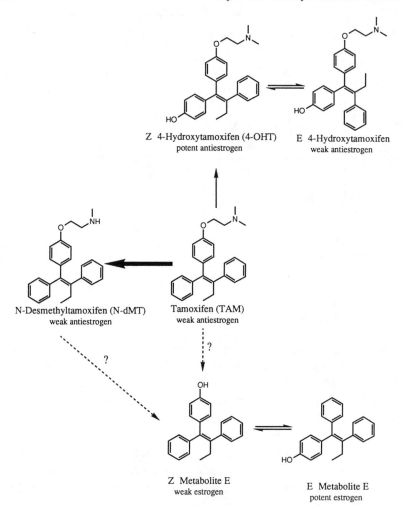

Figure 10.2. Potential pathways of TAM metabolism.

alterations occur in the estrogen-responsive machinery in mammary tumors. These changes cause a subset of the cell population within a tumor to respond to tamoxifen or its principal metabolites as stimulators rather than as inhibitors of growth. Both hypotheses will be discussed in detail below.

In humans tamoxifen (TAM) is converted to two principal metabolites (Fig. 10.2), N-desmethyltamoxifen (N-dMT) and 4-hydroxytamoxifen (4-OHT). At steady state, N-dMT is present at roughly twice the concentration of the parent compound, whereas 4-OHT is present at about 1% of the concentration of tamoxifen (Langan-Fahey et al. 1990). N-dMT is a weak anti-estrogen with potency, efficacy, and affinity for the ER similar to those of tamoxifen. In contrast, 4-OHT is a potent antiestrogen which binds to the ER with an affinity comparable to that of estradiol (Jordan et al. 1977).

Because tamoxifen and all its metabolites are substituted ethylenes, they can exist in either of two isomeric forms, Z or E. Tamoxifen, which does not interconvert between forms in solution, is administered as the Z form. The presence of the electron-withdrawing hydroxyl group on 4-OHT destabilizes the double bond, and in aqueous solution Z 4-OHT can convert to a mixture of the Z and E isomers of the compound. Whereas Z 4-OHT is a potent, high affinity antiestrogen, E 4-OHT is a weak antiestrogen with an activity similar to that of tamoxifen itself (Murphy et al. 1990).

Metabolite E, another hydroxylated derivative of tamoxifen, is also relevant to the metabolic model of tamoxifen-stimulated tumor growth. Metabolite E is formed by the removal of the dimethylaminoethane side chain (Fig. 10.2). Metabolism of tamoxifen via this pathway would result in the formation of the Z isomer of metabolite E, which is a weak, low affinity estrogen (Murphy et al. 1990). As is the case with 4-OHT, the hydroxyl substituent facilitates the isomerization of Z metabolite E to the potent estrogen agonist E metabolite E (Murphy et al. 1990).

The metabolism hypothesis has been extensively investigated and described by Osborne and colleagues (Osborne et al. 1991; Osborne et al. 1992; Wiebe et al. 1992). These investigators have reported that tamoxifen-stimulated variants of MCF-7 tumors, generated as described above, contain significantly lower levels of tamoxifen than does a tamoxifen-sensitive tumor in a comparably dosed animal (Osborne et al. 1991). Further, they reported that the development of tamoxifen-stimulated tumor growth in this model is associated with increased isomerization of Z 4-OHT to the weaker E isomer. Osborne et al. (1992) have also reported similar findings in preliminary studies on breast cancer patients failing to respond to tamoxifen therapy. Patients with progressive disease were reported to have lower tumor tamoxifen concentrations than patients responding to therapy. It is not clear whether or not dose escalation would have been of benefit to the women failing to respond. The authors also reported that in patients failing to respond to therapy, the ratio of E 4-OHT to Z 4-OHT was higher than observed in patients responding to tamoxifen treatment.

Finally, in a preliminary study of five patients with tamoxifen-nonresponsive breast cancer, Wiebe et al. (1992) identified metabolite E in tumor tissue. They did not indicate if metabolite E was present at concentrations sufficient to have any effect in the context of high background concentrations of tamoxifen and its antiestrogenic metabolites. They reported that in a tamoxifen-stimulated MCF-7 tumor from an athymic mouse metabolite E and bisphenol, another potential estrogenic metabolite of tamoxifen, were present. However, neither compound was present at concentrations likely to compete effectively for ER binding with TAM, N-dMT, or Z and E 4-OHT in the amounts that these compounds were present.

On the basis of the available information about the affinities of the various estrogenic and antiestrogenic metabolites of tamoxifen, we reasoned that both formation of metabolite E and isomerization of this metabolite to the potent E isomer (and concomitant isomerization of 4-OHT to the weakly antiestrogenic E isomer) must occur (Fig. 10.2). Therefore, our laboratory decided to address the question of isomerization directly. Using a fixed-ring, nonisomerizable analog of tamoxifen (Fig. 10.3), we found that isomerization is not necessary for tamoxifen to stimulate the growth of MCF-7 TAM tumors. Fixed-ring tamoxifen (FRT; McCague et al. 1986) is an analog of tamoxifen in which the ethyl side chain has been replaced by a propyl group bonded at one end to the ethylene backbone and at the other end to one of the phenyl rings on the other side of the ethylene backbone. This structure prevents isomerization around the double bond. FRT blocks estrogen-stimulated growth of MCF-7 cells *in vitro* at the same concentrations as tamoxifen. As described above, fixed-ring compounds were also used *in vitro* to demonstrate that Z 4-OHT is a potent antiestrogen and that E 4-OHT is a weak, low affinity antiestrogen (Murphy et al. 1990). In addition, fixed-ring analogs of metabolite E were used to show that the E isomer was a potent estrogen, whereas the Z isomer had only weak estrogenic activity.

As shown in Figure 10.4A, both FRT and TAM blocked the estrogen-stimulated growth of MCF-7 tumors implanted into athymic mice (Wolf et al. 1993). In addition, both compounds stimulated the growth of the MCF-7 TAM tumor variant in athymic mice with equal efficacy (Fig. 10.4B). Obviously, in this model isomerization of tamoxifen or its metabolites from the Z to the E isomers cannot occur. Therefore, isomerization is not necessary for tamoxifen-stimulated growth.

Finally, when TAM and FRT concentrations were measured in MCF-7 and MCF-7 TAM tumors taken from tumor-bearing athymic mice, it was found that MCF-7 TAM tumors had concentrations of TAM or FRT equivalent to, if not higher than, concentrations observed in the normal tamoxifen-inhibited MCF-7 tumors (Wolf et al. 1993). These data differ from the report by Osborne et al. (1991) that tamoxifen-stimulated tumors have tamoxifen

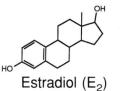

Estradiol (E₂)

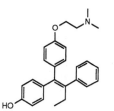

Tamoxifen (TAM)

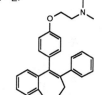

Fixed-Ring Tamoxifen (FRT)

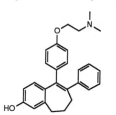

4-Hydroxytamoxifen (4-OHT)

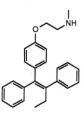

N-Desmethyltamoxifen (N-dMT)

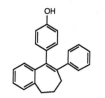

FR Z 4-Hydroxytamoxifen

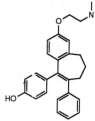

FR E 4-Hydroxytamoxifen

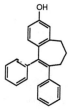

FR Z Metabolite E

FR E Metabolite E

Figure 10.3. Structure of compounds used in the investigation of TAM-stimulated tumor growth.

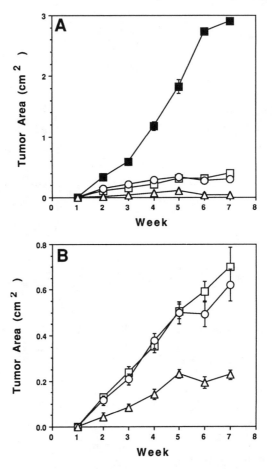

Figure 10.4. Ability of TAM and FRT (A) to inhibit the growth of estradiol-stimulated MCF-7 tumors and (B) to stimulate the growth of MCF-7 TAM tumors *in vivo*. For A, ■ = E_2, □ = TAM + E_2, ○ = FRT + E_2, Δ = control. For B, □ = TAM, ○ = FRT, Δ = control.

levels of approximately 10% that of tamoxifen-inhibited tumors. These data indicate that, although reductions in tumor tamoxifen levels may be associated with tamoxifen-stimulated growth in some cases, reduced intratumoral tamoxifen levels are not *necessary* for tamoxifen-stimulated growth to occur.

Thus the causative mechanism behind the development of tamoxifen-stimulated breast tumor growth in this model remains to be identified. However, recent research has provided some promising clues. Data from the progesterone (Vegeto et al. 1992), androgen (Olea et al. 1990; Schuurmans et al. 1990; Veldscholte et al. 1990, Wilding et al. 1989), and estrogen (Jiang, Langan-Fahey, et al. 1992) receptor models indicate that mutations in a steroid receptor can confer responsiveness to ligands that either are not recognized by or are antagonists for the wild-type receptor. The development of tamoxifen-stimulated tumor growth is a reproducible phenomenon (Osborne et al. 1991; Wolf et al. 1993). It is possible that reproducible alterations which confer a tamoxifen-stimulated phenotype occur in the estrogen receptor or other parts of the estrogen-response mechanism.

IV. *Conclusion and Future Prospects*

A great deal has been accomplished over the past several years leading to the understanding of tamoxifen treatment failure and the development of tamoxifen-resistant or tamoxifen-dependent tumor growth. These accomplishments have been brought about by the work of many researchers. However, the investigation is by no means complete. Work over the next several years in the area of tamoxifen insensitivity will focus on identifying the functional role of mutant steroid receptors in circumventing the normal cellular growth-control pathways. Research will also focus on clarifying the developing realization that control of the cell cycle does not occur by a series of discrete linear steps but rather by an interconnected set of parallel pathways. Experiments will be done to determine which pathways are activated to circumvent the need for an estrogen-occupied ER to activate cell growth.

In the area of tamoxifen-dependent tumor growth, research will focus on finding the causative alterations in tumor cells responsible for this phenotype. In particular, research will focus on identifying reproducible alterations in ERs from tamoxifen-stimulated tumor cells as well as alterations in the entire ER-mediated transcriptional complex. Although the production of novel tamoxifen metabolites and isomers thereof is not necessary for the development of tamoxifen-stimulated growth, these phenomena may be found to play a role in some cases.

Ultimately, this research must be linked to the clinic, by finding ways to use the information about treatment resistance to design new, specific therapies which will benefit the patient who has experienced disease recurrence while taking tamoxifen.

References

Arteaga, C. L., and C. K. Osborne. 1989. Growth inhibition of human breast cancer cells *in vitro* with an antibody against the type I somatomedin receptor. *Cancer Research* 49:6237–6241.

Butta, A., K. MacLennan, K. C. Flanders, N. P. M. Sacks, I. Smith, A. McKinna, M. Dowsett, L. M. Wakefield, M. B. Sporn, M. Baum, and A. A. Coletta. 1992. Induction of transforming growth factor ß1 in human breast cancer *in vivo* following tamoxifen treatment. *Cancer Research* 52:4261–4264.

Cole, M. P., C. J. Jones, and I. D. Todd. 1971. A new antioestrogenic agent in late breast cancer. An early clinical appraisal of ICI 46,474. *British Journal of Cancer* 25:270–275.

Colletta, A. A., L. M. Wakefield, F. V. Howell, K. E. van Roozendaal, D. Danielpour, S. R. Ebbs, M. B. Sporn, and M. Baum. 1990. Anti-oestrogens induce the secretion of active transforming growth factor beta from human fetal fibroblasts. *British Journal of Cancer* 62:405–409.

Colletti, R. B., J. D. Roberts, J. T. Devlin, and K. C. Copeland. 1989. Effect of tamoxifen on plasma insulin-like growth factor I in patients with breast cancer. *Cancer Research* 49:1882–1884.

Dotzlaw, H., M. Alkhalaf, and L. C. Murphy. 1992. Characterization of estrogen receptor variant mRNAs from human breast cancers. *Molecular Endocrinology* 6:773–785.

Early Breast Cancer Trialists' Collaborative Group. 1992. Systemic treatment of early breast cancer by hormonal, cytotoxic, or immune therapy. 133 randomised trials involving 31,000 recurrences and 24,000 deaths among 75,000 women. *Lancet* 339:1–15 and 71–85.

Friedl, A., V. C. Jordan, and M. Pollak. 1993. Effect of tamoxifen on insulin-like growth factor–1 levels in breast cancer patients. *European Journal of Cancer.* 29A:1368–1372.

Fuqua, S. A., S. D. Fitzgerald, G. C. Chamness, A. K. Tandon, D. P. Mcdonnell, Z. Nawaz, B. W. O'Malley, and W. L. McGuire. 1991. Variant human breast tumor estrogen receptor with constitutive transcriptional activity. *Cancer Research* 51:105–109.

Fuqua, S. A., S. D. Fitzgerald, D. C. Allred, R. M. Elledge, Z. Nawaz, D. P. McDonnell, B. W. O'Malley, G. L. Greene, and W. L. McGuire. 1992. Inhibition of estrogen receptor action by a naturally occurring variant in human breast tumors. *Cancer Research* 52:483–486.

Gottardis, M. M., and V. C. Jordan. 1988. Development of tamoxifen-stimulated growth of MCF-7 tumors in athymic mice after long-term antiestrogen administration. *Cancer Research* 48:5183–5187.

Gottardis, M. M., S. P. Robinson, and V. C. Jordan. 1988. Estradiol-stimulated growth of MCF-7 tumors implanted in athymic mice: a model to study the tumoristatic action of tamoxifen. *Journal of Steroid Biochemistry* 30:311–314.

Gottardis, M. M., S. Y. Jiang, M. H. Jeng, and V. C. Jordan. 1989. Inhibition of tamoxifen-stimulated growth of an MCF-7 tumor variant in athymic mice by novel steroidal antiestrogens. *Cancer Research* 49:4090–4093.

Gottardis, M. M., S. P. Robinson, P. G. Satyaswaroop, and V. C. Jordan. 1988. Contrasting actions of tamoxifen on endometrial and breast tumor growth in the athymic mouse. *Cancer Research* 48:812–815.

Gottardis, M. M., R. J. Wagner, E. C. Borden, and V. C. Jordan. 1989. Differential ability of antiestrogens to stimulate breast cancer cell (MCF-7) growth *in vivo* and *in vitro*. *Cancer Research* 49:4765–4769.

Graham II, M. L., N. L. Krett, L. A. Miller, K. K. Leslie, D. F. Gordon, W. M. Wood, L. L. Wei, and K. B. Horwitz. 1990. T47D$_{co}$ cells, genetically unstable and containing estrogen receptor mutations, are a model for the progression of breast cancers to hormone resistance. *Cancer Research* 50:6208–6217.

Horwitz, K. B., and W. L. McGuire. 1975. Predicting response to endocrine therapy in human breast cancer: a hypothesis. *Science* 189:726–727.

Huff, K. K., D. Kaufman, K. H. Gabbay, E. M. Spencer, M. E. Lippman, and R. B. Dickson. 1986. Secretion of an insulin-like growth factor–I–related protein by human breast cancer cells. *Cancer Research* 46:4613–4619.

Iino, Y., D. M. Wolf, S. M. Langan-Fahey, D. A. Johnson, M. Ricchio, M. E. Thompson, and V. C. Jordan. 1991. Reversible control of oestradiol-stimulated growth of MCF-7 tumours by tamoxifen in the athymic mouse. *British Journal of Cancer* 64:1019–1024.

Jiang, S. Y., D. M. Wolf, J. M. Yingling, C. Chang, and V. C. Jordan. 1992. An estrogen receptor positive MCF-7 clone that is resistant to antiestrogens and estradiol. *Molecular and Cellular Endocrinology* 90:77–86.

Jiang, S. Y., S. M. Langan-Fahey, A. L. Stella, R. McCague, and V. C. Jordan. 1992. Point mutation of estrogen receptor (ER) in the ligand binding domain changes the pharmacology of antiestrogens in ER-negative breast cancer cells stably expressing cDNAs for ER. *Molecular Endocrinology* 6:2167–2174.

Jordan, V. C. 1993. Should all women with a diagnosis of breast cancer be treated with tamoxifen? *Postgraduate Surgery* (in press).

Jordan, V. C., M. M. Collins, L. Rowsby, and G. Prestwich. 1977. A monohydroxylated metabolite of tamoxifen with potent antioestrogenic activity. *Journal of Endocrinology* 75:305–316.

Jordan, V. C., M. F. Wolf, D. M. Mirecki, D. A. Whitford, and W. V. Welshons. 1988. Hormone receptor assays: clinical usefulness in the management of carcinoma of the breast. *Critical Reviews in Clinical Laboratory Sciences* 26:97–152.

Karey, K. P., and D. A. Sirbasku. 1988. Differential responsiveness of human breast cancer cell lines MCF-7 and T47D to growth factors and 17 beta-estradiol. *Cancer Research* 48:4083–4092.

Knabbe, C., M. E. Lippman, L. M. Wakefield, K. C. Flanders, A. Kasid, R. Derynk, and R. B. Dickson. 1987. Evidence that transforming growth factor–ß is a hormonally regulated negative growth factor in human breast cancer cells. *Cell* 48:417–428.

Langan-Fahey, S. M., D. C. Tormey, and V. C. Jordan. 1990. Tamoxifen metabolites in patients on long-term adjuvant therapy for breast cancer. *European Journal of Cancer* 26:883–888.

McCague, R., R. Kuroda, G. LeClerq, and S. Stoessel. 1986. Synthesis and estrogen receptor binding of 6,7-dihydro-8-phenyl-9-[4-[2-(dimethylamino)ethoxy]phenyl]5H-benzocyclo-heptene, a non-isomerizable analogue of tamoxifen. X-ray crystallographic studies. *Journal of Medicinal Chemistry* 29:2053–2058.

McGuire, W. L., G. C. Chamness, and S. A. Fuqua. 1991. Estrogen receptor variants in clinical breast cancer. *Molecular Endocrinology* 5:1571–1577.

Murphy, C. S., S. M. Langan-Fahey, R. McCague, and V. C. Jordan. 1990. Structure-function relationships of hydroxylated metabolites of tamoxifen that control the proliferation of estrogen-responsive T47D breast cancer cells *in vitro*. *Molecular Pharmacology* 38:737–743.

Murphy, L. C., and H. Dotzlaw. 1989. Variant estrogen receptor mRNA species detected in human breast cancer biopsy samples. *Molecular Endocrinology* 3:687–693.

Nayfield, S. G., J. E. Karp, L. G. Ford, F. A. Dorr, and B. S. Kramer. 1991. Potential role of tamoxifen in prevention of breast cancer. *Journal of the National Cancer Institute* 83:1450–1459.

Olea, N., K. Sakabe, A. M. Soto, and C. Sonnenschein. 1990. The proliferative effect of "anti-androgens" on the androgen-sensitive human prostate tumor cell line LNCaP. *Endocrinology* 126:1457–1463.

Osborne, C. K., E. B. Coronado, and J. P. Robinson. 1987. Human breast cancer in the athymic nude mouse: cytostatic effects of long term antiestrogen therapy. *European Journal of Cancer and Clinical Oncology* 23:1189–1196.

Osborne, C. K., K. Hobbs, and G. M. Clark. 1985. Effect of estrogens and antiestrogens on growth of human breast cancer cells in athymic nude mice. *Cancer Research* 45:584–590.

Osborne, C. K., E. Coronado, D. C. Allred, V. Wiebe, and M. DeGregorio. 1991. Acquired tamoxifen resistance: correlation with reduced breast tumor levels of tamoxifen and isomerization of trans-4-hydroxytamoxifen. *Journal of the National Cancer Institute* 83:1477–1482.

Osborne, C. K., V. J. Wiebe, W. L. McGuire, D. R. Ciocca, and M. DeGregorio. 1992. Tamoxifen and the isomers of 4-hydroxytamoxifen in tamoxifen-resistant tumors from breast cancer patients. *Journal of Clinical Oncology* 10:304–310.

Pollak, M., J. Costantino, C. Polychronakos, S. A. Blauer, H. Guyda, C. Redmond, B. Fisher, and R. Margolese. 1990. Effect of tamoxifen on serum insulin-like growth factor I levels in stage I breast cancer patients. *Journal of the National Cancer Institute* 82:1693–1697.

Powles, T. J., C. R. Tillyer, A. L. Jones, S. E. Ashley, J. Treleaven, J. B. Davey, and J. A. McKinna. 1990. Prevention of breast cancer with tamoxifen—an update on the Royal Marsden Hospital pilot programme. *European Journal of Cancer* 26:680–684.

Powles, T. J., J. R. Hardy, S. E. Ashley, G. M. Farrington, D. Cosgrove, J. B. Davey, M. Dowsett, J. A. McKinna, A. G. Nash, H. D. Sinnett, C. R. Tillyer, and J. Treleaven. 1989. A pilot trial to evaluate the acute toxicity and feasibility of tamoxifen for prevention of breast cancer. *British Journal of Cancer* 60:126–131.

Satyaswaroop, P. G., R. J. Zaino, and R. Mortel. 1984. Estrogen-like effects of tamoxifen on human endometrial carcinoma transplanted into nude mice. *Cancer Research* 44:4006–4010.

Schuurmans, A. L., J. Bolt, J. Veldscholte, and E. Mulder. 1990. Stimulatory effects of anti-androgens on LNCaP human prostate tumor cell growth, EGF-receptor level and acid phosphatase secretion. *Journal of Steroid Biochemistry and Molecular Biology* 37:849–853.

Shafie, S. M., and F. H. Grantham. 1981. Role of hormones in the growth and regression of human breast cancer cells (MCF-7) transplanted into athymic nude mice. *Journal of the National Cancer Institute* 67:51–56.

Sporn, M. B., A. B. Roberts, L. M. Wakefield, R. K. Assoian. 1986. Transforming growth factor ß: Biological function and chemical structure. *Science* 233:532–534.

van der Burg, B., L. Isbrücker, A. J. van Selm-Miltenburg, S. W. de Laat, and E. J. van Zoelen. 1990. Role of estrogen-induced insulin-like growth factors in the proliferation of human breast cancer cells. *Cancer Research* 50:7770–7774.

van der Burg, B., G. R. Rutteman, M. A. Blankenstein, S. W. de Laat, and E. J. van Zoelen. 1988. Mitogenic stimulation of human breast cancer cells in a growth factor-defined medium: synergistic action of insulin and estrogen. *Journal of Cellular Physiology* 134:101–108.

Vegeto, E., G. F. Allan, W. T. Schrader, M. J. Tsai, D. P. McDonnell, and B. W. O'Malley. 1992. The mechanism of RU486 antagonism is dependent on the conformation of the carboxy-terminal tail of the human progesterone receptor. *Cell* 69:703–713.

Veldscholte, J., M. M. Voorhorst-Ogink, J. Bolt–de Vries, H. C. J. van Rooij, J. Trapman, and E. Mulder. 1990. Unusual specificity of the androgen receptor in the human prostate tumor cell line LNCaP: high affinity for progestagenic and estrogenic steroids. *Biochimica et Biophysica Acta* 1052:187–194.

Walker, K. J., J. M. Price-Thomas, W. Candlish, and R. I. Nicholson. 1991. Influence of the antiestrogen tamoxifen on normal breast tissue. *British Journal of Cancer* 64:764–768.

Wiebe, V. J., C. K. Osborne, W. L. McGuire, and M. W. DeGregorio. 1992. Identification of estrogenic tamoxifen metabolite(s) in tamoxifen-resistant human breast tumors. *Journal of Clinical Oncology* 10:990–994.

Wilding, G., M. Chen, and E. P. Gelmann. 1989. Aberrant response *in vitro* of hormone-responsive prostate cancer cells to antiandrogens. *Prostate* 14:103–115.

Wolf, D. M., and V. C. Jordan. 1992. Gynecologic complications associated with long-term adjuvant tamoxifen therapy for breast cancer. *Gynecologic Oncology* 45:118–128.

Wolf, D. M., S. M. Langan-Fahey, C. P. Parker, R. McCague, and V. C. Jordan. 1993. Investigation of the mechanism of tamoxifen-stimulated breast tumor growth using non-isomerizable analogs of tamoxifen and metabolites. *Journal of the National Cancer Institute* 85:806–812.

Yee, D., S. Paik, G. S. Lebovic, R. R. Marcus, R. E. Favoni, K. J. Cullen, M. E. Lippman, and N. Rosen. 1989. Analysis of insulin-like growth factor I gene expression in malignancy: evidence for a paracrine role in human breast cancer. *Molecular Endocrinology* 3:509–517.

11

A New Approach to Breast Cancer Therapy—Total Estrogen Ablation with Pure Antiestrogens

A. E. WAKELING

 I. INTRODUCTION 220
 II. RATIONALE FOR THERAPY WITH PURE ANTIESTROGENS 221
 III. STRATEGY FOR DISCOVERY OF NOVEL ANTIESTROGENS 222
 IV. PROPERTIES OF PURE ANTIESTROGENS 223
  A. PHARMACOLOGY 223
  B. EFFECTS ON HUMAN BREAST CANCER CELLS 225
  C. BIOCHEMISTRY 226
 V. FROM LEAD COMPOUND TO DRUG CANDIDATE 229
 VI. SUMMARY 230
  REFERENCES 231

I. *Introduction*

THE primary strategy for the treatment of breast cancer has been based on altering the endocrine environment of the tumor, specifically to attenuate the growth-stimulatory effects of estrogens. A wide range of hormone ablative or additive therapies has been evaluated. Older procedures like oophorectomy and adrenalectomy, or high-dose estrogen or androgen therapy, have largely been replaced by more specific medical treatments designed to reduce the synthesis or action of estrogens, for example, by the use of luteinizing hormone–releasing hormone (LHRH) analogs, aromatase inhibitors, and antiestrogens (see Fig. 11.1). Most recently, the antiestrogen tamoxifen (ICI 46,474: Nolvadex* tamoxifen citrate) has emerged as the treatment of choice. This compound is well tolerated, simple to administer, provides effective palliation of advanced breast cancer, and, when used in adjuvant therapy, delays recurrence and improves survival (Jackson et al. 1991; Early Breast Cancer Trialist's Collaborative Group 1992).

An important common feature of the above medical treatments is that none achieves *complete* removal of the tumor growth stimulatory actions of endogenous estrogens or of estrogens arising, directly or indirectly, from dietary sources. It may be thought that such concerns do not apply in the case of tamoxifen treatment, because this agent blocks the cellular actions of estrogens by direct competition with the natural ligand(s) at the level of the estrogen receptor (ER) (Jordan and Murphy 1990). Thus, the impressive clinical efficacy of tamoxifen might seem to render unlikely the possibility that alternative, more effective antiestrogens could be discovered. However, the properties of some new pure antiestrogens may yet challenge this conclusion. The rationale for seeking such compounds and their discovery and potential to achieve complete estrogen ablation are described in this chapter. Particular emphasis is placed on how pure antiestrogens differ from tamoxifen and what these differences may presage in the clinical context.

---

*Nolvadex is a trademark, property of Imperial Chemical Industries, PLC.

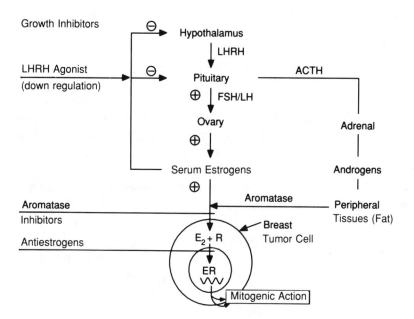

Figure 11.1. Endocrine control of breast cancer.

II. *Rationale for Therapy with Pure Antiestrogens*

Estrogen stimulation of tumor growth is mediated by the binding of estrogens to ER in the cell nucleus, to activate the transcription of a specific subset of genes characterized by the presence of specific DNA sequences in their control regions, termed estrogen response elements (Beato 1989). Tamoxifen similarly forms a nuclear-ER complex, competitive with estrogens. This complex attenuates, but does not always block completely, the growth-stimulatory mechanisms controlled by endogenous estradiol-ER. This is exemplified by pharmacological studies with tamoxifen. In the absence of endogenous estrogens, the effects of tamoxifen may be equivalent to or similar to, but of a smaller magnitude than, those of estradiol (full or partial agonist, respectively). When endogenous estrogens are present, tamoxifen may cause a partial or complete blockade of normal stimulatory responses (partial or complete antagonist). This inherent variation is observed in both experimental animals (Macnab et al. 1984) and man (Jordan and Murphy 1990) at the gene, cell, and organ level (Wakeling and Slater 1981; Wakeling

1987a). The rationale for seeking novel antiestrogens was based on the recognition of the biochemical mechanism underlying the pharmacological actions of tamoxifen, namely, that ER-specific ligands which could compete effectively with estradiol *without inducing any estrogen-like actions,* that is *pure antiestrogens,* might be of value (Wakeling 1985, 1991).

Two important *potential* clinical advantages of pure antiestrogens in comparison with partial agonist/antagonist antiestrogens like tamoxifen were recognized. First, *complete* blockade of all stimulatory actions of estrogens in breast cancer patients may result in a more rapid, complete, and longer-lasting tumor remission. Second, pure antiestrogens *may* have an improved toxicology profile because of the absence of estrogen-like stimulatory actions. Such effects of tamoxifen lead to developmental abnormalities of the reproductive tract in rodents (Tucker et al. 1984) and, in patients, may underlie undesirable actions on the endometrium (Nayfield et al. 1991). Thus, pure antiestrogens may be more likely than partial agonists to satisfy drug regulatory requirements for therapeutic use in nonmalignant estrogen-responsive conditions like endometriosis, fibroids, and benign breast disease. Such uses would represent a significant extension of the therapeutic use of antiestrogens beyond their current principal use in the treatment of malignancy.

III. *Strategy for Discovery of Novel Antiestrogens*

The two key elements of the search for pure antiestrogens were, first, a novel medicinal chemistry strategy to identify new ER ligands and, second, robust and reliable biological test systems. The strategy chosen for initial chemistry is described elsewhere (Bowler et al. 1989) and involved synthesis of estradiol analogs bearing C7 substituents, which retain a high affinity for ER, an essential feature recognized in our drug target profile (Wakeling 1990). Intrinsic potency could be monitored accurately *in vitro* by receptor-binding assays (Wakeling 1987b) and antiestrogenic activity determined by the inhibition of the growth of estrogen-sensitive human breast cancer (MCF-7) cells (Wakeling 1989). Additionally, we had much experience of facile and reproducible testing for both agonist and antagonist activity *in vivo* using a uterotropic-antiuterotropic assay in immature rats (Wakeling et al. 1983). Synthesis of novel 7α-alkylamide analogs of estradiol provided, amongst the first examples, compounds with mixed agonist-antagonist activity (Bowleret al. 1989). However, compounds devoid of estrogenic activity but capable, when administered together with estradiol, of blocking completely the uterotropic effect

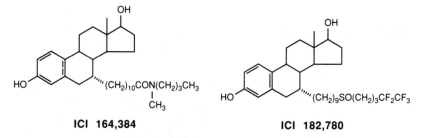

ICI 164,384   ICI 182,780

Figure 11.2. Structures of pure antioestrogens.

of the natural hormone in rodents were also described (Wakeling and Bowler 1987; Bowler et al. 1989). Most important, such compounds were also shown to block the uterotropic action of tamoxifen (Wakeling and Bowler 1987). This work exemplified for the first time the pharmacological effects expected of a pure antiestrogen.

Structure-activity analysis revealed the importance of the position, length, and flexibility of the C7 sidechain (Bowler et al. 1989). For example, it was shown that receptor binding and biological activity reside almost exclusively in the 7α rather than the 7ß isomers. Pure antagonist activity is constrained to compounds with an overall chain length of 16–18 atoms, and tertiary rather than secondary amides are preferred. The most potent pure antagonist amongst the alkylamides was N-n-butyl-N-methyl-11-(3,17ß-dihydroxy estra-1,3,5(10)-trien-7α-yl)undecanamide, ICI 164,384 (Fig. 11.2). Subsequent work in this and other laboratories, using a wide variety of *in vitro* and *in vivo* assays for estrogen action and its inhibition, has served to confirm the unique properties of these steroidal pure antiestrogens (see Wakeling 1991 for a review).

IV. *Properties of Pure Antiestrogens*

A. PHARMACOLOGY

The key difference between compounds like ICI 164,384 and tamoxifen is the fact that ICI 164,384 is devoid of estrogenic activity. Thus, the tropic effects of estrogens can be blocked completely rather than partly. The most instructive demonstration of this difference is the ability of ICI 164,384 to antagonize the uterotropic action of tamoxifen as well as that of estrogens (Wakeling and Bowler 1987). Because this complete absence of stimulatory activity may be of particular significance to future clinical uses of pure antiestrogens, other relevant studies are highlighted here.

In ovariectomized, pubescent female rats, hormone replacement by estradiol, or by tamoxifen, supported the normal extent and time scale of mammary ductal growth. In this assay of breast development, tamoxifen would therefore be classified as a full estrogen. In contrast, ICI 164,384 was devoid of stimulatory activity and blocked both estrogen- and tamoxifen-induced growth (Nicholson et al. 1988). Pure antiestrogens are thus likely to minimize the possibility of tumor flare, which occurs in some patients beginning Nolvadex treatment and is thought to reflect an estrogenic action of tamoxifen (Reddel and Sutherland 1984). However, studies of normal breast tissue from patients receiving tamoxifen have failed to reveal any growth stimulatory effect (Walker et al. 1991). In another sensitive bioassay of estrogenic activity, the treatment of neonatal female rats with ICI 164,384, in contrast with estradiol and tamoxifen, did not accelerate the onset of puberty or lead to abnormalities in the development of the reproductive tract (Wakeling and Bowler 1988). These assays demonstrating the lack of estrogen-like stimulatory activity, in both the breast and uterus, minimize the concerns about potential toxicological effects which have prevented the widespread use of Nolvadex in the treatment of nonmalignant conditions of the breast and uterus (Diver et al. 1986).

The corollary of the absence of estrogenic activity in pure antiestrogens is that total estrogen ablation should be achievable. This has been demonstrated in intact female rats where ICI 164,384 treatment results in an ovariectomy-like regression of the uterus (Wakeling and Bowler 1988). In those studies, ICI 164,384 had no effect on indices of estrogen action at the hypothalamic-pituitary axis, for example, on LH secretion. This argues that a peripherally selective action of pure antiestrogens might be achieved in patients. Thus, an antitumor or antiuterine effect may be achievable without disruption of the hypothalamic-pituitary-ovarian axis. Translated to the clinical setting, pure antiestrogens would thus provide a particularly desirable pharmacological action in premenopausal patients.

The majority of breast cancer patients are postmenopausal, so effects on the hypothalamic-pituitary-ovarian axis are largely irrelevant. However, to the same extent, the question of total estrogen ablation is relevant in such patients. Studies with mammary carcinoma in rats, treated with a combination of an LHRH analog (Zoladex*) to mimic cessation of ovarian function and ICI 164,384, showed that the antiestrogen reduced further the size of the uterus and provided a more rapid rate of tumor involution compared with the effect of the LHRH analog alone (Nicholson et al. 1990).

---

*Zoladex is a trademark, the property of Imperial Chemical Industries, PLC.

A question of particular significance to the therapeutic potential of pure antiestrogens is whether tumors resistant to Nolvadex will be cross-resistant to these new agents. This question has been addressed in nude mice bearing xenografts of human breast cancer cells treated long-term with tamoxifen. Tamoxifen initially attenuates tumor growth by a cytostatic mechanism (Osborne et al. 1987) but tumor growth may subsequently resume (Gottardis and Jordan 1988). This model reflects a common course of the disease in patients. Studies in nude mice transplanted with these "tamoxifen resistant" tumors have shown that their continued growth requires the presence of tamoxifen (or estrogen) (Gottardis and Jordan 1988). Furthermore, in those tumors requiring tamoxifen to sustain growth, treatment with ICI 164,384 produced a marked growth inhibition (Gottardis et al. 1989). Similar observations have been made with a human endometrial-derived tumor (Gottardis et al. 1990). These observations argue that one form of tamoxifen resistance is in fact the development of a dependence on the "agonist" estrogen-like action of the drug, and that such tumors may be effectively treated with a pure antiestrogen.

Careful review of patient data for clinical parallels to these animal model studies provides evidence that some tumors may "see" the antiestrogen as an agonist. In these patients apparent resistance, that is, the resumption of tumor growth after an initial response to Nolvadex, may in fact be a manifestation of the existance or development of responsiveness to the estrogenic component of tamoxifen's activity (Howell et al. 1990). A most interesting recent development which may explain both the animal model and clinical observations is the report by Osborne et al. (1991), which attributes the acquired tamoxifen resistance to reduced uptake and altered metabolism of tamoxifen in the tumor. A part of the alterations in drug metabolism may be an increased formation of estrogenic metabolites (Osborne et al. 1991). These changes have been described to date only in human tumors grown in nude mice. Similar measurements in tumors from patients relapsing on Nolvadex treatment are awaited.

B. Effects on Human Breast Cancer Cells

The 50% inhibitory concentrations of tamoxifen and ICI 164,384 on MCF-7 human breast cancer cells were 1 μM and 2 nM, respectively, and growth inhibition was reversed fully by estradiol (Wakeling and Bowler 1988). The specificity of this growth inhibition is emphasized by studies with ER-negative MDA-MB-231 human breast cancer cells in which ICI 164,384 had no effect (Thompson et al. 1989; Wakeling 1991). A particularly interesting distinction between the action of partial agonists like tamoxifen and the pure antagonists emerged from the early studies with MCF-7 cells. Qualitatively, the effects of both types of antiestrogen on ER-containing cells were similar, in that cell proliferation was blocked in the G_1 phase of the cell cycle (Wakeling et al. 1989; Musgrove et al. 1989). However, it was also clear that the efficacy, as well as the potency, of ICI 164,384 was markedly greater than that of tamoxifen. Under identical experimental conditions, the proportion of cells exposed to antiestrogens which remained capable of DNA synthesis was reduced to 7% by ICI 164,384, compared with 19% for tamoxifen (Wakeling et al. 1989). That this was not simply a reflection of potency differences was demonstrated by substituting, for tamoxifen, nonsteroidal antiestrogens with a higher receptor-binding affinity, like 4-hydroxytamoxifen (Wakeling 1989) or hydroxyclomiphene (Musgrove et al. 1989). This difference in efficacy was attributed to the estrogenic activity of the nonsteroidal antiestrogens (Wakeling et al. 1989), which can induce proliferation in these tumor cells (Katzenellenbogen et al. 1987), an exact parallel with their uterotropic activity. The "residual" stimulatory activity of tamoxifen, absent in pure antiestrogens, can be synergistically amplified in the presence of other growth factors like insulin (Wakeling et al. 1989) and IGF-I (Stewart et al. 1990). The stimulatory effects of tamoxifen on tumor cells *in vitro* are also manifest in assays of invasive activity. Like estradiol, tamoxifen, but not ICI 164,384, increased the rate at which MCF-7 cells penetrated a model basement membrane (Thompson et al. 1989). Translation of these observations to a clinical setting argues that the pure antiestrogens are likely to be more effective antiproliferative and antimetastatic agents than tamoxifen.

C. BIOCHEMISTRY

An important feature of the action of antiestrogens is their capacity to compete effectively with estradiol for binding to ER. ICI 164,384 is much more effective than tamoxifen in this respect. Both antiestrogens compete with estradiol in a competitive, concentration-dependent manner, but the relative binding affinity of ICI 164,384 for ER is substantially higher than that of tamoxifen (0.19 and 0.025, respectively, cf. estradiol, 1; Wakeling and Bowler 1987).

The key to explaining the molecular mode of estrogen action, and the effects of antagonists, lies in defining the mechanisms which are interposed between the initial ligand recognition event and the activation of the transcription of hormone-responsive genes. Identification of the genes encoding ER and other steroid receptors, together with the description of specific sequences of DNA-termed hormone response elements (HREs), which bind the hormone receptor complex and control the efficiency of transcription (Beato 1989; Tsai et al. 1991), has allowed the application of molecular genetic techniques to this problem. Original studies which defined three functionally important domains of ER (Kumar et al. 1986) have proved to reflect a general consensus (Green and Chambon 1988). Each receptor has a centrally located DNA-binding domain which shows a high degree of sequence homology across receptor classes and is responsible for HRE recognition, a less well-conserved C-terminal ligand-binding domain, and an N-terminal domain widely variant in size and sequence between receptors. In terms of the *efficiency* of transcriptional activation induced by ligand-ER complex binding to estrogen response elements (EREs), specific sequences termed transcriptional activation functions (TAFs) are thought to be important (Webster et al. 1988; Lees et al. 1989; Tora et al. 1989). TAF-1, located in the N-terminus of ER, can function independently of the ligand-binding domain, and hence of the ligand. The activity of TAF-1 is variable in different cells, and its efficiency in activating transcription also varies between promotors. TAF-2, located in the C-terminal ligand-binding domain, is thought to be functionally active only for ligand-ER complexes containing the natural hormone (Green and Chambon 1988).

The role of TAFs in transmitting ligand-receptor "signals" following binding of different antiestrogens has been analyzed (Berry et al. 1990). In tamoxifen-receptor complexes, TAF-2 was disabled but TAF-1 retained functional activity. Thus, one hypothesis to explain the remarkable variations of biological responses arising from tamoxifen-receptor complexes attributes the diversity to the continued activity of TAF-1. Variations in the strength of the estrogen-like signals at the organ and cellular level thus attributed beg the question of what controls the efficiency of TAF-1. It is assumed that this requires the concurrent presence of other *cell specific* transcription factors, the identity of which remains to be elucidated. Similarly, differences in the efficiency with which specific estrogen-responsive genes respond to tamoxifen in individual cells presumably reflect the strength of interaction between TAF-1 and particular promotors (Green and Chambon 1988). The effects of ICI 164,384–ER complexes on transcriptional activation are the subject of controversy. Berry et al. (1990) showed that, in contrast with tamoxifen, the ICI 164,384–receptor complexes failed to promote transcription. Because it was also shown that ICI 164,384 did not inhibit the activity of TAF-1, it is implied that ER complexed with ICI 164,384 did not bind to DNA (Berry et al. 1990). These studies are in agreement with previous work which showed that ICI 164,384 did not promote receptor binding to DNA (Wilson et al. 1990; Fawell, White, et al. 1990). If this "poisoning" of the receptor's ability to recognize DNA proves correct it would conform to the mechanistic objective in our original definition of pure antiestrogens. Other studies, however, do indicate that ICI 164,384 can promote receptor binding to DNA (Martinez and Wahli 1989; Lees et al. 1989; Sabbah et al. 1991; Pham et al. 1991) and are supported by observations that, in some experimental conditions, very weak agonist effects of ICI 164,384 can be detected (Weaver et al. 1988; Wakeling et al. 1989; Pasqualini et al. 1990; Jamil et al. 1991).

A necessary prerequisite for DNA recognition is the ligand-induced dissociation of a 90 kDa heat shock protein (HSP 90) (Denis et al. 1988), which is a component common to the native, ligand-free steroid receptors (Joab et al. 1984). Dissociation of HSP 90 is thought to allow receptors to dimerize (Miller et al. 1985). The homodimeric receptor complex binds tightly to DNA (Kumar et al. 1986). Further analysis of ER has shown that domains controlling HSP 90 binding and receptor dimerization overlap in the hormone-binding region of the receptor (Fawell, Lees, et al. 1990; Chambraud et al. 1990). It was suggested that hormone antagonists fail to promote dissociation of HSP 90 and would therefore prevent dimerization and DNA recognition (Baulieu 1989). Recent studies by Fawell, White, et al. (1990) with ICI 164,384 support this hypothesis. Dimerization of the estrogen receptor was severely impaired by the pure antagonist. Other investigators have reached opposite conclusions (Sabbah et al. 1991; Pham et al. 1991). These apparently conflicting conclusions may be reconciled by assuming that the dimerization function is not absolutely required for DNA binding, but merely enhances ERE-binding affinity (Pham et al. 1991). Whatever the molecular mechanism, there is no dispute that the net result of pure antiestrogen binding is a receptor complex with severely attenuated transcriptional activity.

Although there remains some uncertainty about whether there is an absolute distinction between pure and partial agonist antiestrogens in terms of their biochemical mode of action, it is clear that the former compounds are much less efficient than the latter in promoting the changes in receptor conformation necessary for DNA binding and subsequent activation of transcription. Because the affinity of pure antiestrogens for the receptor is comparable to that of estradiol, and substantially greater than that of tamoxifen (Wakeling and Bowler 1987), how is the high binding energy dissipated in a biologically nonproductive manner? The first clue to this puzzle has emerged from studies of the fate of the receptor in cells following treatment with ICI 164,384. ICI 164,384 dramatically reduced receptor concentration in the mouse uterus to 5% of control levels 4 hours after treatment (Gibson et al. 1991). Because cycloheximide did not affect this response and no change in receptor mRNA was detected, it appears that the receptor-pure antiestrogen complex becomes more "fragile" and perhaps more susceptible to the normal processes involved in receptor degradation. It remains to be seen whether the binding energy released is actively involved in enhancing receptor degradation, but the half-life of the ICI 164,384–ER complex appears to be substantially less than that of the estradiol-ER complex or that of the tamoxifen-ER complex, which is not significantly different when compared with estradiol (Eckert et al. 1984). In the case of the tamoxifen-ER complex, the lower energy available from the binding reaction may simply reduce the efficiency of activation and be insufficient to promote more rapid receptor degradation.

V. From Lead Compound to Drug Candidate

Complete estrogen ablation *in vivo* was difficult to achieve with ICI 164,384, and, for this reason, ICI 164,384 did not merit serious consideration as a drug candidate. Thus, more potent compounds were sought which retained the advantageous pharmacological profile of ICI 164,384 compared with the tamoxifen-like partial agonists. A new compound, 7α-[9-(4,4,5,5,5-pentafluoro pentylsulfinyl)nonyl]estra-1,3,5(10)-triene-3,17ß-diol, ICI 182,780 (Fig. 11.1), was selected for intensive study. ICI 182,780 differs from ICI 164,384 in two key features of the 7α sidechain: the amide moiety of ICI 164,384 was replaced by a sulphinyl group, and the terminal alkyl function was fluorinated to reduce the potential for metabolic attack (Bowler et al. 1989). The pharmacology of ICI 182,780 is described elsewhere (Wakeling et al. 1991). Briefly, the key advantage of ICI 182,780, compared with ICI 164,384, is a significant increase of potency.

In vitro, ICI 182,780 has a 4–5-fold greater affinity for ER (ICI 182,780 = 0.89 vs ICI 164,384 = 0.19, cf. estradiol = 1) and, in experiments with MCF-7 human breast cancer cells, 50% inhibitory concentrations of 0.29 and 1.3 nM were observed for ICI 182,780 and ICI 164,384, respectively. *In vivo,* a comparison of potency in the rat uterotropic-antiuterotropic test showed that ICI 182,780 is devoid of stimulatory activity and is 10-fold more potent than ICI 164,384 (50% effective doses of 0.06 and 0.9 mg/kg, respectively). The 2-fold difference in apparent potency improvement between *in vitro* and *in vivo* assays is thought to reflect differences in absorption and/or distribution and metabolism between ICI 182,780 and ICI 164,384. Like ICI 164,384, ICI 182,780 retains the key pharmacological differences from tamoxifen, namely, greater efficacy against human breast cancer cells, absence of *any* stimulatory estrogen-like actions, and peripherally selective action *in vivo* (Wakeling et al. 1991).

The relatively low oral bioavailability of ICI 182,780 (Wakeling et al. 1991) required the development of parenteral formulations with a sustained duration of action to enhance the potential clinical utility of the drug. This was achieved by dispersion of the drug in oil. Sustained antitumor efficacy was then demonstrated in human breast cancer xenografts in nude mice, where a single injection of ICI 182,780 was at least as effective as daily treatment with tamoxifen over a 1-month period (Wakeling et al. 1991). These studies allowed selection of ICI 182,780 as a drug candidate to test the hypothesis that total estrogen ablation, achieved by treatment with a pure antiestrogen, may offer improved clinical efficacy in breast cancer therapy.

VI. *Summary*

New steroidal antiestrogens, exemplified by ICI 164,384 and ICI 182,780, offer for the first time the opportunity to test clinically the hypothesis that total blockade of estrogen action may have advantages over current medical therapies for breast cancer. The experimental data which distinguish these novel pure antiestrogens from established agents like Nolvadex have been described and provide a pharmacological rationale for the belief that a therapeutic advantage for these new agents may emerge from clinical trials. In particular, the complete absence of agonist activity consequent to binding and inactivation of ER by these new agents leads to more profound antiproliferative and antimetastatic effects on breast cancer cells and is likely to minimize the development of tumor antiestrogen resistance characteristic of partial agonists. The clinical consequences of these properties may emerge as a more rapid, a more complete, and/or a longer-lasting tumor remission. Additionally, reduction of estrogen-associated toxicities, and peripherally selective antiestrogenic activity, may allow the use of pure antiestrogens in the treatment of nonmalignant breast and uterine diseases.

References

Baulieu, E. E. 1989. Contragestation and other clinical applications of RU 486, an antiprogesterone at the receptor. *Science* 245:1352–1357.

Beato, M. 1989. Gene regulation by steroid hormones. *Cell* 56:335–344.

Berry, M., D. Metzger, and P. Chambon. 1990. Role of two trans activating domains in the cell-type and promotor–context dependent agonistic activity of the antioestrogen 4-hydroxytamoxifen. *European Molecular Biology Organisation Journal* 9:2811–2818.

Bowler, J., T. J. Lilley, J. D. Pittam, and A. E. Wakeling. 1989. Novel steroidal pure antiestrogens. *Steroids* 54:71–99.

Chambraud, B., M. Berry, G. Redeuilh, P. Chambon, and E. E. Baulieu. 1990. Several regions of human estrogen receptor are involved in the formation of receptor–heat shock protein 90 complexes. *Journal of Biological Chemistry* 265:20686–20691.

Denis, M., L. Poellinger, A. C. Wikstom, and J. A. Gustafsson. 1988. Requirement of hormone for thermal conversion of the glucocorticoid receptor to a DNA-binding state. *Nature* 333:686–688.

Diver, J. M., I. M. Jackson, and J. D. Fitzgerald. 1986. Tamoxifen and non-malignant indications. *Lancet* 1:733.

Eckert, R. L., A. Mullick, E. A. Rorke, and B. S. Katzenellenbogen. 1984. Estrogen receptor synthesis and turnover in MCF-7 breast cancer cells measured by a density shift technique. *Endocrinology* 114:629–637.

Early Breast Cancer Trialists' Collaborative Group. 1992. Systemic treatment of early breast cancer by hormonal, cytotoxic or immune therapy. 133 randomised trials involving 31,000 recurrences and 24,000 deaths among women. *Lancet* 339:1–15.

Fawell, S. E., J. A. Lees, R. White, and M. G. Parker. 1990. Characterization and colocalization of steroid binding and dimerization activities in the mouse estrogen receptor. *Cell* 60:953–962.

Fawell, S. E., R. White, S. Hoare, M. Sydenham, M. Page, and M. G. Parker. 1990. Inhibition of estrogen receptor–DNA binding by the "pure" antiestrogen ICI 164,284 appears to be mediated by impaired receptor dimerization. *Proceedings of the National Academy of Sciences* 87:6883–6887.

Gibson, M. K., L. A. Nemmers, W. C. Beckman, Jr., V. L. Davis, S. W. Curtis, and K. S. Korach. 1991. The mechanism of ICI 164,384 antiestrogenicity involves rapid loss of estrogen receptor in uterine tissue. *Endocrinology* 129:2000–2010.

Green, S., and P. Chambon. 1988. Nuclear receptors enhance our understanding of transcription regulation. *Trends in Genetics* 4:309–314.

Gottardis, M. M., and V. C. Jordan. 1988. Development of tamoxifen stimulated growth of MCF-7 tumors in athymic mice after long-term antiestrogen administration. *Cancer Research* 48:5183–5187.

Gottardis, M. M., S. Y. Jiang, M. H. Jeng, and V. C. Jordan. 1989. Inhibition of tamoxifen-stimulated growth of an MCF-7 tumor variant in athymic mice by novel steroidal antiestrogens. *Cancer Research* 49:4090–4093.

Gottardis, M. M., M. E. Ricchio, P. G. Satyaswaroop, and V. C. Jordan. 1990. Effect of steroidal and nonsteroidal antiestrogens an the growth of a tamoxifen-stimulated human endometrial carcinoma (EnCa101) in athymic mice. *Cancer Research* 50:3189–3192.

Howell, A., D. J. Dodwell, I. Laidlaw, H. Anderson, and E. Anderson. 1990. Tamoxifen as an agonist for metastatic breast cancer. In *Endocrine therapy of breast cancer,* vol. 4, ed. A. Goldhirsch, 49–58. Berlin: Springer-Verlag.

Jackson, I. M., S. Litherland, and A. E. Wakeling. 1991. Tamoxifen and other antiestrogens. In *Medical management of breast cancer,* ed. T. J. Powles and I. E. Smith, 51–59. London: Martin Dunitz.

Jamil, A., J. D. Croxtall, and J. O. White. 1991. The effect of antioestrogens on cell growth and progesterone receptor concentration in human endometrial cancer cells (Ishikawa). *Journal of Molecular Endocrinology* 6:215–221.

Joab, I., C. Radanyi, M. Renoir, T. Buchou, M. G. Catelli, N. Binart, J. Mester, and E. E. Baulieu. 1984. Common non-hormone binding component in non-transformed chick oviduct receptors of four steroid hormones. *Nature* 308:850–853.

Jordan, V. C., and C. S. Murphy. 1990. Endocrine pharmacology of antiestrogens as antitumor agents. *Endocrine Reviews* 11:578–610.

Katzenellenbogen, B. S., K. L. Kendra, M. J. Norman, and Y. Berthois. 1987. Proliferation, hormonal responsiveness, and estrogen receptor content of MCF-7 human breast cancer cell grown in the short-term and long-term absence of estrogens. *Cancer Research* 47:4355–4360.

Kumar, V., S. Green, A. Straub, and P. Chambon. 1986. Localisation of the oestradiol-binding and putative DNA-binding domains of the human oestrogen receptor. *European Molecular Biology Organisation Journal* 5:2231–2236.

Lees, J. A., S. E. Fawell, and M. G. Parker. 1989. Identification of two transactivation domains in the mouse oestrogen receptor. *Nucleic Acids Research* 17:5477–5488.

Macnab, M. W., R. J. Tallarida, and R. Joseph. 1984. An evaluation of tamoxifen as a partial agonist and by classical receptor theory—an explanation of the dual action of tamoxifen. *European Journal of Pharmacology* 103:321–326.

Martinez, E., and W. Wahli. 1989. Cooperative binding of estrogen receptor to imperfect estrogen-responsive DNA elements correlates with their synergistic hormone-dependent enhancer activity. *European Molecular Biology Organisation Journal* 8:3781–3791.

Miller, M. A., A. Mullick, G. L. Greene, and B. S. Katzenellenbogen. 1985. Characteristics of the subunit nature of nuclear estrogen receptors by the chemical cross-linking and dense amino acid labeling. *Endocrinology* 117:515–522.

Musgrove, E. A., A. E. Wakeling, and R. L. Sutherland. 1989. Points of action of estrogen antagonists and a calmodulin antagonist within the MCF-7 human breast cancer cell cycle. *Cancer Research* 49:2398–2404.

Nayfield, S. G., J. E. Karp, L. G. Ford, F. A. Dorr, and B. S. Kramer. 1991. Potential role of tamoxifen in the prevention of breast cancer. *Journal of the National Cancer Institute* 83:1450–1459.

Nicholson, R. I., K. E. Gotting, J. Gee, and K. J. Walker. 1988. Actions of oestrogens and antioestrogens on rat mammary gland development: relevance to breast cancer prevention. *Journal of Steroid Biochemistry* 30:95–103.

Nicholson, R. I., K. J. Walker, N. Bouzubar, R. J. Wills, J. M. Gee, N. K. Rushmere, and P. Davies. 1990. Estrogen deprivation in breast cancer. Clinical, experimental, and biological aspects. *Annals of the New York Academy of Sciences* 595:316–327.

Osborne, C. K., E. B. Coronado, and J. P. Robinson. 1987. Human breast cancer in athymic nude mouse: cytostatic effects of long-term antiestrogen therapy. *European Journal of Cancer and Clinical Oncology* 23:1189–1196.

Osborne, C. K., E. Coronado, D. C. Allred, V. Wiebe, and M. DeGregorio. 1991. Acquired tamoxifen resistance: correlation with reduced breast tumor levels of tamoxifen and isomerization of trans-4-hydroxytamoxifen. *Journal of the National Cancer Institute* 83:1477–1482.

Pasqualini, J. R., N. Giambiagi, C. Gelly, and G. Chetrite. 1990. Antiestrogen action in mammary cancer and in fetal cells. *Journal of Steroid Biochemistry* 37:343–348.

Pham, T. A., J. F. Elliston, Z. Nawaz, D. P. McDonnell, M. J. Tsai, and B. W. O'Malley. 1991. Antiestrogens can establish nonproductive receptor complexes and alter chromatin structure at target enhancers. *Proceedings of the National Academy of Sciences* 88:3125–3129.

Reddel, R. R., and R. L. Sutherland. 1984. Tamoxifen stimulation of human breast cancer cell proliferation *in vitro:* a possible model for tamoxifen tumour flare. *European Journal of Cancer and Clinical Oncology* 20:1419–1424.

Sabbah, M., F. Gouilleux, B. Sola, G. Redeuilh, and E. E. Baulieu. 1991. Structural differences between hormone and antihormone estrogen receptor complexes bound to the hormone response element. *Proceedings of the National Academy of Sciences* 88:390–294.

Stewart, A. J., M. D. Johnson, F. E. May, and B. R. Westley. 1990. Role of insulin-like growth factors and the type I insulin-like growth factor receptor in the estrogen-stimulated proliferation of human breast cancer cells. *Journal of Biological Chemistry* 265:21172–21178.

Thompson, E. W., D. Katz, T. B. Shima, A. E. Wakeling, M. E. Lippman, and R. B. Dickson. 1989. ICI 164,384, a pure antagonist of estrogen-stimulated MCF-7 cell proliferation and invasiveness. *Cancer Research* 49:6929–6934.

Tora, L., J. White, C. Brou, D. Tasset, N. Webster, E. Scheer, and P. Chambon. 1989. The human estrogen receptor has two independent nonacidic transcriptional activation functions. *Cell* 59:477–487.

Tsai, S. Y., M. Y. Tsai, and B. W. O'Malley. 1991. The steroid receptor superfamily: transactivators of gene expression. In *Nuclear hormone receptors,* ed. M. G. Parker, 103–124. London: Academic Press.

Tucker, M. J., H. K. Adams, and J. S. Patterson. 1984. Tamoxifen. In *Safety testing of new drugs,* ed. A. E. M. Mclean and M. Weatherall, 125–161. London: Academic Press.

Wakeling, A. E. 1985. Antioestrogens in oncology. Past, present and prospects. In *Current clinical practice,* Series No. 31, ed. F. Pannuti, 43–53. Amsterdam: Excerpta Medica.

Wakeling, A. E. 1987a. Pharmacology of antioestrogens. In *Pharmacology and clinical uses of inhibitors of hormone secretion and action,* ed. B. J. A. Furr and A. E. Wakeling, 1–19. London: Bailliere Tindall.

Wakeling, A. E. 1987b. Anti-hormones and other steroid analogues. In *Steroid hormones: a practical approach,* ed. B. Green and R. E. Leake, 219–236. Oxford: IRL Press.

Wakeling, A. E. 1989. Comparative studies on the effects of steroidal and nonsteroidal oestrogen antagonists on the proliferation of human breast cancer cells. *Journal of Steroid Biochemistry* 34:183–188.

Wakeling, A. E. 1990. Therapeutic potential of pure antioestrogens in the treatment of breast cancer. *Journal of Steroidal Biochemistry and Molecular Biology* 37:771–775.

Wakeling, A. E. 1991. Steroidal pure antiestrogens. In *Regulatory mechanisms in breast cancer,* ed. M. E. Lippman and R. Dickson, 239–257. Boston: Kluwer.

Wakeling, A. E., and J. Bowler. 1987. Steroidal pure antiestrogens. *Journal of Endocrinology* 112:R7–R10.

Wakeling, A. E., and J. Bowler. 1988. Novel antioestrogens without partial agonist activity. *Journal of Steroid Biochemistry* 31:645–653.

Wakeling, A. E., and S. R. Slater. 1981. Biochemical and biological aspects of antioestrogen action. In *Mechanisms of steroid action,* ed. G. P. Lewis and M. Ginsberg, 159–171. London: Macmillan.

Wakeling, A. E., M. Dukes, and J. Bowler. 1991. A potent specific pure antiestrogen with clinical potential. *Cancer Research* 51:3867–3873.

Wakeling, A. E., E. Newboult, and S. W. Peters. 1989. Effects of antioestrogens on the proliferation of MCF-7 human breast cancer cells. *Journal of Molecular Endocrinology* 2:225–234.

Wakeling, A. E., K. M. O'Connor, and E. Newboult. 1983. Comparison of the biological effects of tamoxifen and a new antioestrogen (LY 117018) on the immature rat uterus. *Journal of Endocrinology* 99:447–453.

Walker, K. J., J. M. Price-Thomas, W. Candlish, and R. I. Nicholson. 1991. Influence of the antioestrogen tamoxifen on normal breast tissue. *British Journal of Cancer* 64:764–768.

Weaver, C. A., P. A. Springer, and B. S. Katzenellenbogen. 1988. Regulation of pS2 gene expression by affinity labeling and reversibly binding estrogens and antiestrogens: comparison of effects on the native gene and on pS2-chloramphenicol acetyltransferase fusion genes transfected into MCF-7 human breast cancer cells. *Molecular Endocrinology* 2: 936–945.

Webster, N. J., S. Green, J. R. Jin, and P. Chambon. 1988. The hormone-binding domains of the estrogen and glucocorticoid receptors contain an inducible transcription activation function. *Cell* 54:199–207.

Wilson, A. P., P. J. Weatherill, R. I. Nicholson, P. Davies, and A. E. Wakeling. 1990. A comparative study of the interaction of the steroidal pure antioestrogen, ICI,164,384, with the molybdate-stabilized oestrogen receptor. *Journal of Steroid Biochemistry* 35:421–428.

Editor's Note (Added in Proof): Studies in the laboratory demonstrate that ICI 164,384 causes a rapid decrease in the receptor levels of MCF-7 breast cancer cells (Davois et al. 1992). Further studies suggest that ICI 182,780 causes the destruction of newly synthesized estrogen receptor in the cytoplasm before the receptor is "shuttled" to the nuclear compartment (Davois et al. 1993). The net effect is that ICI 182,780 destroys receptors in target tissues so that no estrogen-like responses can be produced.

   A preliminary clinical study with ICI 182,780 (DeFriend et al. 1994) with 6 mg and 18 mg IM daily for 1 week demonstrates decreases in tumor Ki67 proliferation index, progesterone receptors and an almost complete disappearance of estrogen receptors. Studies in both ovariectomized (Dukes et al. 1992) and intact adult female monkeys (Dukes et al. 1993) demonstrate complete blockade of the uteratrophic effects of estradiol by ICI 182,780.

References

Davois, S., P. S. Danielian, R. White and M. G. Parker. 1992. Antiestrogen ICI 164,384 reduces cellular estrogen receptor content by increasing its turnover. *Proceedings of the National Academy of Science* (United States of America) 89:4037–4041.

Davois S., R. White, M. G. Parker. 1993. The antiestrogen ICI 182,780 disrupts estrogen receptor nucleocytoplasmic shuttling. *Journal of Cell Science* 106:1377–1388.

DeFriend D. J., A. Howell, R. I. Nicholson, E. Anderson, M. Dowsett, R. E. Mansel, R. W. Blamey, N. J. Bundred, J. F. Robertson, C. Saunders, M. Baum, P. Walton, F. Sutcliffe and A. E. Wakeling. 1994. Investigation of a pure new antiestrogen (ICI 183,780) in women with primary breast cancer. *Cancer Research* 54:408–414.

Dukes M., D. Miller, A. E. Wakeling and J. C. Waterton. 1992. Antiuterotrophic effects of a pure antioestrogen ICI 182,780: magnetic resonance imaging of the uterus in ovariectomized monkeys. *Journal of Endocrinology* 135:239–247.

Dukes M. J. C. Waterton and A. E. Wakeling. 1993. Antiuterotrophic effects of the pure antioestrogen ICI 182,780 in adult female monkeys (Macaca Nemestrina): quantitative magnetic resonance imaging. *Journal of Endocrinology* 138:203–210.

12

Symptomatic Side Effects of Tamoxifen Therapy

MICHAEL FRITSCH AND DOUGLAS M. WOLF

I. INTRODUCTION 236
II. POTENTIAL SIDE EFFECTS OF TAMOXIFEN THERAPY 237
   A. ACUTE EFFECTS 237
   B. LONG-TERM EFFECTS 241
III. SUMMARY 247
   REFERENCES 247

I. *Introduction*

Tamoxifen was initially used for the treatment of advanced breast cancer in postmenopausal women (Ingle et al. 1981; Muss et al. 1988; Van Veelsen et al. 1986; Alonso-Munoz et al. 1988; Smith et al. 1981). The drug proved to be as efficacious as diethylstilbestrol (DES) in producing tumor regression for advanced disease. However, tamoxifen therapy has been associated with a substantial reduction in side effects compared with DES (Ingle et al. 1981). The success rate and low incidence of side effects have led to the use of tamoxifen as an adjuvant treatment for node-positive (Early Breast Cancer Trialists' Collaborative Group 1988) and node-negative (Fisher et al. 1989) breast cancer in postmenopausal women. Tamoxifen is currently the endocrine treatment of choice for women with any stage of breast cancer.

A recent overview analysis of all randomized clinical trials demonstrates that tamoxifen treatment can improve recurrence-free and overall survival in almost all subsets of women with breast cancer (Early Breast Cancer Trialists' Collaborative Group 1992). Tamoxifen has been shown to benefit women of all ages (pre- and postmenopausal), women with node-positive and node-negative disease, as well as women with estrogen receptor (ER) positive and negative tumors. Statistical analysis reveals that in younger women tamoxifen in addition to chemotherapy may provide an added benefit. One of the most important results of this overview was the finding that long-term tamoxifen therapy (>2 years) was significantly better than short-term therapy (<2 years). Tamoxifen was also shown to reduce the incidence of contralateral breast cancer, suggesting that this therapy may potentially be useful in preventing breast cancer. Given the possibility that large numbers of women might be taking tamoxifen for long periods of time, it is important to consider potential side effects of the drug. In this chapter we discuss possible beneficial actions of tamoxifen as well as the potential acute and long-term adverse effects of tamoxifen therapy and treatments to ameliorate these side effects.

II. *Potential Side Effects of Tamoxifen Therapy*

A. ACUTE EFFECTS

Tamoxifen is a nonsteroidal triphenylethylene derivative that possesses both partial agonist and partial antagonist properties (Furr and Jordan 1984). The side effects of this agent are related to its differential antiestrogenic and estrogenic properties in various target tissues. Table 12.1 summarizes the potential acute adverse effects that have been reported in patients receiving tamoxifen. Several studies (Ingle et al. 1981; Fisher et al. 1989; Pritchard et al. 1980; NATO 1983, 1985; Cummings et al. 1985; Buchanan 1986; Love 1988; Powles et al. 1989; Paterson et al. 1990; Love, Cameron, et al. 1991) have compared the side effects observed in patients treated with tamoxifen with the side effects observed in patients on an alternative therapy or given a placebo treatment. Table 12.1 shows the range of the percentage of patients reporting a given side effect while receiving tamoxifen. Interestingly, the only adverse effect consistently reported by patients receiving tamoxifen that was significantly greater than that reported by patients receiving placebo was vasomotor instability (hot flushes). All the other potential side effects listed in Table 12.1 occur in very few patients or occur in patients receiving placebo with a frequency similar to that in patients receiving tamoxifen. Thus, tamoxifen has very few acute side effects that should lead to cessation of treatment. In fact, fewer than 5% of patients stop tamoxifen therapy because of acute side effects of the drug, including hot flushes, vaginitis, depression, and nausea (NATO 1985; Ribeiro and Swindell 1985; Breast Cancer Trials Committee 1987; Love 1989).

Hot flushes probably represent an antiestrogenic effect of tamoxifen. Vasomotor instability is a characteristic symptom of menopause related to decreasing levels of estrogen. In premenopausal women on tamoxifen therapy, the serum levels of estrogens may actually increase (Manni and Pearson 1980), but at the molecular level tamoxifen acts as a competitive inhibitor of estrogen action by binding to the ER and blocking estrogen binding to the receptor. Therefore, within a target cell exposed to tamoxifen there is an apparent decrease in estrogen activity at the receptor level, and this can lead to symptoms similar to those observed in women with low levels of estrogens such as in the perimenopausal period. The incidence of hot flushes in postmenopausal patients treated with tamoxifen does not increase as much as in premenopausal patients receiving tamoxifen (Fisher et al. 1989; Love 1991). About 50% of patients who experienced hot flushes at menopause will develop hot flushes while on tamoxifen therapy (Rostom and Gershuny 1992). The exact neuroendocrine pathway leading to hot flushes is not completely understood.

Table 12.1. Percentage ranges of patients with acute adverse side effects from tamoxifen

Fatigue	5–70
Vasomotor instability (hot flushes)	17–67
Insomnia	0–54
Headache	9–37
Depression	1–33
Altered menses (amenorrhea, oligomenorrhea, menstrual disorders, vaginal discharge, vaginal bleeding)	1–31
Pain (bone or musculoskeletal)	2–30
Fluid retention (edema)	2–25
Nausea	3–21
Anorexia	1–16
Leukopenia	1–15
Skin rash	4–13
Vomiting	1–12
Diarrhea	8–10
Ovarian cysts	3–5
Constipation	2–4
Weight gain	4
Hypercalcemia	3–4
Abdominal cramps	1–3
Thrombocytopenia	1–2
Phlebitis	<1
Dizziness, light-headedness	<1

From Ingle et al. 1981; Fisher et al. 1989; Pritchard et al. 1980; NATO 1983, 1985; Cummings et al. 1985; Buchanan et al. 1986; Love 1988; Powles et al. 1989; Paterson et al. 1990; Love, Cameron, et al. 1991.

The treatment for hot flushes in perimenopausal women is estrogen replacement therapy (Stuenkel 1989). Obviously estrogen replacement cannot be given to women with breast cancer who are on tamoxifen therapy because of the tumor growth–promoting effects of estrogens on ER-positive breast cancers (Jordan and Murphy 1990). Estrogens given at high enough doses can reverse the antitumor action of tamoxifen (Iino et al. 1991). If hot flushes are severe enough so that a patient is considering discontinuing tamoxifen therapy, there are alternative treatments to decrease the intensity and severity of the hot flushes. Decreasing the dosage of tamoxifen from 10 mg twice a day could be considered, but there are no data to support the continued beneficial therapeutic effect of tamoxifen on controlling breast cancer growth at doses of less than 20 mg per day. However, the circulating levels of tamoxifen could be determined to ensure an adequate therapeutic range if the dose were decreased. An alternative treatment for hot flushes is the coadministration of a progestin. Oral medroxyprogesterone acetate (MPA) at 20 mg per day decreases hot flushes better than placebo (Bullock et al. 1975; Schiff et al. 1980). Alternatively, injection of Depo-Provera (DMPA) at 150 mg every 3 months can also decrease the incidence of hot flushes. Although progestins are capable of reducing hot flushes, medroxyprogesterone acetate has also been shown to decrease the effectiveness of tamoxifen in some cases (Mouridsen et al. 1979). Other agents have also been shown to reduce hot flushes including the alpha-adrenergic agonist clonidine (Clayden et al. 1974; Nagamani 1987). A clonidine patch using 10 mg weekly reduces hot flushes in 70% of patients. Clonidine is also a relatively safe medication with few serious side effects at these low doses. However, the combination of tamoxifen therapy and clonidine has not yet been studied.

A frequently reported (10–20%) adverse effect of tamoxifen therapy is nausea, although the same incidence is reported in control groups (Ingle et al. 1981; Fisher et al. 1989; Pritchard et al. 1980; NATO 1983, 1985; Cummings et al. 1985; Buchanan 1986; Love 1988; Powles et al. 1989; Paterson et al. 1990; Love, Cameron, et al. 1991). Patients experiencing nausea and vomiting while on tamoxifen should be counseled on the importance of continuing the medication. Physicians can recommend taking the tamoxifen tablets with meals. If doses greater than 20 mg per day are being taken, the dosage can be safely reduced to 10 mg BID without affecting the beneficial effects of tamoxifen on recurrence-free and overall survival (Early Breast Cancer Trialists' Collaborative Group 1992). There is no evidence that doses greater than 20 mg per day provide any added benefit.

Tamoxifen can lead to gynecological side effects in both pre- and postmenopausal women. Gynecological symptoms have been reported to occur more frequently in tamoxifen-treated patients than in the control group (Love, Cameron, et al. 1991; Fornander et al. 1991). The effects of tamoxifen on the female reproductive tract tend to be estrogenic in nature. Patients experiencing leukorrhea, endometrial hyperplasia (Gal et al. 1991; Neven 1990), polyps (Corley et al. 1992), or endometriosis (Buckley 1990) have been reported (Leake 1991). A recent case report also describes the rapid growth of a leiomyoma in a patient receiving tamoxifen (Dilts et al. 1992). Although some premenopausal women become amenorrheic during tamoxifen therapy, most women continue to have normal or only mildly altered menstrual cycles (Love 1991). In both pre- and postmenopausal women vaginal discharge, vaginal bleeding, and vaginitis have been reported. Patients with vaginitis may benefit from androgen cream (Love 1989). Gynecological symptoms are usually mild and seldom warrant cessation of therapy.

Patients with advanced breast cancer may develop bone or tumor pain shortly after starting tamoxifen therapy. The pain is due to sudden tumor flare following the initiation of tamoxifen treatment and is probably related to the partial agonist properties of tamoxifen (Cech et al. 1986; Brooks and Lippman 1985; Stoll 1985, 1980; Plotkin et al. 1978). Patients experiencing pain from tumor flare may require analgesics (Hanks 1985). A rare but potentially life-threatening complication of tamoxifen therapy in patients with skeletal metastases is severe hypercalcemia (Gibson 1990; Larsen et al. 1990). The serum calcium level should be monitored closely in patients with skeletal metastases after starting tamoxifen therapy. Pain and tumor flare generally subside rapidly even if the patient continues tamoxifen therapy.

Although leukopenia and thrombocytopenia have been observed in up to 1–15% of patients on tamoxifen therapy, it remains unclear whether these occur with a higher incidence than in control groups. Since these adverse reactions are potentially serious, routine complete blood counts should be performed to monitor white blood cell and platelet counts in patients receiving tamoxifen, especially during the first few months of therapy.

There are several case reports of potentially serious side effects that have occurred in patients during tamoxifen therapy, including purpuric vasculitis (Drago et al. 1990), factor VIII deficiency (Barlas 1986), hepatocellular necrosis and agranulocytosis (Ching et al. 1992), and organic delusional syndrome (Ron et al. 1992). A cause and effect relationship for these has not been established, because these effects are very rare. However, patients that develop central nervous system symptoms such as headache, dizziness, light-headedness, confusion, weakness, or drowsiness should stop tamoxifen therapy and be carefully evaluated. Although rare, some patients develop severe depression while on tamoxifen therapy. If a patient has symptoms of a major depressive disorder, tamoxifen should be stopped (NATO 1985; Love 1988).

Thrombosis is an uncommon but serious complication of tamoxifen therapy. Venous and arterial thrombosis occur more frequently in patients receiving chemotherapy plus tamoxifen than in patients receiving only chemotherapy (Saphner et al. 1991). Patients with any evidence of thromboembolic disorders (shortness of breath or painful swelling in the legs) should cease tamoxifen therapy and be treated for these disorders. Tamoxifen has been associated with decreased levels of antithrombin III (Jordan et al. 1987b; Love, Surawicz, and Williams 1992), but these are not clinically significant reductions, except possibly in the case of a patient with a previous history of a clotting disorder. However, previous clotting disorders in patients with breast cancer should probably not be considered as a contraindication of tamoxifen administration. Such patients should be closely monitored with the potential for this risk in mind.

The occurrence of male breast cancer is relatively rare, about one-hundreth of the incidence observed in women. Because of the low incidence, large controlled studies of the effectiveness of tamoxifen for male breast cancer have been difficult to perform. The majority of studies using tamoxifen for the treatment of male breast cancer (Ribeiro and Swindell 1992; Ribeiro 1985; Adami et al. 1985; Kantarjian et al. 1983; Patterson et al. 1980) or prostate cancer (Glick et al. 1982; Spremulli et al. 1982) have shown no unusual side effects in males. Most of the reported side effects in males include nausea and vomiting with occasional hot flushes, tumor flares, or thrombocytopenia. Despite a recent case report describing priapism in a male patient on tamoxifen therapy for an undefined adenocarcinoma (Fernando and Tobias 1989), tamoxifen appears to be safe in both males and females for the treatment of breast cancer.

Tamoxifen is a relatively nontoxic drug. Studies of the acute toxicities of a tamoxifen overdose in animals showed that respiratory difficulties and convulsions could lead to death (Furr and Jordan 1984). However, the LD50 for tamoxifen is high in all species tested, suggesting that fatal overdoses of tamoxifen are unlikely to occur. Acute overdoses in humans have not been reported. Therefore, treatment for an acute overdose of tamoxifen should be symptomatic.

Tamoxifen can interact with other medications. Tamoxifen can lead to an increase in the anticoagulant action of coumarin-like medications, requiring a lower dose of coumarin during tamoxifen treatment (Lodwick et al. 1987; Tenni et al. 1989; Ritchie and Grant 1989). The prothrombin time of patients receiving both agents should be carefully monitored. Estrogens should not be coadministered with tamoxifen, because they may interfere with tamoxifen's therapeutic effect (Iino et al. 1991).

B. Long-Term Effects

Most of the short-term complications associated with tamoxifen administration are mild. Tamoxifen treatment for advanced breast cancer is not likely to be a major concern with respect to most late-occurring adverse effects, because the treatment is primarily palliative. The case is somewhat different when tamoxifen is used as an adjuvant treatment, because women with stage I (node-negative) or stage II (node-positive) breast cancer can expect to survive for many years and possibly decades. Therefore, the less immediate and possibly much more dangerous effects potentially associated with long-term tamoxifen treatment become a matter of significant concern.

An antiestrogen might be expected to have effects on every estrogen target tissue in the body. These include the breasts, uterus, ovaries, pituitary, bone, and liver. It is interesting to note that tamoxifen does not appear to have adverse effects on two areas that an antiestrogen might be expected to affect negatively, i.e., bone maintenance and serum lipid levels.

Tamoxifen does not cause any reduction in bone density (Powles et al. 1990; Love et al. 1988; Fentiman et al. 1989; Kalef-Ezra et al. 1992), and in two clinical trials postmenopausal patients receiving tamoxifen actually experienced a beneficial effect on bone density compared with patients receiving no endocrine treatment (Turken et al. 1989; Love, Mazess, et al. 1992). No comparisons have been made between the bone-sparing effects of tamoxifen versus exogenous estrogens in postmenopausal women. However, since women with breast cancer are a group of patients that is uniformly ineligible for postmenopausal estrogen replacement therapy, any bone-sparing effect due to tamoxifen is an added benefit to its tumoristatic action.

Patients treated with tamoxifen also experience significant reductions in total serum cholesterol, LDL cholesterol, and apolipoprotein B levels (Powles et al. 1989; Love et al. 1990; Love, Weibe, et al. 1991). These effects are all associated with reductions in the risk of cardiovascular disease, and in one study, a significant reduction in the incidence of fatal myocardial infarction was observed in the tamoxifen-treated group compared with controls (McDonald and Stewart 1991).

In a laboratory model, tamoxifen is capable of promoting the growth of chemically initiated liver tumors in rats (Yager et al. 1986; Ghia and Mereto 1989; Yager and Shi 1991; Dragan et al. 1991). Administration of high doses of tamoxifen to rats may also contribute to the initiation of hepatocellular carcinoma (Gau 1986; ICI Pharmaceuticals 1990). Tamoxifen induces liver tumors in rats (Greaves et al. 1993; Hard et al. 1993) and produces DNA adducts in the liver of rats and other species (Han and Liehr 1992; White et al. 1992). However liver tumors are only noted in rats. It should be pointed out that the doses used for the rat studies are about 40 times the daily per kg dose used to treat patients. The dose per kg used to treat patients is the same as the antitumor dose used in rats i.e., 250 mg/kg. The dose used to produce liver tumors in rats is 10 mg/kg. There are few clinical data available concerning hepatic complications in women receiving tamoxifen. In an adjuvant tamoxifen trial containing more than 900 women in each (tamoxifen or placebo) arm, Fornander and others have reported that two of the women in the tamoxifen-treated group developed hepatocellular carcinoma, compared with none in the control group (Fornander et al. 1989). This result was not statistically significant, but given the rarity of hepatocellular carcinoma in the general population, it should not be ignored, especially since a trend is being established for the administration of tamoxifen to large numbers of clinically disease-free women in prevention studies. An elevated incidence of hepatocellular carcinoma would clearly be an unacceptable side effect for stage I patients and disease-free women taking the drug as part of a prevention trial. Clinicians treating patients with tamoxifen should carefully evaluate any signs or symptoms of hepatic complications that might indicate the presence of hepatocellular carcinoma.

Many of the effects of tamoxifen outside the breast appear to be due to its estrogenic, rather than antiestrogenic, effects. In the case of bone maintenance and serum lipids, this is beneficial. However, an estrogenic (i.e., proliferative) effect on the endometrium could be detrimental. Persistent stimulation of the endometrium can lead to hyperplasia and possibly to the development of endometrial carcinoma. The relationship between tamoxifen use and endometrial cancer remains controversial. Tamoxifen has been successfully used as a treatment for endometrial carcinoma (Bonte et al. 1981; Broens et al. 1980; Swenerton 1980). However, evidence gathered in both the laboratory and clinic have demonstrated that tamoxifen can have proliferative effects on the endometrium and possibly act as a tumor promoter. Using the athymic mouse model, researchers have shown that estrogen receptor–positive endometrial tumors can be stimulated to grow in the presence of tamoxifen, even though ER-positive breast tumors simultaneously implanted on the opposite flank are growth inhibited (Gottardis et al. 1988).

Tamoxifen has also been implicated in the development of endometrial tumors in patients. In one study with an accrual of over 1800 postmenopausal women who received either tamoxifen or placebo after primary surgery for breast cancer, 13 patients in the tamoxifen-treated group developed endometrial cancer compared with 2 in the placebo-treated group (Fornander et al. 1989). This study also showed that the incidence of endometrial cancer was correlated with the duration of tamoxifen administration. Early analysis of a trial underway in the United States supports these results. In this study, conducted by the Southwest Oncology Group (SWOG), 4 of 641 patients treated for 1 year with tamoxifen developed endometrial cancer, compared with no cases of endometrial cancer in the 325 patients treated with adjuvant chemotherapy (Sunderland and Osborne 1991). A study by Andersson et al. (1991) describes a trend toward an increased incidence of endometrial cancer in tamoxifen-treated women. A case-control study (Hardell 1990; Hardell 1988a,b) has indicated an increase of endometrial cancer in women receiving tamoxifen for breast cancer. This risk was exacerbated in women receiving both pelvic irradiation and tamoxifen.

The dose of tamoxifen used in the largest study discussed above (Fornander et al. 1989) was 40 mg/day, which is twice that commonly used in the United States. This does not imply that tamoxifen at lower doses is without effect on the reproductive organs. Case studies have reported an association between tamoxifen treatment and endometriosis, endocervical polyps, and endometrial polyps (Corley et al. 1992; De Muylder et al. 1991; Nuovo et al. 1989; Neven et al. 1989; Ford et al. 1988). Also, the ratio of proliferative to atrophic uterine mucosae in postmenopausal women taking tamoxifen is higher than that seen in comparable controls (Neven et al. 1989). Administration of a progestin in conjunction with tamoxifen might be expected to alleviate tamoxifen-associated effects on the endometrium. However, it is unclear whether or not a periodic progestin will interfere with the beneficial effects tamoxifen therapy has on disease-free and overall survival in breast cancer patients, which is the primary objective of tamoxifen treatment. It has been suggested (Gusberg 1990) that careful patient monitoring using serial endometrial biopsies may be an appropriate nonpharmacological means of warding off the problem of tamoxifen-associated endometrial cancer. It is unlikely that this approach would be acceptable to patients with node-negative disease or in prevention studies. An alternative to serial biopsies would be to consider an annual uterine evacuation and also to take great care to counsel patients to report any abnormal vaginal bleeding. Patients reporting abnormal bleeding would require immediate evaluation.

There are other factors to consider, however, before it can be concluded that the estrogenic effects of tamoxifen are contributing to the incidence of endometrial carcinoma. Horwitz and Feinstein (1986) argue that the observed increase in endometrial carcinoma attributed to estrogens (and presumably tamoxifen) may be due to increased detection of lesions that would otherwise remain as silent tumors. They support this conjecture by reporting that the incidence of "silent" endometrial cancers diagnosed at autopsy is roughly 5 times the incidence seen in the living population. It is possible that an estrogen (or partial estrogen agonist such as tamoxifen) could act on these silent tumors, and the resultant appearance of abnormal bleeding or other symptoms would bring about an increase in the rate of diagnosis of endometrial carcinoma compared with that seen for untreated women.

Schwartzbaum et al. (1987) have investigated the effects of a previous history of estrogen use on survival after diagnosis of endometrial cancer. They report that the probability of surviving 5 years after a diagnosis of endometrial cancer is 0.89 for previous estrogen users, but only 0.53 for nonusers. These data support the hypothesis that estrogens may promote earlier detection of occult tumors by causing abnormal bleeding or other symptoms prior to the development of metastases. Proper and timely gynecological examinations are essential for women receiving adjuvant tamoxifen therapy.

Tamoxifen induces ovarian steroidogenesis in premenopausal women (Shutt et al. 1973; Groom and Griffiths 1976; Senior et al. 1978; Tanaka et al. 1978; Manni et al. 1979; Sherman et al. 1979; Rose and Davis 1980; Fukushima et al. 1982; Kokko et al. 1982; Fukishima and Maeyama 1983; Tajima 1984; Sawka et al. 1986; Jordan et al. 1987a; Ravdin et al. 1988; Jordan et al. 1991), elevating serum estradiol levels to as high as 2500 pg/ml (Manni and Pearson 1980). Chronically elevated estrogen levels normally cause decreased follicle-stimulating hormone (FSH) and luteinizing hormone (LH) production. Treatment with tamoxifen might be expected to elevate gonadotrophin levels by blocking negative feedback. However, FSH and LH levels remain largely unchanged (Groom and Griffiths 1976; Manni et al. 1979; Sherman et al. 1979; Sawka et al. 1986; Ravdin et al. 1988), which indicates that tamoxifen may act directly on the ovary to increase steroidogenesis, and the balance between its agonist and antagonist activities maintains pituitary gonadotrophin secretion at near normal levels in the face of elevated serum estradiol levels.

Increased ovarian steroidogenesis does not appear to interfere with the antiproliferative action of tamoxifen on a breast tumor, provided serum tamoxifen levels are kept sufficiently high (Iino et al. 1991). It is unclear whether or not this hypersecretory state might lead to adverse ovarian pathology, but tamoxifen has been associated with an increased incidence of fibroid ovaries and ovarian cysts (Powles et al. 1989).

Many premenopausal women receiving tamoxifen continue to have normal menstrual cycles and may continue to be at risk for pregnancy. Tamoxifen administration is contraindicated during pregnancy according to the manufacturer. No reports have been published on the adverse effects of neonatal exposure of humans to tamoxifen; but there have been several studies using rodent models to investigate this issue. Tamoxifen induces hypertrophy and progesterone receptor synthesis in the uterus and vagina of guinea pig perinates (Pasqualini et al. 1986). Tamoxifen causes adenosis-like lesions of the vagina and cervix in neonatally treated mice, involution of the musculature and suppression of gland genesis in the uterus, and formation of an excessively fibrous uterus dominated by a mesenchymal stroma (Iguchi et al. 1989). Neonatal exposure to tamoxifen has also been linked to bladder herniation in adult mice (Iguchi et al. 1986). Rats exposed neonatally to tamoxifen develop gross reproductive tract abnormalities, which include early vaginal opening, absence of estrous cycles, and atrophic uteri and ovaries in adult rats. In addition, the oviducts of these animals show severe squamous metaplasia and abscess formation (Chamness et al. 1979). One study reported the effects tamoxifen had on developing human reproductive tracts implanted into nude mice (Cunha et al. 1987). This showed that tamoxifen administration beyond an equivalent gestational age of 16 weeks was associated with inappropriate proliferation and maturation of squamous vaginal epithelium. Tamoxifen also delayed the development of endometrial and cervical glands and inhibited segregation of uterine mesenchyme into endometrial stromal and myometrial layers. Tamoxifen was also associated with the presence of hyperplastic and disorganized epithelium in the fallopian tubes. All these data support the absolute necessity of discouraging pregnancy in premenopausal women receiving tamoxifen. It is therefore the responsibility of the clinician to advise premenopausal women with intact ovaries and uterus to use some form of barrier contraception during tamoxifen therapy.

Tamoxifen suppresses lactation in laboratory animals (Furr and Jordan 1984). There are reports of suppression of lactation in humans (Furr and Jordan 1984). Even if a woman receiving tamoxifen therapy is able to lactate, she should avoid breast feeding because the effects of tamoxifen on the newborn are unclear.

Other potential long-term adverse reactions to tamoxifen therapy include ocular effects. Triphenylethylenes, including tamoxifen and clomiphene, can cause cataracts in rats (Furr and Jordan 1984). Cases of retinopathy (Kaiser-Kupfer et al. 1981; Vinding and Nielsen 1983; Kaiser-Kupfer and Lippman 1978; Griffiths 1987; Bentley et al. 1992), optic neuritis (Pubesgaard and von Eyben 1986), and keratopathy (Kaiser-Kupfer and Lippman 1978) have been reported in patients receiving tamoxifen. Retinopathy was initially reported in patients receiving very high doses of tamoxifen, but recent reports suggest retinopathy can also occur at the usual low dose of 20 mg/day (Griffiths 1987; Gerner 1989; Pavlidis et al. 1992). Two prospective studies have demonstrated no adverse ocular effects associated with low-dose tamoxifen therapy (Beck and Mills 1979; Longstaff et al. 1989), whereas a recent prospective study has demonstrated reversible ocular toxicity associated with long-term, low-dose tamoxifen therapy (Pavlidis et al. 1992). Whether tamoxifen at 20 mg/day can lead to ocular toxicity is not yet resolved, but any change in a woman's visual acuity during tamoxifen therapy should be carefully evaluated.

III. *Summary*

Tamoxifen has proved to be a safe and effective adjuvant treatment for patients with breast cancer. The acute toxicities of tamoxifen only rarely lead to cessation of therapy, and some of these side effects could potentially be treated without compromising the tumoristatic actions of the drug. Long-term tamoxifen therapy is associated with some rare but potentially serious adverse effects, and patients should be carefully monitored for the development of symptoms related to these side effects. Long-term tamoxifen therapy is also associated with a number of beneficial effects besides its tumoristatic action on the original breast cancer. These benefits include a decrease in the development of contralateral breast cancer, the maintenance of bone density in postmenopausal women, and a decrease in cardiovascular disease.

The low incidence of side effects associated with tamoxifen treatment and the documented benefits of tamoxifen in numerous trials (Early Breast Cancer Trialists' Collaborative Group 1992) have led to the proposal that tamoxifen might be effective as a preventive agent in women at high risk for the development of breast cancer (Cuzick et al. 1986; Jordan 1990; Baum et al. 1991; Nayfield et al. 1991; Jordan 1992a,b; Bernstein et al. 1992). Adjuvant trials in node-positive women have demonstrated that the cessation of tamoxifen therapy due to acute side effects is low. However, this group of patients is highly motivated to continue therapy, because they have a potentially life-threatening disease. In preventive studies a high degree of compliance will be necessary to ensure a beneficial outcome, yet these women will not have as great an incentive to continue the medication if side effects occur. A recent study of tamoxifen versus placebo in postmenopausal node-negative patients has demonstrated that the perceived side effects of tamoxifen are much more severe than previously thought (Love, Cameron, et al. 1991). Since the perceived side effects will dictate compliance, especially in prevention trials, physicians should be willing to discuss all potential side effects with patients and explain the risks and benefits of tamoxifen therapy to ensure continuation of therapy.

References

Adami, H. O., L. Holmberg, B. Malker, and L. Ries. 1985. Long-term survival in 406 males with breast cancer. *British Journal of Cancer* 52:99–103.
Alonso-Munoz, M. C., M. B. Ojeda-Gonzalez, M. Beltran-Fabregat, J. Dorca-Ribugent, L. Lopez-Lopez, J. Borras-Balada, F. Cardenal-Alemany, X. Gomez-Batiste, J. Fabregat-

Mayol, and P. Viladiu-Quemada. 1988. Randomized trial of tamoxifen versus aminoglutethimide and versus combined tamoxifen and aminoglutethimide in advanced postmenopausal breast cancer. *Journal of Immunology* 45:350–353.

Andersson, M., H. H. Storm, and H. T. Mouridsen. 1991. Incidence of new primary cancers after adjuvant tamoxifen therapy and radiotherapy for early breast cancer. *Journal of the National Cancer Institute* 83:1013–1017.

Barlas, A. H. 1986. Acquired factor VIII deficiency in an elderly woman on tamoxifen. *Journal of the American Geriatric Society* 34:318–320.

Baum, M., Y. Ziv, and A. A. Colletta. 1991. Can we prevent breast cancer? *British Journal of Cancer* 64:205–207.

Beck, M., and P. V. Mills. 1979. Ocular assessment of patients treated with tamoxifen. *Cancer Treatment Reports* 63:1833–1834.

Bentley, C. R., G. Davies, and W. A. Aclimandos. 1992. Tamoxifen retinopathy: a rare but serious complication. *British Medical Journal* 304:495–496.

Bernstein, L. R., K. Ross, and B. E. Henderson. 1992. Prospects for the primary prevention of breast cancer. *American Journal of Epidemiology* 135:142–152.

Bonte, J., P. Ide, G. Billiet, and P. Wynants. 1981. Tamoxifen as a possible chemotherapeutic agent in endometrial adenocarcinoma. *Gynecologic Oncology* 11:140–161.

Breast Cancer Trials Committee, Scottish Cancer Trials Office. 1987. Adjuvant tamoxifen in the management of operable breast cancer: the Scottish trial. *Lancet* 2:171–175.

Broens, J., H. T. Mouridsen, and H. M. Soerensen. 1980. Tamoxifen in advanced endometrial carcinoma. *Cancer Chemotherapy and Pharmacology* 4:213.

Brooks, B. J., and M. E. Lippman. 1985. Tamoxifen flare in advanced endometrial carcinoma. *Journal of Clinical Oncology* 3:222–223.

Buchanan, R. B., R. W. Blamey, K. R. Durrant, A. Howell, A. G. Paterson, P. E. Preece, D. C. Smith, C. J. Williams, and R. G. Wilson. 1986. A randomized comparison of tamoxifen with surgical oophorectomy in premenopausal patients with advanced breast cancer. *Journal of Clinical Oncology* 4:1326–1330.

Buckley, C. H. 1990. Tamoxifen and endometriosis. *British Journal of Obstetrics and Gynaecology* 97:645–646.

Bullock, J. L., F. M. Massey, and R. D. Gambrell, Jr. 1975. Use of medroxyprogesterone acetate to prevent menopausal symptoms. *Obstetrics and Gynecology* 46:165–168.

Cech, P., J. B. Block, L. A. Cone, and R. Stone. 1986. Tumor lysis syndrome after tamoxifen flare. *New England Journal of Medicine* 315:263–264.

Chamness, G. C., G. A. Bannayan, L. A. Landry Jr., P. J. Sheridan and W. L. McGuire. 1979. Abnormal reproductive development in rats after neonatally administered antiestrogen (tamoxifen). *Biology of Reproduction* 21:1087–1090.

Ching, C. K., P. G. Smith, and R. G. Long. 1992. Tamoxifen-associated hepatocellular damage and agranulocytosis. *Lancet* 339:940.

Clayden, J. R., J. W. Bell, and P. Pollard. 1974. Menopausal flushing: double-blind trial of a nonhormonal medication. *British Medical Journal* 1:409–412.

Corley, D., J. Rowe, M. T. Curtis, W. M. Hogan, J. S. Noumoff, and V. A. Livolsi. 1992. Postmenopausal bleeding from unusual endometrial polyps in women on chronic tamoxifen therapy. *Obstetrics and Gynecology* 79:111–116.

Cummings, F. J., R. Gray, T. E. Davis, D. C. Tormey, J. E. Harris, G. G. Falkson, and J. Arseneau. 1985. Adjuvant tamoxifen treatment of elderly women with stage II breast cancer. A double-blind comparison with placebo. *Annals of Internal Medicine* 103:324–329.

Cunha, G. R., O. Taguchi, R. Namikawa, Y. Nishizuka, and S. J. Robboy. 1987. Teratogenic effects of clomiphene, tamoxifen, and diethylstilbestrol on the developing human female genital tract. *Human Pathology* 18:1132–1143.

Cuzick, J., D. Y. Wang, and R. D. Bulbrook. 1986. The prevention of breast cancer. *Lancet* 1:83–86.

De Muylder, X., P. Neven, M. DeSomer, Y. Van Belle, G. Vanderick, and E. De Muylder. 1991. Endometrial lesions in patients undergoing tamoxifen therapy. *International Journal of Gynaecology and Obstetrics* 36:127–130.

Dilts, P. V., M. P. Hopkins, A. E. Chang, and R. L. Cody. 1992. Rapid growth of leiomyoma in patients receiving tamoxifen. *American Journal of Obstetrics and Gynecology* 166:167–168.

Dragan, Y. P., Y. D. Xu, and H. C. Pitot. 1991. Tumor promotion as a target for estrogen/antiestrogen effects in rat hepatocarcinogenesis. *Preventive Medicine* 20:15–26.

Drago, F., M. Arditi, and A. Rebora. 1990. Tamoxifen and purpuric vasculitis. *Annals of Internal Medicine* 112:965–966.

Early Breast Cancer Trialists' Collaborative Group. 1988. Effects of adjuvant tamoxifen and of cytotoxic therapy on mortality in early breast cancer. An overview of 61 randomized trials among 28,896 women. *New England Journal of Medicine* 319:1681–1692.

Early Breast Cancer Trialists' Collaborative Group. 1992. Systemic treatment of early breast cancer by hormonal, cytotoxic, or immune therapy. 133 randomised trials involving 31,000 recurrences and 24,000 deaths among 75,000 women. *Lancet* 339:1–15 and 71–85.

Fentiman, I. S., M. Caleffi, A. Rodin, B. Murby, and I. Fogelman. 1989. Bone mineral content of women receiving tamoxifen for mastalgia. *British Journal of Cancer* 60:262–264.

Fernando, I. N., and J. S. Tobias. 1989. Priapism in patients on tamoxifen. *Lancet* 1:436.

Fisher, B., J. Costantino, C. Redmond, R. Poisson, D. Bowman, J. Couture, N. V. Dimitrov, N. Wolmark, D. L. Wickerham, E. R. Fisher, R. D. Margolese, C. Sutherland, A. Glass, R. Foster, and R. Caplan. 1989. A randomized clinical trial evaluating tamoxifen in the treatment of patients with node-negative breast cancer who have estrogen-receptor-positive tumors. *New England Journal of Medicine* 320:479–484.

Ford, M. R., M. J. Turner, C. Wood, and W. P. Soutter. 1988. Endometriosis developing during tamoxifen therapy. *American Journal of Obstetrics and Gynecology* 158:1119.

Fornander, T., L. E. Rutqvist, and N. Wilking. 1991. Effects of tamoxifen on the female genital tract. *Annals of the New York Academy of Sciences* 622:469–476.

Fornander, T., L. E. Rutqvist, B. Cedermark, U. Glas, A. Mattsson, C. Silfversward, L. Skoog, A. Somell, T. Theve, N. Wilking, J. Askergren, and M. L. Hjalmer. 1989. Adjuvant tamoxifen in early breast cancer: occurrence of new primary cancers. *Lancet* 1:117–120.

Fukushima, T., and M. Maeyama. 1983. Action of tamoxifen on folliculogenesis in the menstrual cycle of infertile patients. *Fertility and Sterility* 40:210–214.

Fukushima, T., C. Tajima, K. Fukuma, and M. Maeyama. 1982. Tamoxifen in the treatment of infertility associated with luteal phase deficiency. *Fertility and Sterility* 37:755–761.

Furr, B. J., and V. C. Jordan. 1984. The pharmacology and clinical uses of tamoxifen. *Pharmacology and Therapeutics* 25:127–205.

Gal, D., S. Kopel, M. Bashevkin, J. Lebowicz, R. Lev, and M. L. Tancer. 1991. Oncogenic potential of tamoxifen on endometria of postmenopausal women with breast cancer—preliminary report. *Gynecologic Oncology* 42:120–123.

Gau, T. C. 1986. Open letter to all U.S. medical oncologists describing the toxicological findings in rats with high dose tamoxifen treatment. Stuart Pharmaceutical, a division of ICI Americas, Wilmington, Delaware.

Gerner, E. W. 1989. Ocular toxicity of tamoxifen. *Annals of Ophthalmology* 21:420–423.

Ghia, M., and E. Mereto. 1989. Induction and promotion of gamma glutamyltranspeptidase-positive foci in the liver of female rats treated with ethinyl estradiol, clomiphene, tamoxifen and their associations. *Cancer Letters* 46:195–202.

Gibson, T. C. 1990. Severe hypercalcaemia and tamoxifen "flare." *British Journal of Clinical Practice* 44:716–717.

Glick, J. H., A. Wein, K. Padavic, W. Negendank, D. Harris, and H. Brodovsky. 1982. Phase II trial of tamoxifen in metastatic carcinoma of the prostate. *Cancer* 49:1367–1372.

Gottardis, M. M., S. P. Robinson, P. G. Satyaswaroop, and V. C. Jordan. 1988. Contrasting actions of tamoxifen on endometrial and breast tumor growth in the athymic mouse. *Cancer Research* 48:812–815.

Greaves, P., R. Goonetillebe, G. Nunn, J. Topham and T. Orton. 1993. Two year carcinogenicity study of tamoxifen in Adderly Park Wistar-derived rats. *Cancer Research* 53:3919–3924.

Griffiths, M. F. 1987. Tamoxifen retinopathy at low dosage. *American Journal of Ophthalmology* 104:185–186.

Groom, G. V., and K. Griffiths. 1976. Effect of the antioestrogen tamoxifen on plasma levels of luteinizing hormone, follicle-stimulating hormone, prolactin, oestradiol and progesterone in normal premenopausal women. *Journal of Endocrinology* 70:421–428.

Gusberg, S. B. 1990. Tamoxifen for breast cancer: associated endometrial cancer. *Cancer* 65:1463–1464.

Han, Y., and J. G. Liehr. 1992. Induction of covalent DNA adducts in rodents by tamoxifen. *Cancer Research* 52:1360–1363.

Hanks, G. W. 1985. Drug treatments for relief of pain due to bone metastases. *Journal of the Royal Society of Medicine* 78 (Supplement 9):26–30.

Hard, G. C., M. J. Intropoulos, K. Jordan, L. Radi, O. P. Kalkenberg, A. R. Imondi, and G. M. Williams. 1993. Major differences in the hepatocarcinogenicity and DNA adduct forming ability between toremifere and tamoxifen in female Crl:CD(BR)rats. *Cancer Research* 53:4534–4541.

Hardell, L. 1988a. Tamoxifen as a risk factor for carcinoma of corpus uteri. *Lancet* 2:563.

Hardell, L. 1988b. Pelvic irradiation and tamoxifen as risk factors for carcinoma of corpus uteri. *Lancet* 2:1432.

Hardell, L. 1990. Tamoxifen as a risk factor for endometrial cancer. *Cancer* 66:1661.

Horwitz, R. I., and A. R. Feinstein. 1986. Estrogens and endometrial cancer. Responses to arguments and current status of an epidemiologic controversy. *American Journal of Medicine* 81:503–507.

ICI Pharmaceuticals. 1990. Unpublished toxicology data. London.

Iguchi, T., M. Hirokawa, and N. Takasugi. 1986. Occurrence of genital tract abnormalities and bladder hernia in female mice exposed neonatally to tamoxifen. *Toxicology* 42:1–11.

Iguchi, T., R. Todoroki, S. Yamaguchi, and N. Takasugi. 1989. Changes in the uterus and vagina of mice treated neonatally with antiestrogens. *Acta Anatomica* 136:146–154.

Iino, Y., D. M. Wolf, S. M. Langan-Fahey, D. A. Johnson, M. Ricchio, M. E. Thompson, and V. C. Jordan. 1991. Reversible control of oestradiol-stimulated growth of MCF-7 tumours by tamoxifen in the athymic mouse. *British Journal of Cancer* 64:1019–1024.

Ingle, J. N., D. L. Ahmann, S. J. Green, J. H. Edmonson, H. F. Bisel, L. K. Kvols, W. C. Nichols, E. T. Creagon, R. G. Hahn, J. Rubin, and S. Frytak. 1981. Randomized clinical trial of diethylstilbestrol versus tamoxifen in postmenopausal women with advanced breast cancer. *New England Journal of Medicine* 304:16–21.

Jordan, V. C. 1990. Tamoxifen for the prevention of breast cancer. In *Cancer prevention,* ed. V. T. DeVita, S. Hellman, and S. A. Rosenberg, 1–12. Philadelphia: J. B. Lippincott Company.

Jordan, V. C. 1992a. Overview from the international conference on long-term tamoxifen therapy for breast cancer. *Journal of the National Cancer Institute* 84:231–234.

Jordan, V. C. 1992b. The strategic use of antiestrogens to control the development and growth of breast cancer. *Cancer* 70:977–982.

Jordan, V. C., and C. S. Murphy. 1990. Endocrine pharmacology of antiestrogens as antitumor agents. *Endocrine Reviews* 11:578–610.

Jordan, V. C., N. F. Fritz, and D. C. Tormey. 1987a. Endocrine effects of adjuvant chemotherapy and long-term tamoxifen administration on node-positive patients with breast cancer. *Cancer Research* 47:624–630.

Jordan, V. C., N. F. Fritz, and D. C. Tormey. 1987b. Long-term adjuvant therapy with tamoxifen: effects on sex-hormone-binding globulin and antithrombin III. *Cancer Research* 47:4517–4519.

Jordan, V. C., N. F. Fritz, S. Langan-Fahey, M. Thompson, and D. C. Tormey. 1991. Alteration of endocrine parameters in premenopausal women with breast cancer during long-term adjuvant therapy with tamoxifen as a single agent. *Journal of the National Cancer Institute* 83:1488–1491.

Kaiser-Kupfer, M. I., and M. E. Lippman. 1978. Tamoxifen retinopathy. *Cancer Treatment Reports* 62:315–320.

Kaiser-Kupfer, M. I., C. Kupfer, and M. M. Rodrigues. 1981. Tamoxifen retinopathy. A clinicopathologic report. *Ophthalmology* 88:89–93.

Kalef-Ezra, J., D. Glaros, G. Klouvas, J. Hatzikonstantinou, A. Karantanas, K. C. Siamopoulos, and N. Pavlidis. 1992. New evidence that tamoxifen does not induce osteoporosis: a nuclear activation analysis and absorptiometry study. *British Journal of Radiology* 65:417–420.

Kantarjian, H., H. Y. Yap, G. Hortobagyi, and G. Blumenschein. 1983. Hormonal therapy for metastatic male breast cancer. *Archives of Internal Medicine* 143:237–240.

Kokko, E., O. Jänne, A. Kauppila, and R. Vihko. 1982. Effects of tamoxifen, medroxyprogesterone acetate, and their combination on human endometrial estrogen and progestin receptor concentrations, 17 beta-hydroxysteroid dehydrogenase activity, and serum hormone concentrations. *American Journal of Obstetrics and Gynecology* 143:382–388.

Larsen, W., G. Fellowes, and L. S. Rickman. 1990. Life-threatening hypercalcemia and tamoxifen. *American Journal of Medicine* 88:440–442.

Leake, R. E. 1991. Side effects of adjuvant tamoxifen. *British Medical Journal* 303:1061.

Lodwick, R., B. McConkey, and A. M. Brown. 1987. Life-threatening interaction between tamoxifen and warfarin. *British Medical Journal* 295:1141.

Longstaff, S., H. Sigurdsson, M. O'Keeffe, S. Ogston, and P. Preece. 1989. A controlled study of the ocular effects of tamoxifen in conventional dosage in the treatment of breast carcinoma. *European Journal of Cancer and Clinical Oncology* 25:1805–1808.

Love, R. R. 1988. The Wisconsin tamoxifen study: toxicity in node-negative postmenopausal women. *Cancer Investigation* 6:601–605.

Love, R. R. 1989. Tamoxifen therapy in primary breast cancer: biology, efficacy, and side effects. *Journal of Clinical Oncology* 7:803–815.

Love, R. R. 1991. Antiestrogen chemoprevention of breast cancer: critical issues and research. *Preventive Medicine* 20:64–78.

Love, R. R., T. S. Surawicz, and E. C. Williams. 1992. Antithrombin III level, fibrinogen level, and platelet count changes with adjuvant tamoxifen therapy. *Archives of Internal Medicine* 152:317–320.

Love, R. R., L. Cameron, B. L. Connell, and H. Leventhal. 1991. Symptoms associated with tamoxifen treatment in postmenopausal women. *Archives of Internal Medicine* 151:1842–1847.

Love, R. R., R. B. Mazess, D. C. Tormey, H. S. Barden, P. A. Newcomb, and V. C. Jordan. 1988. Bone mineral density in women with breast cancer treated with adjuvant tamoxifen for at least two years. *Breast Cancer Research and Treatment* 12:297–302.

Love, R. R., P. A. Newcomb, D. A.. Wiebe, T. S. Surawicz, V. C. Jordan, P. P. Carbone, and D. L. DeMets. 1990. Effects of tamoxifen therapy on lipid and lipoprotein levels in postmenopausal patients with node-negative breast cancer. *Journal of the National Cancer Institute* 82:1327–1332.

Love, R. R., R. B. Mazess, H. S. Barden, S. Epstein, P. A. Newcomb, V. C. Jordan, P. P. Carbone, and D. L. DeMets. 1992. Effects of tamoxifen on bone mineral density in postmenopausal women with breast cancer. *New England Journal of Medicine* 326:852–856.

Love, R. R., D. A. Weibe, P. A. Newcomb, L. Cameron, H. Leventhal, V. C. Jordan, J. Feyzi, and D. L. DeMets. 1991. Effects of tamoxifen on cardiovascular risk factors in postmenopausal women. *Annals of Internal Medicine* 115:860–864.

McDonald, C. C., and H. J. Stewart. 1991. Fatal myocardial infarction in the Scottish adjuvant tamoxifen trial. The Scottish Breast Cancer Committee. *British Medical Journal* 303:435–437.

Manni, A., and O. H. Pearson. 1980. Antiestrogen-induced remissions in premenopausal women with stage IV breast cancer: effects on ovarian function. *Cancer Treatment Reports* 64:779–785.

Manni, A., J. E. Trujillo, J. S. Marshall, J. Brodkey, and O. H. Pearson. 1979. Antihormone treatment of stage IV breast cancer. *Cancer* 43:444–450.

Mouridsen, H. T., K. Ellemann, W. Mattson, T. Palshof, J. L. Daehnfeldt, and C. Rose. 1979. Therapeutic effect of tamoxifen versus tamoxifen combined with medroxyprogesterone acetate in advanced breast cancer in postmenopausal women. *Cancer Treatment Reports* 63:171–175.

Muss, H. B., H. B. Wells, E. H. Paschold, W. R. Black, M. R. Cooper, R. L. Capizzi, R. Christian, J. M. Cruz, D. V. Jackson, B. L. Powell, R. Richards, D. R. White, P. J. Zekan, C. L. Spurr, E. Pope, D. Case, and T. M. Morgan. 1988. Megestrol acetate versus tamoxifen in advanced breast cancer: 5-year analysis—a phase III trial of the Piedmont Oncology Association. *Journal of Clinical Oncology* 6:1098–1106.

Nagamani, M., M. E. Kelver, and E. R. Smith. 1987. Treatment of menopausal hot flushes with transdermal administration of clonidine. *American Journal of Obstetrics and Gynecology* 156:561–565.

Nayfield, S. G., J. E. Karp, L. G. Ford, F. A. Dorr, and B. S. Kramer. 1991. Potential role of tamoxifen in prevention of breast cancer. *Journal of the National Cancer Institute* 83:1450–1459.

Neven, P. 1990. Endometrial hyperplasia in an oophorectomized woman receiving tamoxifen therapy. *British Journal of Obstetrics and Gynaecology* 97:190–192.

Neven, P., X. De Muylder, Y. Van Belle, G. Vanderick, and E. De Muylder. 1989. Tamoxifen and the uterus and endometrium. *Lancet* 1:375–376.

Nolvadex Adjuvant Trial Organisation (NATO). 1983. Controlled trial of tamoxifen as adjuvant agent in the management of early breast cancer. Interim analysis at four years. *Lancet* 1:257–261.

Nolvadex Adjuvant Trial Organisation (NATO). 1985. Controlled trial of tamoxifen as a single adjuvant agent in the management of early breast cancer. Analysis at six years. *Lancet* 1:836–840.

Nuovo, M. A., G. J. Nuovo, R. M. McCaffrey, R. U. Levine, B. Barron, and B. Winkler. 1989. Endometrial polyps in postmenopausal patients receiving tamoxifen. *International Journal of Gynecological Pathology* 8:125–131.

Pasqualini, J. R., B. L. Nguyen, C. Sumida, N. Giambiagi, and C. Mayrand. 1986. Tamoxifen and progesterone effects in target tissues during the perinatal period. *Journal of Steroid Biochemistry* 25:853–857.

Paterson, A. H., J. Hanson, K. I. Pritchard, E. Sansregret, S. Dahrouge, R. S. McDermot, S. Fine, D. F. White, M. Trudeau, D. J. Stewart, and W. Ungar. 1990. Comparison of antiestrogen and progesterone therapy for initial treatment and consequences of their combination for second-line treatment of recurrent breast cancer. *Seminars in Oncology* 17:52–62.

Patterson, J. S., L. A. Battersby, and B. K. Bach. 1980. Use of tamoxifen in advanced male breast cancer. *Cancer Treatment Reports* 64:801–804.

Pavlidis, N. A., C. Petris, E. Briassoulis, G. Klouvas, C. Psilas, J. Rempapis, and G. Petroutsos. 1992. Clear evidence that long-term, low-dose tamoxifen treatment can induce ocular toxicity. *Cancer* 69:2961–2964.

Plotkin, D., J. L. Lechner, W. E. Jung, and P. J. Rosen. 1978. Tamoxifen flare in advanced breast cancer. *Journal of the American Medical Association* 240:2644–2646.

Powles, T. J., C. R. Tillyer, A. L. Jones, S. E. Ashley, J. Treleaven, J. B. Davey, and J. A. McKinna. 1990. Prevention of breast cancer with tamoxifen—an update on the Royal Marsden Hospital pilot programme. *European Journal of Cancer* 26:680–684.

Powles, T. J., J. R. Hardy, S. E. Ashley, G. M. Farrington, D. Cosgrove, J. B. Davey, M. Dowsett, J. A. McKinna, A. G. Nash, H. D. Sinnett, C. R. Tillyer, and J. Treleaven. 1989. A pilot trial to evaluate the acute toxicity and feasibility of tamoxifen for prevention of breast cancer. *British Journal of Cancer* 60:126–131.

Pritchard, K. I., D. B. Thomson, R. E. Myers, D. J. Sutherland, B. G. Mobbs, and J. W. Meakin. 1980. Tamoxifen therapy in premenopausal patients with metastatic breast cancer. *Cancer Treatment Reports* 64:787–796.

Pubesgaard, T., and F. E. von Eyben. 1986. Bilateral optic neuritis evolved during tamoxifen treatment. *Cancer* 58:383–386.

Ravdin, P. M., N. F. Fritz, D. C. Tormey, and V. C. Jordan. 1988. Endocrine status of premeno-pausal node-positive breast cancer patients following adjuvant chemotherapy and long-term tamoxifen. *Cancer Research* 48:1026–1029.

Ribeiro, G. 1985. Male breast carcinoma—a review of 301 cases from the Christie Hospital and Holt Radium Institute, Manchester. *British Journal of Cancer* 51:115–119.

Ribeiro, G., and R. Swindell. 1985. The Christie Hospital tamoxifen (Nolvadex) adjuvant trial for operable breast carcinoma: seven year results. *European Journal of Cancer and Clinical Oncology* 24:1817–1821.

Ribeiro, G., and R. Swindell. 1992. Adjuvant tamoxifen for male breast cancer (MBC). *British Journal of Cancer* 65:252–254.

Ritchie, L. D., and S. M. Grant. 1989. Tamoxifen-warfarin interaction: the Aberdeen hospitals drug file. *British Medical Journal* 298:1253.

Ron, I. G., M. J. Inbar, Y. Barak, S. Stier, and S. Chaitchik. 1992. Organic delusional syndrome associated with tamoxifen treatment. *Cancer* 69:1415–1417.

Rose, D. P., and T. E. Davis. 1980. Effects of adjuvant chemohormonal therapy on the ovarian and adrenal function of breast cancer patients. *Cancer Research* 40:4043–4047.

Rostom, A. Y., and A. R. Gershuny. 1992. Adjuvant treatment in breast cancer. *Lancet* 339:424.

Saphner, T., D. C. Tormey, and R. Gray. 1991. Venous and arterial thrombosis in patients who received adjuvant therapy for breast cancer. *Journal of Clinical Oncology* 9:286–294.

Sawka, C. A., K. I. Pritchard, A. H. Paterson, D. B. Thomson, W. E. Shelley, R. E. Myers, B. G. Mobbs, A. Malkin, and J. W. Meakin. 1986. Role and mechanism of action of tamoxifen in premenopausal women with metastatic breast carcinoma. *Cancer Research* 46:3152–3156.

Schiff, I., D. Tulchinsky, D. Cramer, and K. J. Ryan. 1980. Oral medroxyprogesterone in the treatment of postmenopausal symptoms. *Journal of the American Medical Association* 244:1443–1445.

Schwartzbaum, J. A., B. S. Hulka, W. C. Fowler, D. G. Kaufman, and D. Hoberman. 1987. The influence of exogenous estrogen use on survival after diagnosis of endometrial cancer. *American Journal of Epidemiology* 126:851–860.

Senior, B. E., M. L. Cawood, R. E. Oakley, J. M. McKiddie, and D. R. Siddle. 1978. A comparison of the effects of clomiphene and tamoxifen treatment on the concentrations of oestradiol and progesterone in the peripheral plasma of infertile women. *Clinical Endocrinology* 8:381–389.

Sherman, B. M., F. K. Chapler, K. Crickard, and D. Wycoff. 1979. Endocrine consequences of continuous antiestrogen therapy with tamoxifen in premenopausal women. *Journal of Clinical Investigation* 64:398–404.

Shutt, D. A., I. D. Smith, and R. P. Shearman. 1973. Induction of ovulation and plasma changes following treatment with an antioestrogen, tamoxifen. *Journal of the International Research Communication System* 12:85.

Smith, I. E., A. L. Harris, M. Morgan, H. T. Ford, J. C. Gazet, C. L. Harmer, H. White, C. A. Parsons, A. Villardo, G. Walsh, and J. A. McKinna. 1981. Tamoxifen versus aminoglutethimide in advanced breast carcinoma: a randomised crossover trial. *British Medical Journal—Clinical Research* 283:1432–1434.

Spremulli, E., P. DeSimone, and J. Durant. 1982. A phase II study of Nolvadex (tamoxifen) in the treatment of advanced prostatic adenocarcinoma. *American Journal of Clinical Oncology* 5:149–153.

Stoll, B. A. 1980. The significance of tumor "stimulation" by tamoxifen. In *Endocrine treatment of breast cancer,* vol. 17, ed. B. Henningson, F. Linder, and C. Steichele, 149–150. New York: Springer-Verlag.

Stoll, B. A. 1985. Mechanisms in endocrine therapy of bone metastases. *Journal of the Royal Society of Medicine* 78 (Supplement 9):11–14.

Stuenkel, C. A. 1989. Menopause and estrogen replacement therapy. *Psychiatric Clinics of North America* 12:133–152.

Sunderland, M. C., and C. K. Osborne. 1991. Tamoxifen in premenopausal patients with metastatic breast cancer: a review. *Journal of Clinical Oncology* 9:1283–1297.

Swenerton, K. D. 1980. Treatment of advanced endometrial adenocarcinoma with tamoxifen. *Cancer Treatment Reports* 64:805–811.

Tajima, C. 1984. Endocrine profiles in tamoxifen-induced conception cycles. *Fertility and Sterility* 42:548–553.

Tanaka, M., K. Abe, S. Ohnami, I. Adachi, K. Yamguchi, and S. Miyakawa. 1978. Tamoxifen in advanced breast cancer: response rate, effect on pituitary hormone reserve and binding affinity to estrogen receptor. *Japanese Journal of Clinical Oncology* 8:141–148.

Tenni, P., D. L. Lalich, and M. J. Byrne. 1989. Life-threatening interaction between tamoxifen and warfarin. *British Medical Journal* 298:93.

Turken, S., E. Siris, D. Seldin, E. Flaster, G. Hyman, and R. Lindsay. 1989. Effects of tamoxifen on spinal bone density in women with breast cancer. *Journal of the National Cancer Institute* 81:1086–1088.

Van Veelsen, H., P. H. Willemse, T. Tjabbes, M. J. Schweitzer, and D. T. Sleijfer. 1986. Oral high-dose medroxyprogesterone acetate versus tamoxifen. A randomized crossover trial in postmenopausal patients with advanced breast cancer. *Cancer* 58:7–13.

Vinding, T., and N. V. Nielsen. 1983. Retinopathy caused by treatment with tamoxifen in low dosage. *Acta Ophthalmologica* 61:45–50.

White, I. N. H., F. de Mattees, A. Davis, L. L. Smith, C. Crojton Sleigh, S. Venitt, A. Hewer and D. H. Phillips. 1992. Gerotoxic potential of tamoxifen and analogues in female Fisher F344/n rats, DBA/2 and C57BL/6 mice and in human MCL-5 cells. *Carcinogenesis* (Lond.) 13:2197–2203.

Yager, J. D., and Y. E. Shi. 1991. Synthetic estrogens and tamoxifen as promoters of hepatocarcinogenesis. *Preventive Medicine* 20:27–37.

Yager, J. D., B. D. Roebuck, T. L. Paluszcyk, and V. A. Memoli. 1986. Effects of ethinyl estradiol and tamoxifen on liver DNA turnover and new synthesis and appearance of gamma glutamyl transpeptidase–positive foci in female rats. *Carcinogenesis* 7:2007–2014.

Editor's Note (Added in Proof): Tamoxifen is associated with a doubling of the risk of developing endometrial carcinoma (Fisher et al. 1994). The incidence rate is 2 per 1000 per year for women taking 10 mg b.i.d. Deaths have been observed from endometrial carcinoma in NSABP Study B_{14} that are associated with tamoxifen administration. Tamoxifen does not control the growth of pre-existing endometrial carcinoma and patients must be screened before starting therapy, and with periodic evaluations during tamoxifen therapy. Spotting and bleeding *must* be rapidly followed up with an evaluation of endometrial carcinoma. Tamoxifen is however not associated with more aggressive high grade endometrial carcinoma (Fisher et al. 1994, von Leeuwen et al. 1994).

References

Fisher B., J. P. Costantino, C. K. Redmond, E. R. Fisher, D. L. Wickerham, W. M. Cronin and other NSABP contributors. 1994. Endometrial cancer in tamoxifen-treated breast cancer patients: findings from the NSABP B_{14}. *Journal of the National Cancer Institute* 86:527–537.

Van Leeuwen F. E., J. Benraadt, J. W. W. Coebergh, L. A. L. M. Kiemeney, C. H. Gimbrere, R. Otter, L. J. Shouten, R. A. M. Damhuis, M. Bontenbal, F. W. Diepenhorst, A. W. van-den-Belt-Dusebout, H. van Tinton. 1994. Risk of endometrial cancer after tamoxifen treatment of breast cancer. *Lancet* 343:448–52.

13

The Prevention of Breast Cancer with Tamoxifen

Monica Morrow and V. Craig Jordan

I. Introduction 258
II. Tamoxifen as Current Therapy 259
III. The Prevention of Breast Cancer: Biological Rationale 260
IV. Additional Beneficial Effects of Tamoxifen 261
V. Whom to Select for Intervention? 263
   A. Age 263
   B. Family History 263
   C. Reproductive Factors and Hormone Use 264
   D. Benign Breast Disease 265
   E. Lobular Carcinoma *in Situ* 266
   F. Problems with the Identification of High-Risk Women 268
VI. Current Trials 269
VII. The Concerns To Be Monitored 270
VIII. Conclusion 273
   References 274

I. Introduction

URING the past decade clinical trial organizations have established treatment protocols for the control of advanced and primary breast cancer. Although effective therapeutic agents have been identified and survival advantages have been noted, 44,000 women in the United States die annually from breast cancer, making it clear that new therapeutic strategies need to be formulated.

A strategy of chemoprevention, i.e., the administration of a target site–specific agent to prevent the development of breast cancer, is an important new alternative approach. Naturally, any selected agent must have proven efficacy and be nontoxic to the healthy women who may be required to take the intervention for many years. Currently two types of pharmacological agents are being considered: the retinoids and antiestrogens. The retinoids (Moon and Mehta 1990) offer the potential to control the replication of both estrogen-dependent and -independent disease, but, although there is a wealth of preclinical information to support their use as preventives, very little clinical experience is available about potential long-term toxicities or efficacy in humans. On the face of it, antiestrogens (Lerner and Jordan 1990) might be expected only to reduce breast cancer incidence by one-third, because this is the known response rate in advanced disease. However, it is reasoned that early intervention will have a more pronounced effect because of the essential role of estrogen in the promotion of breast cancer (Fig. 13.1).

This chapter will review the potential for tamoxifen to prevent breast cancer. There is extensive clinical information available about the side effects and worth of tamoxifen in the treatment of breast cancer (Furr and Jordan 1984; Legha 1988), and laboratory studies have demonstrated the ability of tamoxifen to prevent rodent mammary carcinogenesis (Jordan 1983). However, unlike the rodent models that were reviewed in Chapter 1, where all animals develop tumors, it is not possible to identify women who *will* develop breast cancer. Although women at increased risk can be selected for an intervention, the majority will never develop breast cancer. The potential benefits and toxicities of tamoxifen will be discussed to clarify the risk-benefit assessment for the target population.

258

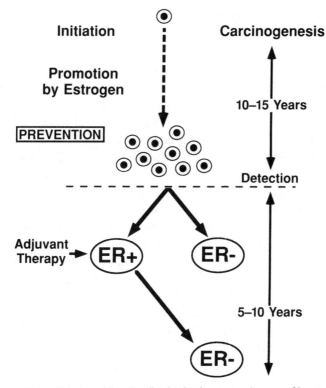

Figure 13.1. A model to describe the development and course of breast cancer with current therapeutic strategies. At detection the primary tumor is classified as estrogen receptor (ER) positive or negative. Adjuvant therapy with tamoxifen has proven worth to increase the survival of postmenopausal women with node-negative or node-positive disease. The antiestrogen is more effective in ER-positive patients. The goal of current strategies is to prevent the development of breast cancer and reduce incidence. Estrogen is considered to be an essential promoter of breast carcinogenesis, so the administration of tamoxifen to high-risk women could reduce incidence by more than 50%. ER-negative disease is both aggressive and difficult to manage. This preemptive strategy could also reduce the incidence of ER-negative disease, because it is believed to be derived by genetic drift from ER-positive cells.

II. *Tamoxifen as Current Therapy*

Multiple clinical trials have demonstrated the safety and effectiveness of adjuvant tamoxifen therapy in the treatment of breast cancer. A summary of the results of treatment in 30,000 women (Early Breast Cancer Trialists'

Collaborative Group 1992) by the Early Breast Cancer Clinical Trials Group has reported the following conclusions: (1) Doses of tamoxifen greater than 20 mg per day provide no added benefit. (2) Long-term tamoxifen is better than short-term tamoxifen for both recurrence and survival. (3) The proportional risk reduction from tamoxifen is approximately equal for node-positive and node-negative disease. However, the absolute risk reduction is greater for node-positive patients because of the higher likelihood of recurrence in this group. (4) Patients with ER-positive tumors benefit more from tamoxifen than patients with ER-negative tumors, although patients with ER-negative tumors treated with tamoxifen experience significantly fewer recurrences than placebo-treated patients. (5) The effects of tamoxifen are independent of the effects of chemotherapy, and patients may benefit more from a combined chemo- and endocrine therapy approach. (6) Women over 50 years of age benefit more from tamoxifen than women under 50 years of age. This effect may not be strictly related to menopausal status. Women under 50 years of age do show a significant reduction in recurrence from tamoxifen mono-therapy. (7) Tamoxifen therapy also leads to a reduction in contralateral breast cancers and cardiovascular deaths. This overview analysis of randomized clinical trials with tamoxifen provides the statistical information necessary to demonstrate the worth of this drug as an anticancer agent, and to identify the subgroups of patients most likely to benefit from the drug.

III. The Prevention of Breast Cancer: Biological Rationale

The successful use of tamoxifen for the treatment of breast cancer, and the low reported incidence of side effects observed with the more than 4.5 million women years of clinical experience, has acted as a catalyst to support the use of tamoxifen in normal women at risk for developing breast cancer. The experimental evidence (Chapter 1) suggesting that tamoxifen may be effective as a chemopreventive agent is supported by data on the reduced incidence of second primary breast cancers in women with stage I and II breast cancer treated with adjuvant tamoxifen. In the Stockholm trial (Fornander et al. 1989) 1846 postmenopausal women under age 71 were randomized to no endocrine therapy or 2 or 5 years of tamoxifen at a dose of 40 mg daily. At a median follow-up of 7 years, a 40% reduction in the incidence of contralateral breast cancers was observed in the tamoxifen-treated women when compared with controls. No differences in contralateral cancer incidence were observed between women treated for 2 or 5 years with tamoxifen (Rutqvist et al. 1991).

Table 13.1. Cumulative frequency of contralateral breast cancer during adjuvant therapy for breast cancer

Trial	Dose	Duration	Tamoxifen-treated cancers (N)		Controls cancer (N)	
Copenhagen	20 mg	1 yr	3	(164)	4	(153)
CRC	20 mg	2 yrs	7	(947)	18	(965)
ECOG	20 mg	2 yrs	1	(91)	3	(90)
NATO	20 mg	2 yrs	15	(564)	17	(567)
NSABP	20 mg	5 yrs	23	(1419)	32	(1419)
Scottish	20 mg	5 yrs	9	(661)	12	(651)
Stockholm	40 mg	2–5 yrs	18	(931)	32	(915)
Toronto-Edmonton	20 mg	2 yrs	3	(198)	3	(202)
Total			79	(4975)	121	(4971)
			(1.6%)		(2.4%)	

Adapted from Nayfield et al. 1991.

Tamoxifen at a dose of 20 mg daily has also been shown to decrease breast cancer risk. In National Surgical Adjuvant Breast and Bowel Project protocol B14 (Fisher et al. 1989), 2892 pre- and postmenopausal women with node-negative breast cancer were treated with tamoxifen or placebo for at least 5 years. At a mean follow-up of 59 months, a 50% reduction in contralateral breast cancer was seen in the tamoxifen-treated women. Similar reductions were observed in the Cancer Research Campaign Trial (CRC Adjuvant Breast Trial Working Party 1988) and the Scottish trial (Breast Cancer Trials Committee 1987), and the published data are summarized in Table 13.1.

The overview analysis (Early Breast Cancer Trialists' Collaborative Group 1992) presented information on the incidence of contralateral breast cancer in about two-thirds of the patients in the tamoxifen trials. Contralateral breast cancer was reported in 184/9135 (2.0%) of controls compared with 122/9128 (1.3%) of patients treated with tamoxifen (an odds reduction of 39%, $p < 0.00001$).

IV. Additional Beneficial Effects of Tamoxifen

Table 13.2 summarizes the potential benefits and concerns raised about long-term tamoxifen treatment. The majority of possible beneficial and adverse side effects are related primarily to tamoxifen's partial estrogenic properties. However, other adverse reactions with unknown mechanisms have also been described. These concerns will be discussed later in this chapter.

Estrogens play an important role in maintaining bone density in women, and estrogen replacement therapy is efficacious in preventing the develop-

Table 13.2. Potential beneficial and adverse side effects of long-term tamoxifen therapy

Beneficial effects
Reduction in contralateral breast cancer
Maintenance of bone density
Reduction in serum cholesterol: decrease in myocardial infarction
Adverse effects
Thromboembolic disorders
Endometrial stimulation
Liver carcinogenesis
Ophthalmic toxicities
Ovarian stimulation
Teratogenesis

ment of osteoporosis following menopause. The long-term antiestrogenic properties of tamoxifen could potentially facilitate the development of osteoporosis. However, tamoxifen is not a pure antiestrogen (Furr and Jordan 1984), and animal models have demonstrated estrogenic actions of tamoxifen on bone (Jordan, Phelps, and Lindgren 1987; Turner et al. 1987). Clinical studies have confirmed that tamoxifen does not lead to osteoporosis (Love et al. 1988; Turken et al. 1989; Fornander et al. 1990), with patients showing no decrease in bone mineral density following 2 years of adjuvant tamoxifen. One study (Chapter 3) shows that spinal bone density is maintained in patients receiving 2 years of tamoxifen therapy (Love et al. 1992).

Estrogen is also known to decrease low density lipoprotein (LDL) cholesterol and increase high density lipoprotein (HDL) cholesterol. High levels of LDL and low levels of HDL in men have been associated with a higher incidence of cardiovascular disease. It has been proposed that the effect of estrogen in premenopausal women on LDL and HDL levels may account for the lower incidence of myocardial infarctions observed in these women compared with age-matched men. After menopause, the incidence of coronary artery disease in women parallels that in men of the same age. Therefore, long-term tamoxifen might increase the risk for premature coronary heart disease because of its antiestrogenic properties. However, tamoxifen appears to be more estrogen-like in this respect, resulting in lower levels of cholesterol in women (Bertelli et al. 1988; Bruning et al. 1988; Love et al. 1990, 1991). Most of the effect is observed in the LDL fraction, because HDL cholesterol tends to remain unchanged during tamoxifen therapy. The recent overview analysis of clinical trials involving tamoxifen did indicate a decrease (25%) in vascular-related deaths in tamoxifen-treated patients when compared with patients not receiving tamoxifen (Early Breast Cancer Trialists' Collaborative

Group 1992). The Scottish trial (McDonald and Stewart 1991) has also demonstrated a significant reduction ($p = 0.0087$) in fatal myocardial infarctions in tamoxifen-treated patients (10/200) compared with the control group (25/251). The Stockholm adjuvant study of tamoxifen has demonstrated a lower rate of hospital visits for cardiovascular problems in patients taking tamoxifen. Five years of tamoxifen is superior to two years of treatment (Rutqvist and Mattsson, 1993). These additional beneficial effects of tamoxifen give added impetus to its use as a preventive agent in high-risk women.

V. Whom to Select for Intervention?

A number of factors which increase the risk of breast cancer development have been identified. These include both endogenous characteristics such as age, family history, and reproductive history, and anatomic factors such as the presence of benign breast disease. As breast cancer prevention becomes a clinical reality, an understanding of the magnitude of the increase in risk conferred by each of these factors, as well as their interactions with each other, assumes increasing importance. Only with a precise determination of an individual's risk status can a risk-benefit evaluation of a preventive therapy be made.

A. AGE

Breast cancer remains the most common malignancy in American women, although it is second to lung cancer as a cause of death. The American Cancer Society estimated that 180,000 new cases would occur in 1992, accounting for 32% of the malignancies occurring in females (Boring et al. 1992). Everyone is familiar with the American Cancer Society statistic that 1 in 9 women will develop breast cancer in her lifetime. However, this figure represents the risk of developing breast cancer from birth to age 110. One-half of a woman's risk of breast cancer development occurs after age 65 (Seidman et al. 1985). For the average woman, the risk of developing breast cancer in the 20-year interval between age 35 and 55 is about 2.5%. If a woman survives to age 65, her risk of breast cancer development in the next 20 years increases to 5.5% (Seidman et al. 1985). Thus, any determination of a woman's risk status must take into account her age.

B. FAMILY HISTORY

Family history is probably the most widely recognized breast cancer risk factor. Only 5% of carefully studied breast cancer patients are felt to have a pedigree consistent with hereditary breast cancer, although 10–20% will have a family history of breast cancer (Lynch et al. 1976). The risk of developing breast cancer is increased 1.5–3.0 times when a mother or a sister has the disease, and risk may be greater when a sibling is affected than when a mother is affected (Ottman et al. 1983; Anderson 1974). In some studies, risk increases with the number of affected first-degree relatives (Bain et al. 1980; Sattin et al. 1985), so that a family history of both a mother and a sister with breast cancer carries a relative risk of 5.6, compared with relative risks of 2.5 (sister) or 1.8 (mother) for single relatives (Bain et al. 1980). There is agreement that bilateral premenopausal breast cancer is associated with the highest risk of breast cancer development (Ottman et al. 1983; Anderson 1974, Anderson and Badzioch 1985). Anderson (Anderson and Badzioch 1985) observed a 9-fold increase in risk in relatives of women with bilateral, premenopausal breast cancer compared with a 1.5-fold excess in relatives of women with unilateral, postmenopausal breast cancer. For women whose relatives have unilateral breast carcinoma, the significance of its occurrence premenopausally or postmenopausally is unclear. Anderson (1974) noted higher risks for relatives of women with unilateral cancer occurring before the menopause, but this finding was not confirmed in other studies (Ottman et al. 1983). It is important to recognize that the lifetime risk of breast cancer for a 30-year-old woman with both a mother and a sister with bilateral breast cancer is reported to be 25% (Anderson and Badzioch 1985), with a corresponding risk of 7%–14% (Ottman et al. 1983; Anderson and Badzioch 1985) if a sister has unilateral breast carcinoma. Thus, the cumulative probability of breast cancer development for most women with a family history of the disease is under 30%.

C. Reproductive Factors and Hormone Use

Numerous studies have linked breast cancer incidence to the age of menarche, menopause, and first pregnancy. Age at menarche is consistently associated with breast cancer risk (MacMahon et al. 1973, 1982; Henderson et al. 1985; Trichopoulos et al. 1984; Bernstein et al. 1987). A review of case control studies suggests that a 20% decrease in breast cancer risk is seen for each year after age 12 that menarche is delayed (MacMahon et al. 1973). The late onset of menarche is associated with a delay in the establishment of regular ovulatory cycles, which is felt by some authors to have an additional protective effect (Henderson et al. 1985; Bernstein et al. 1987), although there is dispute on this point (MacMahon et al. 1982; Trichopoulos et al. 1984). A woman's level of physical activity, even when moderate, impacts on the likelihood that ovulatory cycles will occur and thus may alter breast cancer risk (Bernstein et al. 1987).

Similarly, age at menopause is a factor in breast cancer risk. The relative risk of developing breast cancer for a woman with natural menopause before age 45 is 0.73 compared with a woman with natural menopause between the ages of 45 and 54 (Thomas and Lilienfeld 1976). Oophorectomy prior to age 50 decreases breast cancer risk, with an increasing magnitude of risk reduction as the age at oophorectomy decreases (Trichopoulos et al. 1972). From this data, it seems likely that the total duration of menstrual life is an important factor in breast cancer risk, although the mechanisms through which risk is altered remain uncertain.

Parity and age at first birth are other endogenous hormonal factors which influence breast cancer risk. Nulliparous women have a relative risk of 1.4 compared with those who have born children (MacMahon et al. 1970). It has become increasingly apparent that the effect of term pregnancy on breast cancer risk varies with the age at first birth, with women whose first term pregnancy occurs after age 30 having a 2–5-fold increase in breast cancer risk compared with women having a first term pregnancy before age 18 or 19 (Trichopoulos et al. 1983; Brinton et al. 1983). Abortion, whether spontaneous or induced, prior to full-term pregnancy has no protective effect (Trichopoulos et al. 1972) and in several studies has actually been shown to increase breast cancer risk (Pike et al. 1981; Hadjimichael et al. 1986).

In contrast with the consistent finding of the importance of endogenous hormonal factors in breast cancer risk, the data on exogenous hormone usage are less clear. In a review of 27 studies of oral contraceptive use and breast cancer (Henderson 1990), only 2 studies showed an increase in risk for the entire study population. These data suggest that if oral contraceptives increase overall breast cancer risk, the magnitude of the increase is small. The use of postmenopausal estrogen replacement therapy may be associated with a small increase in breast cancer risk in the range of 1.5–2.0 for moderate-dose conjugated estrogen therapy for periods of 10–20 years (Henderson 1990). Little information is available on the effect of long-term, low-dose therapy such as is currently employed.

D. Benign Breast Disease

The importance of benign breast disease as a risk factor for breast carcinoma has been a subject of controversy. Relative risks ranging from less than 1 to 4.5 have been reported for women with benign breast disease (Morrow 1992). Considerable progress in resolving the confusion surrounding benign breast disease and breast cancer risk has been made in recent years, largely through the work of Dupont and Page (Dupont and Page 1985, 1989; Page et al. 1985). Dupont and Page (1985) reviewed 10,366 benign breast biopsies, and classified them according to strict pathological definitions as nonproliferative lesions, proliferative lesions, or proliferative with atypia. The histological diagnoses grouped under these headings are shown in Table 13.3. The incidence of subsequent invasive breast carcinoma was assessed at a median follow-up of 17 years and compared with reference data from the Third National Cancer Survey. Women with proliferative disease were found to have a relative risk of breast cancer of 1.9, and the subcategory of women with atypical hyperplasia were found to have a relative risk of 4.4. Nonproliferative breast disease was associated with no increased risk of breast cancer. These increases in risk were seen for both pre- and post-menopausal women and were greatest in the first 10 years after biopsy (Dupont and Page 1989). After the 10-year interval, the risk of breast cancer development for women with atypia was halved, and the risk for women with proliferative disease returned to that of the index population. A marked interaction between atypia and a family history of a first-degree relative with breast cancer was also noted in these studies (Dupont and Page 1985; Page et al. 1985). The absolute risk of breast cancer development in women with a positive family history and atypical hyperplasia was 20% at 15 years compared with 8% in women with atypical hyperplasia and a negative family history of breast carcinoma (Dupont and Page 1985). Of note, the study population in the original work of Dupont and Page consisted of women with clinically evident breast lesions, and only 3.6% demonstrated atypical hyperplasia whereas 68% had nonproliferative lesions. The incidence of atypical hyperplasia appears to be somewhat higher in mammographically directed biopsies, with reported incidences of 10–18% (Morrow 1992; Rubin et al. 1988). Thus, although atypical hyperplasia is an important risk factor for breast cancer development, this entity accounts for a small percentage of biopsies done for benign disease.

E. Lobular Carcinoma in Situ

Lobular carcinoma *in situ* (LCIS) was first described by Foote and Stewart in 1941. LCIS was recognized as a multicentric lesion, which is an incidental microscopic finding that cannot be identified clinically or by gross

Table 13.3. Classification of benign breast diseases

Nonproliferative	Proliferative
Adenosis	Hyperplasia, moderate or florid
Cysts, macro or micro	Papilloma with fibrovascular core
Duct ectasia	Atypical hyperplasia, ductal or lobular
Fibroadenoma	
Fibrosis	
Mastitis	
Metaplasia, apocrine or squamous	
Mild hyperplasia	

pathological exam. The authors concluded that LCIS was a premalignant lesion best treated by simple mastectomy. The true incidence of LCIS is difficult to define, because it lacks clinical or mammographic features (Pope et al. 1988), but it is diagnosed in from 0.8% to 8.0% of breast biopsies, with an incidence of 2.5% thought to reflect the frequency of the lesion when all breast biopsies are considered (Schwartz et al. 1984; Wheeler et al. 1974; Frykberg et al. 1987).

The diagnosis of LCIS is associated with a bilateral risk of breast cancer, even if the LCIS is present in only one breast, suggesting that LCIS is a risk factor for breast cancer rather than an actual premalignant lesion. Haagensen reported 211 women with LCIS who were followed for a mean of 14 years with a 17% incidence of invasive carcinoma, equally distributed between the index and the contralateral breast (Haagensen et al. 1978). Rosen et al. (1978) noted a 27% incidence of subsequent invasive carcinoma in 99 patients who were followed a mean of 24 years after the diagnosis of LCIS, again equally distributed between both breasts. Andersen reviewed 228 published cases of LCIS treated by biopsy alone and found that 15.5% developed invasive carcinoma of the ipsilateral breast, and 9.3% had a contralateral carcinoma (Andersen 1977). Estimates of relative risks of breast cancer in women with LCIS range from 6.9 to 12 (Haagensen et al. 1978; Rosen et al. 1978; Andersen 1977). The interval to the development of carcinoma after a diagnosis of LCIS can be quite protracted, with Rosen (Rosen et al. 1978) noting that 38% of the cancers in his series occurred 20 or more years after the diagnosis of LCIS. In contrast with the data presented for atypical hyperplasia, the increased risk of breast cancer seen with LCIS does not diminish with follow-up through 25 years. Efforts to identify features of LCIS associated with a higher likelihood of the development of malignancy have been largely unsuccessful. Haagensen et al. (1978) noted that the relative risk of breast cancer increased from 5.7 for women with LCIS alone to 8.5 in women with both a positive family history and LCIS. Histological features, including the amount of LCIS present, have not been predictive of the subsequent development of invasive carcinoma (Rosen et al. 1978).

F. Problems with the Identification of High-Risk Women

Unfortunately, although it is clear that a diagnosis of atypical hyperplasia or LCIS is associated with an increased risk of breast cancer, considerable variation in the criteria used to classify benign lesions exists. This was emphasized in a recent study by Rosai (1991), in which five pathologists, acknowledged as having special expertise in breast disease, were asked to examine 17 proliferative breast lesions and render a diagnosis. In none of the cases reviewed did all five pathologists agree on the diagnosis, and in only three cases did four of the five concur. Perhaps even more alarming, in one-third of the cases the diagnosis ranged from hyperplasia without atypia to carcinoma *in situ*. This degree of interobserver variability emphasizes the need for caution in classifying women as high risk on the basis of results of a breast biopsy alone. The assessment of risk and the interaction of various risk factors is poorly understood by most clinicians. The classification of a woman as high risk is frequently a cause of anxiety for both the woman and her physician, as evidenced by a British study in which high-risk women underwent 5 times the number of breast biopsies as expected, with a predictive value of only 20% (Roberts et al. 1984). In addition, most reports evaluating risk factors have considered only the factor under study, providing no information on its interaction with other risk variables. Gail and coauthors (1989) have developed a model which integrates the risk associated with a family history of breast carcinoma, age at menarche, age at first birth, and number of breast biopsies to provide an individualized risk estimate over a number of time intervals. For example, from this model it can be calculated that a 40-year-old woman whose menarche occurred at age 12, who has a mother with breast cancer, who first gave birth at age 30, and who has had one breast biopsy, has a 6% chance of developing breast cancer in the next 10 years and a 30-year risk of approximately 20%. The Gail model does not subclassify benign breast disease as atypical hyperplasia, hyperplasia, or nonproliferative, although the authors suggest that a mathematical correction for women known to have atypical hyperplasia might further improve the accuracy of the model. This model is not applicable to women with LCIS or a pedigree consistent with true hereditary breast cancer.

VI. *Current Trials*

At present, there are four ongoing breast cancer prevention studies, three involving tamoxifen and one using the retinoid N-4-hydroxyphenyl retinamide. The first trial, a pilot study, was begun at the Royal Marsden Hospital in 1986 (Powles et al. 1989), and when last reported (Powles et al. 1990) had accrued 435 women who were randomized between tamoxifen 20 mg QID and placebo for 3 years. Two thousand women have now been randomized in the study. High-risk women, for the purposes of this study, were defined as those with at least one first-degree relative who had developed breast cancer under age 40 or bilateral breast cancer at any age, or with at least two first-degree relatives with breast cancer at any age. Risk factors other than family history were not considered. The age range of study participants is from 30 to 66, with a mean of 48 years. At 12 months an 83% compliance rate was noted for women in the tamoxifen arm of the trial; by 2 years that had decreased to approximately 70%. This study was designed as a feasibility trial with the ultimate goal being a large-scale multicenter trial. In March 1992 the Medical Research Council (MRC) of Great Britain voted to restrict entry into the multicenter trial to women over the age of 40 with a 4-fold or greater relative risk of breast cancer. Eligibility criteria, as defined by the MRC, are listed in Table 13.4. Concern over tamoxifen's induction of liver tumors in rats was cited by the council as the major reason for restricting entry into the study. Currently the trial is proceeding with government approval but without financial support from the MRC but with the full and unequivocal support of the Cancer Research Campaign and the Imperial Cancer Research Fund (Anonymous 1992). The MRC is currently re-evaluating their position.

A second study, again randomizing participants to treatment with tamoxifen 20 mg daily or placebo, opened in the United States in May 1992. This study, administered by the National Surgical Adjuvant Breast and Bowel Project (NSABP), has an accrual goal of 16,000 women over the next 2 years (Fig. 13.2). Those eligible for entry into the study include any woman over the age of 60, or women between the ages of 35 and 59 whose 5-year risk of developing breast cancer, as predicted by the Gail model, equals that of a 60-year-old woman. Any woman over age 35 with a diagnosis of LCIS treated by biopsy alone is eligible for study entry. In the absence of LCIS, the risk factors necessary to enter the study vary with age, so that a 35-year-old woman must have a relative risk of 5.07, whereas a 45-year-old female's relative risk must be 1.79 to be eligible for study entry. Eligibility requirements for this trial are summarized in Table 13.5. Treatment will continue for a minimum of 5 years.

Table 13.4. British trial of tamoxifen for breast cancer prevention: recommended eligibility
          criteria

Age:	Over 40
Family history:	First-degree relative (mother, sister, daughter) with bilateral breast cancer
	or
	Two first-degree relatives with breast cancer
Personal history:	Unilateral breast cancer or atypical hyperplasia

The last two chemoprevention trials are being conducted by the National Cancer Institute of Milan, Italy. The first is using N-4-hydroxyphenyl retinamide as the test drug. In this study, high-risk women were defined as those treated for unilateral T1 or T2, node-negative breast carcinomas who did not receive adjuvant chemo- or hormonotherapy. Three thousand women have entered this study, but at present, no published data are available. The second trial is a tamoxifen trial. Twenty thousand women over the age of 45 are being randomized to 20mg tamoxifen daily or a placebo for 5 years. Only hysterectomized women are admitted to the trial. More than one thousand women are already participating.

VII. *The Concerns to Be Monitored*

Most of the potential toxicities and concerns have been reviewed in Chapters 2, 3, and 12, but the major concerns will be summarized here.

The wide acceptance of tamoxifen as an adjuvant treatment of breast cancer is partly due to the low incidence and mild nature of acute adverse effects of the drug. The most common acute side effect associated with tamoxifen is vasomotor instability (hot flashes) (Furr and Jordan 1984). Several other signs and symptoms have been attributed to tamoxifen treatment, but most of these occur at similar rates in placebo-treated patients. These adverse reactions seldom are severe enough to warrant the cessation of therapy.

Tamoxifen's partial estrogenic activity can lead to the same complications as estrogen administration, including increased risks for thrombosis and endometrial carcinoma. The risk of these potential complications must be placed in perspective and weighed against the potential benefit of tamoxifen to prevent breast cancer, cardiovascular deaths, and osteoporosis.

There are several anecdotal reports (Nevasaari et al. 1978; Hendrick and Subraminian 1980; Lipton et al. 1984) of thromboembolic events occurring in association with tamoxifen therapy. However, detailed studies documenting a statistically significant increase in thromboembolic disorders during long-term tamoxifen monotherapy are lacking. Decreased antithrombin III levels

Potential Participants

**>60 years old—with/without risk factors
35–59 years old—with risk factors**

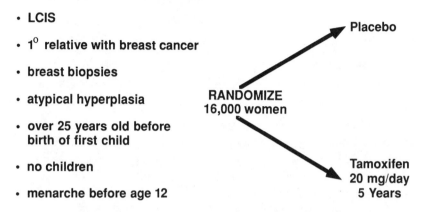

- **LCIS**

- **1⁰ relative with breast cancer**

- **breast biopsies**

- **atypical hyperplasia**

- **over 25 years old before birth of first child**

- **no children**

- **menarche before age 12**

Placebo

**RANDOMIZE
16,000 women**

**Tamoxifen
20 mg/day
5 Years**

Figure 13.2. NSABP–NCI trial to test the worth of tamoxifen to prevent breast cancer in women. Women between the ages of 35 and 59 years will have to present with risk factors to produce a cumulative risk equivalent to the lifetime risk for a 60-year-old woman.

Table 13.5. NSABP trial of tamoxifen for breast cancer prevention: eligibility criteria

Age	Relative risk	Estimated number of women per thousand	Sample profile
35	5.07	3	1 or more first-degree relatives *and* at least 2 breast biopsies
40	2.65	27	2 or more first-degree relatives *or* at least 2 breast biopsies
45	1.79	71	1 or more first-degree relatives *or* at least 2 breast biopsies
50	1.51	93	Same as age 45
55	1.23	125	1 or more first-degree relatives *or* first live birth after age 30

have been observed in postmenopausal women receiving tamoxifen for advanced (Enck and Rios 1984) or node-positive breast cancer (Jordan et al. 1987). However, the decreased antithrombin III levels usually remain within normal limits. Further studies are needed to determine a clear association between tamoxifen therapy and thromboembolic disease.

The long-term stimulatory effects of tamoxifen on the human uterus are unknown, but tamoxifen does produce some estrogen-like effects in postmenopausal women (Furr and Jordan 1984). The relationship between

Table 13.6. Cumulative frequency of uterine cancers during adjuvant
tamoxifen therapy (20 mg daily)

Trial	Tamoxifen-treated cancers (n)		Control cancers (n)	
Copenhagen	2	(164)	0	(153)
ECOG	1	(91)	1	(90)
NATO	0	(564)	0	(567)
NSABP	2	(1419)	0	(1428)
Scottish	4	(661)	2	(651)
Toronto-Edmonton	0	(198)	1	(202)
Total	9	(3097)	4	(3091)
		0.3%		0.2%

endometrial carcinoma and tamoxifen treatment is complex. Data from an animal model show that both tamoxifen and estradiol can stimulate the growth of a human endometrial carcinoma that is ER- and progesterone receptor–positive when grown in athymic mice (Satyaswaroop et al. 1984; Gottardis et al. 1988). Clinically (Killacky et al. 1985; Hardell 1988; Gusberg 1990), cases of endometrial cancer have been reported in patients receiving adjuvant tamoxifen therapy. Studies are currently evaluating the changes in uterine pathophysiology during tamoxifen therapy (Gal et al. 1991). A randomized adjuvant clinical trial from Sweden (Fornander et al. 1989) has demonstrated a significant increase in endometrial carcinoma in patients receiving tamoxifen (13 endometrial tumors in 931 patients) for 2–5 years compared with the control group (2 endometrial tumors in 915 patients). However, the dose of tamoxifen in this study (40 mg QID) was twice that normally prescribed in the United States. It is noteworthy that two large clinical studies of long-term tamoxifen administered at a dose of 20 mg QID have not reported (Breast Cancer Trials Committee 1987; Fisher et al. 1989) an increased incidence of endometrial carcinoma. The incidence of endometrial carcinoma in published trials of adjuvant tamoxifen therapy is summarized in Table 13.6. Similarly, the recent overview analysis (Early Breast Trialists' Collaborative Group 1992) did not show any significant increase in deaths due to endometrial cancer in tamoxifen-treated patients compared with control groups.

Estrogens, while not carcinogenic, are known *promoters* of rat liver carcinogenesis. Tamoxifen has been implicated in the development of hepatocellular cancer in rats when given in high doses (Gau 1986). Tamoxifen produces DNA-adduct formation in rats (Han and Liehr 1992), but the relevance of this observation to the initiation of carcinogenesis even in the rat is unclear. In recent studies (Dragan et al. 1991) we have shown that tamoxifen, at doses much higher than those used clinically, is only a promoter of rat liver carcinogenesis, i.e., like estrogen or oral contraceptives (but much weaker). Clinical data demonstrating an association between liver tumors and tamoxifen treatment in patients are sparse. The Swedish study reported (Fornander et al. 1989) two cases of hepatocellular cancer in the tamoxifen arm of the study and none in the control arm. However, it is interesting to note that tamoxifen has been studied (Ergstrom et al. 1990; Farinati et al. 1990) as a treatment for hepatocellular carcinoma, and, although little benefit was reported, no evidence of tumor stimulation was observed.

High-dose tamoxifen therapy (over 10-fold higher dosages than the current 20 mg per day used in most patients) has been associated with retinal changes in patients (Kaiser-Kupfer and Lippman 1978). Concern has been raised that with decades of tamoxifen treatment these ophthalmic toxicities could be accumulated. A number of reports have documented ocular changes that occur during tamoxifen therapy (Pugesgaard and Von Eyben 1986; Beck and Mills 1979; Gerner 1989; Ashford et al. 1988). At the current doses of tamoxifen there is no clinical evidence that severe ocular changes routinely occur (Longstaff et al. 1989), although retinopathy has been reported recently (Bentley et al. 1992).

Tamoxifen can induce ovarian steroidogenesis in premenopausal women (Sunderland and Osborne 1991). However, the elevated levels of estradiol are not high enough to interfere with the actions of tamoxifen (Sunderland and Osborne 1991; lino et al. 1991). The elevated levels of estradiol do not seem to alter the levels of follicle-stimulating hormone (FSH) or luteinizing hormone (LH), and most premenopausal women receiving tamoxifen continue to have normal menstrual cycles (Jordan et al. 1991). Patients should be strongly advised to use some method of barrier contraception to prevent pregnancy. The avoidance of pregnancy while receiving tamoxifen therapy is important, because the teratogenic effects of tamoxifen in humans are unknown.

VIII. *Conclusion*

We are entering a new era in the treatment of breast cancer. Tamoxifen can reduce the incidence of second primary breast cancers, and as a chemotherapeutic intervention tamoxifen is unique in that it has an appropriate level of estrogen-like properties that could provide benefits to the target population over and above the prevention of breast cancer. The major cause of death for women in their 60s and 70s is cardiovascular disease, and significant morbidity occurs in this age group because of complications from osteoporosis.

An agent like tamoxifen, which may impact on three major diseases of women, provides an unusual opportunity for the clinical community to test its worth in improving women's health. Nevertheless, tamoxifen can be adequately evaluated only in randomized double-blind clinical trials. These trials are in place, and physicians should encourage women to participate and establish a new therapeutic option as rapidly as possible. Tamoxifen should not be used in women at risk for breast cancer outside the context of a clinical trial.

Acknowledgments

We wish to thank Bonnie Rayho and Nancy Jakubovie for typing this manuscript.

References

Andersen, J. 1977. Lobular carcinoma *in situ* of the breast. An approach to rational treatment. *Cancer* 39:2597–2602.

Anderson, D. E. 1974. Genetic study of breast cancer: identification of a high risk group. *Cancer* 34:1090–1097.

Anderson, D. E., and M. D. Badzioch. 1985. Bilaterality in familial breast cancer patients. *Cancer* 56:2092–2098.

Anonymous. 1992. Tamoxifen trial controversy. *Lancet* 339:735.

Ashford, A. R., I. Donev, R. P. Tiwari, and T. J. Garrett. 1988. Reversible ocular toxicity related to tamoxifen therapy. *Cancer* 61:33–35.

Bain, C., F. E. Speizer, B. Rosner, C. Belanger, and C. H. Hennekens. 1980. Family history of breast cancer as a risk indicator for the disease. *American Journal of Epidemiology* 111:301–308.

Beck, M., and P. V. Mills. 1979. Ocular assessment of patients treated with tamoxifen. *Cancer Treatment Reports* 63:1833–1834.

Bentley, C. R., G. Davis, and W. A. Aclimandos. 1992. Tamoxifen retinopathy: a rare but serious complication. *British Medical Journal* 304:495–496.

Bernstein, L., R. K. Ross, R. A. Lobo, R. Hanish, M. D. Krailo, and B. E. Henderson. 1987. The effects of moderate physical activity on menstrual cycle patterns in adolescence: implications for breast cancer prevention. *British Journal of Cancer* 55:681–685.

Bertelli, G., P. Pronzato, D. Amoroso, M. P. Cusimano, P. F. Conte, G. Montagna, S. Bertolini, and R. Rosso. 1988. Adjuvant tamoxifen in primary breast cancer: influence on plasma lipids and antithrombin III levels. *Breast Cancer Research and Treatment* 12:307–310.

Boring, C., T. Squires, and T. Tong. 1992. Cancer statistics. *CA—A Cancer Journal for Clinicians* 42:19–39.

Breast Cancer Trials Committee, Scottish Cancer Trials Office. 1987. Adjuvant tamoxifen in the management of operable breast cancer: the Scottish trial. *Lancet* 2:171–175.

Brinton, L. A., R. Hoover, and J. F. Fraumeni, Jr. 1983. Reproductive factors in the aetiology of breast cancer. *British Journal of Cancer* 47:757–762.

Bruning, P. F., J. M. Bonfrer, A. A. Hart, M. de Jong-Bakker, D. Linders, J. van Loon, and W. J. Nooyen. 1988. Tamoxifen, serum lipoproteins and cardiovascular risk. *British Journal of Cancer* 58:497–499.

CRC Adjuvant Breast Trial Working Party. 1988. Cyclophosphamide and tamoxifen as adjuvant therapies in the management of breast cancer—preliminary analysis by the CRC adjuvant breast trial working party. *British Journal of Cancer* 57:604–604.

Dragan, Y. P., Y-D Xu, and H. C. Pitot. 1991. Tumor promotion as a target for estrogen/antiestrogen effects in rat hepatocarcinogenesis. *Preventive Medicine* 20:15–26.

Dupont, W. D., and D. L. Page. 1985. Risk factors for breast cancer in women with proliferative breast disease. *New England Journal of Medicine* 312:146–151.

Dupont, W. D., and D. L. Page. 1989. Relative risk of breast cancer varies with time since diagnosis of atypical hyperplasia. *Human Pathology* 20:723–725.

Early Breast Cancer Trialists' Collaborative Group. 1992. Systemic treatment of early breast cancer by hormonal, cytotoxic or immune therapy. 133 randomised trials involving 31,000 recurrences and 24,000 deaths among 75,000 women. *Lancet* 339:1–15.

Enck, R. E., and C. N. Rios. 1984. Tamoxifen treatment of metastatic breast cancer and antithrombin III levels. *Cancer* 53:2607–2609.

Engstrom, P. F., B. Levin, C. G. Moertel, and A. Schutt. 1990. A phase II trial of tamoxifen in hepatocellular carcinoma. *Cancer* 65:2641–2643.

Farinati, F., M. Salvagnini, N. de Maria, A. Fornasiero, M. Chiaramonte, L. Rossaro, and R. Naccarato. 1990. Unresectable hepatocellular carcinoma: a prospective controlled trial with tamoxifen. *Journal of Hepatology* 11:297–301.

Fisher, B., J. Costantino, C. Redmond, R. Poisson, D. Bowman, J. Couture, N. V. Dimitrov, N. Wolmark, D. L. Wickerham, E. R. Fisher, R. D. Margolese, C. Sutherland, A. Glass, R. Foster, and R. Caplan. 1989. A randomized clinical trial evaluating tamoxifen in the treatment of patients with node-negative breast cancer who have estrogen-receptor-positive tumors. *New England Journal of Medicine* 320:479–484.

Foote, F., and F. Stewart. 1941. Lobular carcinoma in situ: a rare form of mammary carcinoma. *American Journal of Pathology* 17:491–496.

Fornander, T., L. E. Rutqvist, B. Cedermark, U. Glas, A. Mattsson, C. Silfversward, L. Skoog, A. Somell, T. Theve, N. Wilking, J. Askergren, and M. L. Hjalmar. 1989. Adjuvant tamoxifen in early breast cancer: occurrence of new primary cancers. *Lancet* 1:117–120.

Fornander, T., L. E. Rutqvist, H. E. Sjöberg, L. Blomqvist, A. Mattsson, and U. Glas. 1990. Long-term adjuvant tamoxifen in early breast cancer: effect on bone mineral density in post-menopausal women. *Journal of Clinical Oncology* 8:1019–1024.

Frykberg, E. R., F. Santiago, W. L. Betsill, Jr., and P. H. O'Brien. 1987. Lobular carcinoma *in situ* of the breast. *Surgery, Gynecology and Obstetrics* 164:285–301.

Furr, B. J., and V. C. Jordan. 1984. The pharmacology and clinical uses of tamoxifen. *Pharmacology and Therapeutics* 25:127–205.

Gail, M. H., L. A. Brinton, D. P. Byar, D. K. Corle, S. B. Green, C. Schairer, and J. J. Mulvihill. 1989. Projecting individualized probabilities of developing breast cancer for white females who are being examined annually. *Journal of the National Cancer Institute* 81:1879–1886.

Gal, D., S. Kopel, M. Bashevkin, J. Lebowicz, and M. L. Tancer. 1991. Oncogenic potential of tamoxifen on endometria of postmenopausal women with breast cancer: preliminary report. *Gynecologic Oncology* 42:120–123.

Gau, T. 1986. Open letter to all U.S. medical oncologists describing the toxicological findings in rats with high dose tamoxifen treatment. Stuart Pharmaceuticals, a division of ICI Americas, Wilmington, Delaware.

Gerner, E. W. 1989. Ocular toxicity of tamoxifen. *Annals of Ophthalmology* 21:420–423.

Gottardis, M. M., S. P. Robinson, P. G. Satyaswaroop, and V. C. Jordan. 1988. Contrasting actions of tamoxifen on endometrial and breast tumor growth in the athymic mouse. *Cancer Research* 48:812–815.

Gusberg, S. B. 1990. Tamoxifen for breast cancer: associated endometrial cancer. *Cancer* 65:1463–1464.

Haagensen, C. D., N. Lane, R. Lattes, and C. Bodian. 1978. Lobular neoplasia (so-called lobular carcinoma *in situ*) of the breast. *Cancer* 42:737–769.

Hadjimichael, O. C., C. A. Boyle, and J. W. Meigs. 1986. Abortion before first live birth and risk of breast cancer. *British Journal of Cancer* 53:281–284.

Han, X., and J. G. Liehr. 1992. Induction of covalent DNA adducts in rodents by tamoxifen. *Cancer Research* 52:1360–1363.

Hardell, L. 1988. Tamoxifen as risk factor for carcinoma of corpus uteri. *Lancet* 2:563.

Henderson, B. E., R. K. Ross, H. L. Judd, M. D. Krailo, and M. C. Pike. 1985. Do regular ovulatory cycles increase breast cancer risk? *Cancer* 56:1206–1208.

Henderson, I. C. 1990. What can a woman do about her risk of dying of breast cancer? *Current Problems in Cancer* 14:161–230.

Hendrick, A., and V. P. Subramanian. 1980. Tamoxifen and thromboembolism. *Journal of the American Medical Association* 243:514–515.

Iino, Y., D. M. Wolf, S. M. Langan-Fahey, D. A. Johnson, M. Ricchio, M. E. Thompson, and V. C. Jordan. 1991. Reversible control of oestradiol-stimulated growth of MCF-7 tumours by tamoxifen in the athymic mouse. *British Journal of Cancer* 64:1019–1024.

Jordan, V. C. 1983. Laboratory studies to develop general principles for the adjuvant treatment of breast cancer with antiestrogens: problems and potential for future clinical applications. *Breast Cancer Research and Treatment* 3(Supplement):73–86.

Jordan, V. C., N. F. Fritz, and D. C. Tormey. 1987. Long-term adjuvant therapy with tamoxifen: effects on sex hormone binding globulin and antithrombin III. *Cancer Research* 47:4517–4519.

Jordan, V. C., E. Phelps, and J. U. Lindgren. 1987. Effect of antiestrogens on bone in castrated and intact female rats. *Breast Cancer Research and Treatment* 10:31–35.

Jordan, V. C., N. F. Fritz, S. Langan-Fahey, M. Thompson, and D. C. Tormey. 1991. Alteration of endocrine parameters in premenopausal women with breast cancer during long-term adjuvant therapy with tamoxifen as the single agent. *Journal of the National Cancer Institute* 83:1488–1491.

Kaiser-Kupfer, M. I., and M. E. Lippman. 1978. Tamoxifen retinopathy. *Cancer Treatment Reports* 62:315–320.

Killackey, M. A., T. B. Hakes, and V. K. Pierce. 1985. Endometrial adenocarcinoma in breast cancer patients receiving antiestrogens. *Cancer Treatment Reports* 69:237–238.

Legha, S. S. 1988. Tamoxifen in the treatment of breast cancer. *Annals of Internal Medicine* 109:219–228.

Lerner, L. J., and V. C. Jordan. 1990. Development of antiestrogens and their use in breast cancer: eighth Cain Memorial Award Lecture. *Cancer Research* 50:4177–4189.

Lipton, A., H. A. Harvey, and R. W. Hamilton. 1984. Venous thrombosis as a side effect of tamoxifen treatment. *Cancer Treatment Reports* 68:887–889.

Longstaff, S., H. Sigurdsson, M. O'Keeffe, S. Ogston, and P. Preece. 1989. A controlled study of the ocular effects of tamoxifen in conventional dosage in the treatment of breast carcinoma. *European Journal of Cancer and Clinical Oncology* 25:1805–1808.

Love, R. R., R. B. Mazess, D. C. Tormey, H. S. Barden, P. A. Newcomb, and V. C. Jordan. 1988. Bone mineral density in women with breast cancer treated with adjuvant tamoxifen for at least two years. *Breast Cancer Research and Treatment* 12:297–302.

Love, R. R., P. A. Newcomb, D. A. Wiebe, T. S. Surawicz, V. C. Jordan, P. P. Carbone, and D. L. DeMets. 1990. Effects of tamoxifen therapy on lipid and lipoprotein levels in post-menopausal patients with node-negative breast cancer. *Journal of the National Cancer Institute* 82:1327–1332.

Love, R. R., R. B. Mazess, H. S. Barden, S. Epstein, P. A. Newcomb, V. C. Jordan, P. P. Carbone, and D. L. DeMets. 1992. Effects of tamoxifen on bone mineral density in postmenopausal women with breast cancer. *New England Journal of Medicine* 326:852–856.

Love, R. R., D. A. Wiebe, P. A. Newcomb, L. Cameron, H. Leventhal, V. C. Jordan, J. Feyzi, and D. L. DeMets. 1991. Effect of tamoxifen on cardiovascular risk factors in postmenopausal women. *Annals of Internal Medicine* 115:860–864.

Lynch, H. T., H. A. Guirgis, F. Brodkey, J. Lynch, K. Maloney, L. Rankin, and G. M. Mulcahy. 1976. Genetic heterogeneity and familial carcinoma of the breast. *Surgery, Gynecology and Obstetrics* 142:693–699.

McDonald, C. C., and H. J. Stewart. 1991. Fatal myocardial infarction in the Scottish adjuvant tamoxifen trial. The Scottish Breast Cancer Committee. *British Medical Journal* 303:435–437.

MacMahon, B., P. Cole, and J. Brown. 1973. Etiology of human breast cancer: a review. *Journal of the National Cancer Institute* 50:21–42.

MacMahon, B., P. Cole, T. M. Lin, C. R. Lowe, A. P. Mirra, B. Ravnihar, E. J. Salber, V. G. Valaoras, and S. Yuasa. 1970. Age at first birth and breast cancer risk. *Bulletin of the World Health Organization* 43:209–221.

MacMahon, B., D. Trichopoulos, J. Brown, A. P. Andersen, K. Aoki, P. Cole, F. deWaard, T. Kauraniemi, R. W. Morgan, M. Purde, B. Ravnihar, N. Stromby, K. Westlund, and N. C. Woo. 1982. Age at menarche, probability of ovulation and breast cancer risk. *International Journal of Cancer* 29:13–16.

Moon, R. C., and R. G. Mehta. 1990. Cancer chemoprevention by retinoids: animal models. *Methods in Enzymology* 190:395–406.

Morrow, M. 1992. Pre-cancerous breast lesions: implications for breast cancer prevention trials. *International Journal of Radiation Oncology and Biological Physics* 23:1071–1078.

Nayfield, S. G., J. E. Karp, L. G. Ford, F. A. Dort, and B. S. Kramer. 1991. Potential role of tamoxifen in prevention of breast cancer. *Journal of the National Cancer Institute* 83:1450–1459.

Nevasaari, K., M. Heikkinen, and P. J. Taskinen. 1978. Tamoxifen and thrombosis. *Lancet* 2:946–947.

Ottman, R., M. C. Pike, M. C. King, and B. E. Henderson. 1983. Practical guide for estimating risk for familial breast cancer. *Lancet* 2:556–558.

Page, D. L., W. D. Dupont, L. W. Rogers, and M. S. Rados. 1985. Atypical hyperplastic lesions of the female breast. A long-term follow-up study. *Cancer* 55:2698–2708.

Pike, M C., B. E. Henderson, J. T. Casagrande, I. Rosario, and G. E. Gray. 1981. Oral contraceptive use and early abortion as risk factors for breast cancer in young women. *British Journal of Cancer* 43:72–76.

Pope, T. L., Jr., R. E. Fechner, M. C. Wilhelm, H. J. Wanebo, and E. S. de Paredes. 1988. Lobular carcinoma *in situ* of the breast: mammographic features. *Radiology* 168:63–66.

Powles, T. J., C. R. Tillyer, A. L. Jones, S. E. Ashley, J. Treleaven, J. B. Davey, and J. A. McKinna. 1990. Prevention of breast cancer with tamoxifen—an update on the Royal Marsden Hospital pilot programme. *European Journal of Cancer* 26:680–684.

Powles, T. J., J. R. Hardy, S. E. Ashley, G. M. Farrington, D. Cosgrove, J. B. Davey, M. Dowsett, J. A. McKinna, A. G. Nash, H. D. Sinnett, C. R. Tillyer, and J. Treleaven. 1989. A pilot trial to evaluate the acute toxicity and feasibility of tamoxifen for prevention of breast cancer. *British Journal of Cancer* 60:126–131.

Pugesgaard, T., and F. E. Von Eyben. 1986. Bilateral optic neuritis evolved during tamoxifen treatment. *Cancer* 58:383–386.

Roberts, M. M., V. Jones, R. A. Elton, R. W. Fortt, S. Williams, and I. H. Gravelle. 1984. Risk of breast cancer in women with a history of benign disease of the breast. *British Medical Journal* 288:275–278.

Rosai, J. 1991. Borderline epithelial lesions of the breast. *American Journal of Surgical Pathology* 15:209–221.

Rosen, P. P., C. Kosloff, P. H. Lieberman, F. Adair, and D. W. Braun, Jr. 1978. Lobular carcinoma *in situ* of the breast. Detailed analysis of 99 patients with average follow-up of 24 years. *American Journal of Surgical Pathology* 2:225–251.

Rubin, E., D. W. Visscher, R. W. Alexander, M. M. Urist, and W. A. Maddox. 1988. Proliferative disease and atypia in biopsies performed for nonpalpable lesions directed mammographically. *Cancer* 61:2077–2082.

Rutqvist, L. E., B. Cedermark, U. Glas, A. Mattsson, L. Skoog, A. Somell, T. Theve, N. Wilking, J. Askergren, M. L. Hjalmar, S. Rotstein, L. Perbeck, and U. Ringborg. 1991. Contralateral primary tumors in breast cancer patients in a randomized trial of adjuvant tamoxifen therapy. *Journal of the National Cancer Institute* 83:1299–1306.

Rutqvist, L. E., and A. Mattsson. 1993. Cardiac and thrombo embolic morbidity among postmenopausal women with early stage breast cancer in a randomized trial of adjuvant tamoxifen. *Journal of the National Cancer Institute* 85:1398–1406.

Sattin, R. W., G. L. Rubin, L. A. Webster, C. M. Huezo, P. A. Wingo, H. W. Ory, and P. M. Layde. 1985. Family history and the risk of breast cancer. *Journal of the American Medical Association* 253:1908–1913.

Satyaswaroop, P. G., R. J. Zaino, and R. Mortel. 1984. Estrogen-like effects of tamoxifen on human endometrial carcinoma transplanted into nude mice. *Cancer Research* 44:4006–4010.

Schwartz, G. F., S. A. Feig, A. L. Rosenberg, A. S. Patchefsky, and A. B. Schwartz. 1984. Staging and treatment of clinically occult breast cancer. *Cancer* 53:1379–1384.

Seidman, H., M. H. Mushinski, S. K. Gelb, and E. Silverberg. 1985. Probabilities of eventually developing or dying of cancer—United States, 1985. *CA—A Cancer Journal for Clinicians* 35:36–56.

Sunderland, M. C., and C. K. Osborne. 1991. Tamoxifen in premenopausal patients with metastatic breast cancer: a review. *Journal of Clinical Oncology* 9:1283–1297.

Thomas, D., and A. Lilienfeld. 1976. Geographic, reproductive and sociobiological factors. In *Risk factors in breast cancer,* ed. B. Stoll, 25. Chicago: William Heinemann Medical Books.

Trichopoulos, D., B. MacMahon, and P. Cole. 1972. Menopause and breast cancer risk. *Journal of the National Cancer Institute* 48:605–613.

Trichopoulos, D., S. Yen, J. Brown, P. Cole, and B. MacMahon. 1984. The effect of westernization on urine estrogens, frequency of ovulation, and breast cancer risk. A study of ethnic Chinese women in the Orient and the USA. *Cancer* 53:187–192.

Trichopoulos, D., C. C. Hsieh, B. MacMahon, T. M. Lin, C. R. Lowe, A. P. Mirra, B. Ravnihar, E. J. Salber, V. G. Valaoras, and S. Yuasa. 1983. Age at any birth and breast cancer risk. *International Journal of Cancer* 31:701–704.

Turken, S., E. Siris, D. Seldin, E. Flaster, G. Hyman, and R. Lindsay. 1989. Effects of tamoxifen on spinal bone density in women with breast cancer. *Journal of the National Cancer Institute* 81:1086–1088.

Turner, R. T., G. K. Wakley, K. S. Hannon, and N. H. Bell. 1987. Tamoxifen prevents the skeletal effects of ovarian hormone deficiency in rats. *Journal of Bone and Mineral Research* 2:449–456.

Wheeler, J. E., H. T. Enterline, J. M. Roseman, J. P. Tomasulo, C. H. McIlvaine, W. T. Fitts, Jr., and J. Kirshenbaum. 1974. Lobular carcinoma *in situ* of the breast. Long-term follow-up. *Cancer* 34:554–563.

Appendix
Index

Appendix

A list of current review articles (1992–1994) about tamoxifen treatment and the potential use of tamoxifen as a preventive for breast cancer.

Fisher, B. 1992. The evolution of paradigms for the management of breast cancer: A personal perspective. *Cancer Research* 52:2371–2383.

Jordan, V. C. 1993. Can all postmenopausal women with a diagnosis of breast cancer benefit from tamoxifen maintenance? *Reviews on Endocrine-related Cancer* 43:23–31.

Jordan, V. C. 1993. Current view of the use of tamoxifen for the treatment and prevention of breast cancer. Gaddum Memorial Lecture. *British Journal of Pharmacology* 110:507–517.

Jordan, V. C., and M. Morrow. 1993. An evaluation of strategies to reduce the incidence of breast cancer. *Stem Cell* 11:252–262.

Jordan, V. C., C. J. Parker, and M. Morrow. In press. Update: Breast cancer treatment and prevention with antiestrogens in the 1990's. *Endocrine Reviews Update* 1:82–85.

Love, R. R. 1992. Tamoxifen in axillary node-negative breast cancer: Multisystem benefits and risks. *Cancer Investigation* 10:587–593.

Morrow, M. 1992. Precancerous breast lesions: implications for breast cancer prevention trials. *International Journal of Radiation Oncology and Biology* 23:1071–1078.

Morrow, M., and V. C. Jordan. Molecular mechanisms of resistance to tamoxifen therapy in breast cancer. *Archives of Surgery.*

Morrow, M., and V. C. Jordan. 1992. Prospects for the prevention of breast cancer. In *Breast diseases updated,* ed. J. Harris. Lippincott Healthcare Philadelphia (2):1–12.

Morrow, M., and V. C. Jordan. 1992. The tamoxifen trial for breast cancer: clinical issues. In *Cancer Prevention,* eds. V. T. DeVita, S. A. Rosenburg, and S. Hellman. Lippincot Healthcare Philadelphia:1–10.

Index

Abeloff, M. D., 133–57
Ablation, estrogen, 219–34
Abortion, 265
Adam, Hugh, 8
Adaptation phenomena, 170
Additive effects, 185–86, 192
Adiamycin, 162
Adrenalectomy, 220
Adriamycin, 135, 138, 149, 150, 151, 153
Agarose gels, 183–84
Age: and endocrine therapy for premeno-
  pausal women, 84–86; and NATO, 102,
  106, 107, 110; and chemohormonal therapy,
  169–70, 172–73; and the prevention of
  breast cancer, 260, 263, 264–65
Agonism, 123–24, 205, 222, 225, 229, 245
Aldophosphamide, 190
Alkaline phosphatase levels, 69, 74
Alkylamides, 223
Alkylating agents, 184–92
ALTER therapy, 141–53
Amenorrhea, 140, 144–45, 147, 151, 165, 173
American Cancer Society, 263
Aminoglutethimide, 32, 171
Amoroso, Domenico, 159–80
Androgen therapy, 205, 220–21
Antagonism, 123–24, 125, 226–27; and
  cytotoxic chemotherapy, 182–83, 184,
  186–89; and tamoxifen-resistant growth,
  206–7; and pure antiestrogens, 222–23;
  and side effects of tamoxifen therapy, 245
Anthracycline, 174
Antiestrogens: structure of, 4–5; *in vivo*
  activity of, 8, 10, 32–33, 136, 161, 183–84,
  223, 229–30; *in vitro* activity of, 10, 32–
  33, 45, 136, 161, 171, 184, 189–92, 202,
  210, 222–23, 226, 229–30; antagonistic
  action of, 123–24, 125, 182–83, 184, 186–
  89, 206–7, 222–23, 226–27, 245; agonistic
  action of, 123–24, 205, 222, 225, 229,
  245; and chemohormonal therapy, 163–64;

and cytotoxic chemotherapy, 186–87;
  pure, total estrogen ablation with, 219–34;
  novel, strategy for discovering, 222–23.
  See also specific compounds
Antimetabolites, 192–93
Antiprogestin RU 38486, 205
Antiproliferative effects, 188
Antithrombin III (ATIII) levels, 67, 240,
  270–71
Anxiety, trial, 71, 72, 78
Apolipoproteins, 64, 73
Aromatase inhibitors, 220–21
Atypical hyperplasia, 266, 268

Baum, M., 93–113
Beatson, George, 86–87
Benign breast disease, 222, 265–66
Biopsies, 137, 201, 204; and LCIS, 267; predictive value of, 268
Bisphenol, 32, 33, 210
Blamey, R. W., 83–92
Blood pressure, 76
Boccardo, Francesco, 159–80
Bone density, 19, 58, 59, 76–77, 123, 261–62;
  and osteoporosis, 12, 74, 262, 270, 273;
  and osseous system effects, 67–69; beneficial effects on, 242
Breast cancer: premenopausal, 4, 45–48,
  83–112 *passim*, 135–51 *passim*, 161–75
  passim, 195, 200, 239, 245, 246, 264, 273;
  postmenopausal, 4–19, 39–50 *passim*,
  57–81, 93–112, 116–31, 136–53 *passim*,
  161–75 *passim*, 195, 200, 236–47 *passim*, 271–72; prevention of, 5, 16–18, 58,
  201, 257–59; advanced, 5–19, 195, 200,
  201–2; and age, 16, 84–86, 102–11 *passim*,
  140, 169–70, 172–73, 260, 263, 264–65;
  carcinogen-induced, 58; early, 76, 159–79,
  260; and disease-free intervals, 84, 85, 86,
  98–105, 175, 195, 202; metastatic, 94, 110,
  118, 135, 182, 203, 230; contralateral, 103–

283

Breast cancer (*continued*)
4, 110, 111–12, 125–28, 129, 137, 247, 260–
61; male, 241; risk factors for, 263–69, 271
Breast disease, benign, 222, 265–66

Ca channel, antagonism of, 183, 184
Calmodulin, 183
Cancer Research Campaign (CRC), 93–113,
261, 269
Cappellini, Mario, 159–80
Carboxyl terminus, 205
Carcinogen-induced breast cancer, 58
Cardiovascular disease, 58, 62–67, 73, 75–
76, 242, 260, 262–63, 273; and the Stock-
holm trial, 123–24, 128–29
Case Western Reserve University trial, 170
Castagnetta, Luigi, 159–80
Cataracts, 246
Cells: MCF-7 cells, 10, 28, 32, 44, 48, 183–
92 *passim*, 205–10, 222, 225–26; MDA-
MB-231 cells, 205, 225–26. *See also*
Cellular effects
Cellular effects, 182–94 *passim;* cell cycle
arrest, 119–20; membrane effects, 183,
184, 189, 194; kinetic, 188. *See also*
Cells
Central nervous system, 87
Cerebral spinal fluid (CSF), 37
Chemi, G. R. O., 159–80
Chemohormonal therapy, 159–79
Chemoprophylaxis, 111–12
Chemotherapy, 12–13, 15, 47, 240; CMF, 84,
91, 116, 121, 138, 148–49, 150, 151, 162,
195; and NATO, 106, 109; and the Stock-
holm trial, 116, 117, 119–21; and ECOG,
133–57; CMFP (CMF plus prednisone),
135; CMFPT (CMFP plus tamoxifen),
135–39, 141–53; and chemohormonal
therapy, 159–76; cytotoxic, 181–98
Cholesterol levels, 19, 59–65 *passim*, 75–77;
HDL, 60, 63, 64, 65, 73, 75, 262–63;
LDL, 64, 73, 77, 123, 262–63
Christie Hospital, 7
Chromatography, 29–30, 36
Clomiphene, 5, 246
Clonidine patches, 239
Clonogenicity, 183
Chloramiphene, 5
Clotting disorders, 240–41
CNS symptoms, 147

Coagulation proteins, 58, 73
Cole, Mary, 7
Colony surviving fractions (SFs), 185–88,
189, 192–93
Committee on the Safety of Medicines, 8
Conjugation, 32
Contraceptives, 4, 5–6, 265
Cooperative Group for Chemohormonal
Therapy of Early Breast Cancer
(GROCTA), 159–80
Coumarin, 241
CRC (Cancer Research Campaign), 93–113,
261, 269
CSF (Cerebral spinal fluid), 37
Cycloheximide, 229
Cyclophosphamide, 95–101 *passim*, 111, 135,
137–38, 151, 162, 189–96 *passim*
Cytosolic proteins, 95
Cytostatic effects, 183

Daniel, P., 44
De Sanctis, Corando, 159–80
Deamination, 30–31
Demethylation, 30–31
DES (diethylstilbestrol), 236
Desmethyltamoxifen, 31
Dexamethasone, 188
Diabetes, 37–38, 76
Diethylstilbestrol (DES), 236
Dimethylaminoethane side chain, 209
Disease-free intervals, 84–86, 98–105, 175,
195, 202
DMBA-induced cancer, 7–8, 10–11, 13, 17
DMPA (Depo-Provera), 239
DNA: "ladder" effect of shared, 183–84;
and estrogen ablation with antiestrogens,
221, 226, 227, 228;—adduct formation in
rats, 242, 273–74
Doxorubicin, 150, 193–94, 195–96
Ductal carcinoma, 86

E isomers, 32–33
Early Breast Cancer Trialists' Collaborative
Group (EBCTCG), 76, 169, 260
Eastern Cooperative Oncology Group
(ECOG), 13, 28, 133–57, 261; EST 4181
trial, 13, 28; EST 5181 trial, 13, 28
EnCa 101 tumors, implantation of, 206
Endocrine therapy, 83–92, 159–79

Endometrial cancer, 124–25, 129, 206, 225, 243–45, 254, 255, 272
Endometriosis, 222, 244
Enzymes, microsomal, 190–91
Epidoxorubicin, 162
Epithelial tissue, 84, 87, 111, 125, 201
ER content. *See* Estradiol receptor (ER) content
ERE (estrogen response elements), 227, 228
ERICA (estrogen receptor radio immune assay), 90
Erythrocyte sedimentation rate (ESR), 90
Estradiol, 9–10, 32, 33, 47–48, 89, 90, 188, 273; and tamoxifen-resistant growth, 207, 209, 211; and estrogen ablation with anti-estrogens, 221–24, 226; and side effects of tamoxifen therapy, 245. *See also* Estradiol receptor (ER) content
Estradiol receptor (ER) content, 121–23, 127, 129, 130, 136–51 *passim;* and patient age, 16; and NATO, 94, 95, 98, 109–10; and chemohormonal therapy, 159–79; and cytotoxic chemotherapy, 182–96 *passim;* and tamoxifen-resistant growth, 201–5, 212–13; wild-type, 204–6; and estrogen ablation with antiestrogens, 222–30 *passim;* and side effects of tamoxifen therapy, 236–38, 243; and the prevention of breast cancer, 260, 272
Estrogen: —receptor radio immune assay (ERICA), 90; ablation, 219–34; response elements (ERE), 227, 228. *See also* Estrogen receptor(s)
Estrogen receptor(s), 4, 5–8, 9–10, 84, 86, 90;—positive cancer cells, MCF-7, 10, 28, 32, 44, 48, 183–92 *passim*, 205–10, 222, 225–26; high binding affinity for, 32–33; competition with estradiol for, 47–48; and NATO, 95–96, 110
Ethamoxytriphetol, 5
Ethoxy sidechains, 32
Ethylenes, 209, 210

Factor VIII deficiency, 240
Fahey, Susan M. L. 27–56
Falkson, G., 133–57
Falkson, H. C., 133–57
Family history, 263–64, 266, 269
Farris, Antonio, 159–80

FDA (Food and Drug Administration), 4, 8, 16
Feinstein, A. R., 244
Fertility drugs, 4, 5
Fibrinogen levels, 58, 64, 66, 67, 76
Fibroblasts, 110, 201
Fibroids, 222
Fixed-ring tamoxifen (FRT), 210, 211
Fluorescence levels, 30
5-fluorouracil therapy, 135, 137–38, 162, 182, 192–93, 194, 195
Follicle-stimulating hormone (FSH), 44–48, 87, 89, 245, 273
Food and Drug Administration (FDA), 4, 8, 16
Foote, F., 266
Fritsch, Michael, 235–54
Fritz, Nancy F., 27–56
Fromson, J. M., 8, 29
FRT (fixed-ring tamoxifen), 210, 211
FSH (follicle-stimulating hormone). *See* Follicle-stimulating hormone (FSH)

G_0 phase, 136
G_1 phase, 136, 183, 184, 186
G_2 phase, 183
Gail, M. H., 268, 269
Gallo, Luigi, 159–80
Gilchrist, K., 133–57
Globulin, 111; sex-hormone-binding (SHBG), 44–45, 47
Glucocorticoid treatment, 183–84
Glucuronidated conjugates, 36
Goldie, J. H., 135
Gonadotrophins, 44–48, 245
Gottardis, Marco M., 199–217
Grade III tumors, 84
Gray, R., 133–57
Green, M. D., 136
Griffiths, K., 14
GROCTA (Cooperative Group for Chemo-hormonal Therapy of Early Breast Cancer), 159–80
Groom, G. V., 14
Growth factors, 110, 171; TGF (transforming growth factor) β family, 201; IGFs (insulin-like-growth factors), 201–2, 226

H regime (VATH), 135
Haagensen, C. D., 267
Halotestin, 135, 138, 153

Harper, Michael, 5, 7
Hart, R. D., 135
Heart disease. *See* Cardiovascular disease
Heat shock proteins, 228
Hemorrhagic cystitis, 138
Hepatic microsomal enzymes, 190
Hepatocellular carcinoma, 242–43
Horwitz, R. I., 244
Houghton, J., 93–113
HPLC (high-performance liquid chroma-
  tography), 29–30
HREs (DNA-termed hormone response ele-
  ments), 227
HSP 90 (90 kDa heat shock protein), 228
Huggins, Charles, 7
Hydroxyclomiphene, 226
4-hydroxycyclophosphamide, 189–92
Hydroxylation, 8, 30–32
4-Hydroxy-N-Desmethyltamoxifen, 9, 31, 32
4-Hydroxytamoxifen, 8–9, 29, 32, 33, 36,
  41–44, 205, 208–13, 226
Hypercalcemia, 240
Hyperplasia, 266, 268, 271
Hypothalamic-pituitary axis, 44–45, 223–24

Iacobelli, Stefano, 159–80
ICI 46,474. *See* Tamoxifen
ICI 47,699, 7
ICI 77,949. *See also* Tamoxifen metabolism,
  and Metabolite E
ICI 164,384, 207, 223–30, 234
ICI 182,780, 91, 229–30, 234
IGFs (insulin-like-growth factors), 201–2,
  226
Imperial Cancer Research Fund, 269
Insulin, 201–2, 226
Isomerization, 33, 210
Italy, 13, 58, 159–80

Jordan, V. Craig, 3–26, 27–56, 136, 199–217,
  257–74

Kaplan, E. L., 140
Keratopathy, 246
Kidney dialysis, 37
King's College, 10

L-phenylalanine (L-PAM), 135
Lacassagne, A., 16
Lactation, 87

Laird, N. M., 68
Lancet, 86
LCIS (lobular carcinoma *in situ*), 266–69
LDL (low density lipoproteins), 123, 262–63
Lerner, L. J., 5
Leukemia, 194
Leukopenia, 240
Leukorrhea, 239
LH (luteinizing hormone), 224, 245, 273;
  —releasing hormone analogs (LHRH),
  48, 88, 220–21, 224
Lien, E. A., 44
Lipophilic tricyclic triparanol analogues, 184
Lipoproteins, 58; apolipoproteins, 64, 73;
  LDL (low density lipoproteins), 123,
  262–63
Lippman, Marc, 10
Liver, effect of tamoxifen on, 30–31, 36, 48–
  49, 123–25, 192, 242–43, 273–74
LNCaP (prostate carcinoma cell line), 205
Love, Richard R., 57–81
Lung cancer, 261
Luteinizing hormone (LH). *See* LH (lutein-
  izing hormone)
Lymphocytes, 184
Lymphovascular invasion, 86

Mammograms, 117, 139
Manchester Christie Hospital, 91
Mastectomy, 11–12, 91, 94, 137
MCF-7 cells, 10, 28, 32, 44, 48, 183–92
  passim, 205–10, 222, 225–26, 234
MDA-MB-231 cells, 205, 225–26
Medical Research Council (MRC), 269
Medroxyprogesterone, 32, 188, 238
Meier, P., 140
Melanomas, 44
Melphalan, 182, 184–89, 195
Membrane effects, 183, 184, 189, 194
Menarche, 264, 271
Menometrorhagia, 14
Menopause, 237, 262, 265
Menstrual cycle, 245–46
MER 25, 5
Mesiti, Mario, 159–80
Methanol extracts, 29
Methotrexate, 135, 137–38, 153, 162, 195
Mitotic rates, 84
MMTV (mouse mammary tumor virus),
  17–18

Morrow, Monica, 257–74
Mortality rates, 15–16, 124; and NATO, 106; and cardiovascular disease, 128; and cytotoxic chemotherapy, 182; and the prevention of breast cancer, 258
MRC (Medical Research Council), 269
mRNAs (altered ER messenger), 204, 229
Multi-drug-resistant (MDR) phenotype, 184
Mustacchi, Giorgio, 159–80
Myocardial infarction, 14, 242, 263

N-desmethyltamoxifen, 8–9, 12, 29–30, 32, 36–44, 208–13
N-Didesmethyltamoxifen, 9
N-4-hydroxyphenyl retinamide, 269–70
N-nitrosomethylurea (NMU)-induced tumors, 11, 17
Nafoxidine, 186, 187
National Cancer Institute (Italy), 270
National Cancer Institute (NCI), 106, 201
National Cancer Registry, 116, 124, 127
National Cause-of-Death Registry, 116
National Institutes of Health Consensus Conference, 169, 171
National Surgical Adjuvant Breast and Bowel Project (NSABP), 13, 14, 28, 170, 182, 195–96, 201, 269; protocol B14, 249, 261
NATO (Nolvadex Adjuvant Trial Organisation), 13, 93–113, 129, 261
Nenci, Italo, 159–80
Nicholson, Rob, 7, 89
NMU-induced tumors, 11, 17
Nobel Prize, 87
Nolvadex, 8, 13, 93–113, 128, 261
Nolvadex Adjuvant Trial Organisation (NATO), 13, 93–113, 128, 261
Nottingham City Hospital, 84, 90, 91
NSABP (National Surgical Adjuvant Breast and Bowel Project). *See* National Surgical Adjuvant Breast and Bowel Project (NSABP)

Ocular toxicity, 246
4-OHT, 29, 205, 208–13
Oophorectomy, 16–19, 48, 67, 87–89, 220; and chemohormonal therapy, 173; and the prevention of breast cancer, 265
Optic neuritis, 246
OS (overall survival), 116, 120, 129
Osborne, C. K., 10, 136, 181–98

Osseos system effects, 67–69, 73, 74
Osteocalcin levels, 68, 74
Osteoporosis, 12, 74, 262, 270, 273
Ovarian function, 4, 15–18, 87, 91, 150, 245; and chemotherapy, 47, 49–50, 161; and pure antiestrogens, 223–24
Oxidation, 190

P-450 system, 184, 190–91
P-glycoprotein, 183–84
Pacini, Paolo, 159–80
Palliation, 182
Parathyroid hormone, 69
Parenchyma, 84
Pearson, O. H., 170
Pharmacokinetics, 36–44, 48–49; single dose, 36; steady state, 36–40; and distribution into tissues, 40–44
Phenathrene, 29–30
1-Phenylalanine, 138
Phosphoramide mustard, 190
Photochemical reactions, 29–30
Piffanelli, Adriano, 159–80
Pituitary glands, 44–45, 123, 223–24
Polychemotherapy, 16
Prednisone, 137–38, 148, 153
Pregnancy: and tamoxifen therapy, 245–46, 273; and breast cancer risk, 264, 265, 271
Prevention, 5; biological rationale for, 16–18, 260–61; and tamoxifen as current therapy, 201, 259–61
Progesterone receptor (PgR) data, 89, 121–22, 127, 129; and maintenance tamoxifen, 140, 144; and chemohormonal therapy, 167–68, 174; and tamoxifen-resistant growth, 201, 203–4, 205–6
Progestin, 205, 238
Prolactin levels, 44–45
Protein kinase, 183, 184
Purpuric vasculitis, 240

QID, 272
Queen's Award for Technological Achievement, 8

Randomization, 116, 137–39, 141, 145, 149, 151–53, 162
Recurrence, of breast cancer, 15–16, 84, 260; and RFS (recurrence-free survival) rates, 116–120, 121, 127–28, 130; and TTR (time

Recurrence, of breast cancer (*continued*)
to relapse) rates, 139–40, 141–45, 153; and
GROCTA, 161, 163–66; and chemohormonal therapy, 175; and cytotoxic chemo-
therapy, 182; and tamoxifen-resistant
growth, 200; and estrogen ablation with
antiestrogens, 220
Resistance, to tamoxifen, 199–217; and ta-
moxifen insensitivity, 203–6; models for,
203–13; and tamoxifen-stimulated growth,
206–13
Retinoids, 258
Retinopathy, 246
RFS (recurrence-free survival), 116–120, 121,
127–28, 130. *See also* Recurrence, of
breast cancer
Richardson, Dora, 5
Riley, D., 93–113
RNA, 193, 204, 229
Robinson, Simon P., 27–56
Rosai, J., 268
Rössner, S., 123
Royal Marsden Hospital, 269
RU 38486, 205
Rubagotti, Alessandra, 159–80
Rutqvist, Lars E., 115–31

S phase, 183, 184
Scandinavian Adjuvant Chemotherapy Study
Group, 95
Schieppati, Guiseppe, 159–80
Schwartzbaum, J. A., 244
Sex-hormone-binding globulin (SHBG), 44–
45, 47
SFs (colony surviving fractions), 185–88,
189, 192–93
Sismondi, Piero, 159–80
Smoking, 61, 67
Southwest Oncology Group (SWOG), 195, 243
Spinal fluid, cerebral, 37
Steroid hormones, 18
Steroidogenesis, 50, 245, 273
Stewart, F., 266
Stockholm Adjuvant Tamoxifen Trial, 115–
31, 260, 261, 263
Survival rates, 13–16, 28, 84–88, 139–44,
258, 260; and NATO, 96, 98–101; RFS
(recurrence-free survival) rates, 116–120,
121, 127–28, 130; and chemohormonal
therapy, 175; and tamoxifen-resistant

growth, 202; and endometrial cancer,
244–45
Sutherland, Rob, 10
SWOG (Southwest Oncology Group, 195,
243

TAFS (transcriptional activation functions),
227–28
Tamoxifen: development of, 4–19; side
effects of, 7, 12, 69–75, 77, 145–46, 164–
67, 235–54, 258; half-life of, 8, 32, 36;
resistance to, 12, 13, 39, 199–217, 225;
therapy, duration of, 12–14, 17, 26–50 *passim*, 106, 111, 130, 170, 171, 175, 186–87,
236; photochemical reaction to, 29–30; *cis*
or *trans* configuration of, 32–33; and species variations in animals, 33–36, 48–49;
dosages, 34–36, 116, 123, 130, 137–38,
148–49, 238–39, 243–44, 246, 260, 270,
272, 273; oral administration of, 36, 40;
and peak serum levels, 36–40; pharmacokinetics, 36–44, 48–49; toxicity of,
57–81, 162, 173, 258, 270–73; osseous sys-
em effects, 67–69, 73, 74; —stimulated
tumor growth, 200; *de nova* resistance to,
203, 204. *See also* Tamoxifen metabolism
Tamoxifen metabolism, 8–11, 26–36; and
N-desmethyltamoxifen, 8–9, 12, 29–30,
32, 36–44, 208–13; and 4-Hydroxytamox-
ifen, 8–9, 29, 32, 33, 36, 41–44, 205, 208–
13, 226; and Metabolite Z, 9; and Metabolite Y, 9, 12, 28, 31; and metabolic pathways, 30–33; and Metabolite E, 31, 33,
208–13; and species variation, 33–36; and
pharmacokinetics, 36–44, 48–49; and distribution into tissues, 40–44; and cytotoxic chemotherapy, 191–92; and
antimetabolites, 192–93
Tenovus Institute for Cancer Research, 7, 89
TGF (transforming growth factor) β family,
201
Thio-TEPA therapy, 135, 138
Third National Cancer Survey, 266
Thrombocytopenia, 240, 241
Thromboembolic events, 128, 270–71
Thrombosis, 12, 240
TLC (thin-layer chromatography), 29
Toremifene, 187
Tormey, Douglass C., 12, 27–56, 133–57
Traina, Adele, 159–80

Transcriptional activation functions (TAFs), 227–28
Triglyceride levels, 59, 60, 63–64
Triphenylethylenes, 7, 246
TTR (time to relapse) rates, 139–40, 141–45, 153
Tumor Institute, 162
Tumorigenesis, 17–18

Ultraviolet absorbance, 29–30
United Kingdom, 58, 94, 200–201
University of Wisconsin Comprehensive Cancer Center, 28
Uterine cancers, 272

Villa, Eugenio, 159–80
Vinblastine, 135, 138, 153
Vincristine, 162

Viruses, mouse mammary tumor (MMTV), 17–18
Vitamin D levels, 69

Wakeling, A. E., 219–34
Wallgren, A., 123
Walpole, Arthur L., 4–5, 6, 7
Ware, J. H., 68
Waters, David, 27–56
Wiebe, V. J., 209–10
Wisconsin Tamoxifen Study, 57–81
Wolf, Douglas M., 199–217, 235–54
Worcester Foundation for Experimental Biology, 7

Xenografts, 225, 230

Z 4-Hydroxytamoxifen, 31, 33
Z isomers, 32–33
Zoladex, 48, 88–89, 90–91, 174